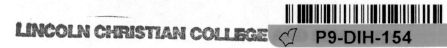

ADHD IN ADOLESCENTS

ADHD in Adolescents
Diagnosis and Treatment

Arthur L. Robin

Foreword by Russell A. Barkley

THE GUILFORD PRESS
New York   London

© 1998 The Guilford Press
A Division of Guilford Publications, Inc.
72 Spring Street, New York, NY 10012
http://www.guilford.com

Printed in the United States of America

This book is printed on acid-free paper.

Last digit is print number: 9   8   7   6   5   4   3   2

Library of Congress Cataloging-in-Publication Data

Robin, Arthur L.
    ADHD in adolescents : diagnosis and treatment / Arthur L. Robin.
       p.   cm.
    Includes bibliographical references and index.
    ISBN 1-57230-391-3 (h.c.) — ISBN 1-57230-545-2 (pbk.)
    1. Attention-deficit disorder in adolescence.   2. Adolescent
psychopathology.   I. Title.
    [DNLM: 1. Attention Deficit Disorder with Hyperactivity—in
adolescence.   2. Attention Deficit Disorder with Hyperactivity—
diagnosis.   3. Attention Deficit Disorder with Hyperactivity—
therapy.   WS 350.8.A8R655a 1998]
RJ506.H9R63   1998
616.85'89'00835—dc21
DNLM/DLC
for Library of Congress   98-36026
                                                                      CIP

To Susan, my eternal love,
who inspires me with creativity, understanding,
wisdom, tenderness, and passion.

Acknowledgments

———————— ○ ————————

I wish to acknowledge a number of very special individuals, without whose support and assistance this book could not have been written. Dr. Thomas Uhde, Chairman of the Department of Psychiatry and Behavioral Neurosciences at Wayne State University, Dr. Alan Gruskin, Chairman of the Department of Pediatrics at Wayne State University, and Mr. Tom Rozek, Senior Executive Vice President for Women and Children's Services in the Detroit Medical Center, supported the sabbatical during which this book was written. Drs. Russell Barkley, Michael Gordon, and Brad Smith served as the reviewers of the original manuscript, and made many suggestions which vastly improved this volume in its final form. Dr. Howard Schubiner shared his wisdom about medication in Chapter 8. Michael Ginsberg and Chris and Pat Edney made invaluable contributions by agreeing to write their stories for Chapter 14. My editors at The Guilford Press, Seymour Weingarten and Rochelle Serwator, helped keep me going and guided the entire process. I also wish to thank the many colleagues, families, and ADHD adolescents who inspired me to develop the ideas in this book, and special thanks to my own children, Melissa and Scott, who kept me honest about parenting ADHD adolescents. Of course, none of this would have been possible without the love and support of my dear wife, Susan, to whom this book is dedicated.

Foreword

○

For much of the last half of this century, clinical wisdom held that children who were quite hyperactive, impulsive, inattentive, passionate, and unruly were likely to outgrow these problems by the time they became adolescents. After all, the best clinical minds at the time (1950s) said so. But on what basis? Largely just clinical observation and anecdote. Much science has been done since then on the longitudinal course and adolescent outcome of such children. Such research tells us, repeatedly, that clinical wisdom was wrong. Now we know better. We know that children who presented to clinics with this behavior pattern and who go on to fulfill all the diagnostic criteria for this pattern's current name, attention-deficit/hyperactivity disorder (ADHD), have a number of risks associated with their disorder and its developmental course. Not the least of these is that they have a 70 to 80 percent chance of continuing to meet clinical diagnostic criteria for the disorder 10 years later, as adolescents.

Along the way, ADHD children and youth are at risk for educational underachievement and underproductivity, retention in grade, suspensions and expulsions from school due to conduct problems, and have a three- to four-fold increase in the likelihood of not completing high school. Many will suffer difficulties with peer relationships. A few will even be friendless. A substantial minority of these children, as teens, are also at considerable risk for early substance experimentation, use, and abuse, as well as lying, stealing, and other antisocial activities. These risks seem mainly to befall those ADHD children who develop conduct disorder by early adolescence. As I and my colleagues have recently documented, these teens are also at serious risk for various negative outcomes associated with their operation of motor vehicles (speeding tickets, accidents, license suspensions and revocations, etc.). And most recently, we have learned that they are at further risk for health and other medical problems, including teen pregnancies and sexually transmitted disease. We have also learned that the families of most ADHD youth, whether conduct-disordered or not, will experience greater stress and conflict than is typically the case with normal teens. These and many other difficulties are nicely, though sadly, documented here by one of the leading clinicians working with ADHD adolescents in the United States today—my good friend, Arthur Robin, PhD.

What Dr. Robin knows from both clinical and first-hand experience is that ADHD is far more than just a problem with paying attention and being impulsive, especially during the adolescent years. He knows, as do I, and as you will discover here, that ADHD most likely represents a developmental disability in that uniquely human domain of functioning—self-regulation. So this is no trivial disorder; it is as disabling of daily adaptive functioning in its own way as are other serious mental disorders, such as autism, mental retardation, and psychosis. Self-regulation is merely a short-hand phrase for a set of evolved cognitive mechanisms or modules that permit humans to sense their past, and from it to develop a sense of the future, all of which occurs before behavior is executed, guiding and informing that behavior all along the way until the goal at which it is aimed is achieved. In doing so, it grants the individual a psychological sense of time and a progressively opening window onto the anticipated future for which the individual must increasingly prepare. Among these mental modules granting us self-regulation is also one that permits the internal regulation of emotion and the development of intrinsic motivation—the capacity to motivate future-directed behavior and overcome the immediate seductions and gratification of the moment. ADHD seems to disrupt all this, leaving ADHD adolescents more at the mercy of the moment than their peers. Teens with ADHD, more than their childhood counterparts, are evidently adrift in time, without the normal tacking mechanisms of internally represented information that serve to regulate and guide behavior toward the future. While such teens may be intelligent and seem otherwise physically normal, they suffer an invisible disability that diminishes their executive control over their own behavior.

All this, and more, you will learn here at the hands of this well-informed and masterful clinician. This book will help you to understand, then, why adolescence poses such a time of conflict for both ADHD youth and their families and educators. Yearning for autonomy and independence yet less capable in the self-governance such autonomy requires, this stage of development is set for disputes and confrontations over the reduced capacity for ADHD youth to assume the responsibility that comes with the privilege of greater independence from parents and other adults. Negotiating this stage will not be easy. There is no more difficult age group of ADHD children with which to work than that of adolescence. And there is no better book than this one to help guide you through and up the ropes.

Dr. Robin teaches us not only about the facts of the disorder, but also about its nature and the proper means of clinically evaluating it. And just as important, if not more so, this text tells us what to do to be of help to these youth, their families, and their educators. The treatment approaches it offers are not those of current popular fashion; they are not glitzy, easy-to-do, or available at the mall's health food store or from the local mystic. If you want style over substance, fashion over efficacy, sizzle over steak, then by all means stop reading right here. This text is not for you. These chapters offer no magic bullet nor quick cure for the disorder. But if what you want is a no-nonsense approach to state-of-the-art diagnosis and treatment, treatment that actually works and has the science to back it up, then this book is for you. The methods to be discussed here take time, knowledge, skill, and effort to implement. Yet these methods represent the work-horses of everyday clinical practice in the scientifically-based treatment arena for ADHD youth. With more than 20 years of clinical service to families of ADHD adolescents, Dr. Robin is the best person I can think of for the job of conveying all this to you. He does so with an insight, wit, wisdom, and sensitivity to the myriad important clinical issues that are not available in other sources. My congratulations to him for crafting this fine clinical text that is sure to give lasting value to its possessor, and my congratulations to you for having the good sense to read it.

RUSSELL A. BARKLEY, PhD
Professor of Psychiatry and Neurology
University of Massachusetts Medical Center

Preface

———————— O ————————

Over the past decade, literally thousands of books, chapters, and articles about Attention-Deficit/Hyperactivity Disorder (ADHD) have been written for physicians, psychologists, educators, parents, children with ADHD, adolescents with ADHD, adults with ADHD, and even specific constituencies such as boy scout leaders. Why, then, do we need a book specifically about diagnosing and treating the adolescent with ADHD? A confluence of several clinical, research, and philosophical streams suggests the need for a book for mental health and health care professionals regarding adolescent ADHD:

1. The follow-up studies reviewed in Chapter 2 of this volume clearly indicate that childhood ADHD often persists into adolescence and adulthood. Researchers and clinicians alike regard ADHD as a life span disorder, and books addressing particular stages of the life span within a life span perspective have only begun to appear.

2. In accordance with this perspective, more and more clinicians are receiving requests to diagnose and treat adolescents with possible ADHD, and they need practical suggestions based on the latest research and clinical experience to respond effectively to these requests within a changing health care system. Such practical advice is available regarding children and adults with ADHD but not exclusively regarding adolescents.

3. Research confirms that the developmental tasks for individuals in the second decade of life are unique and challenging, and the impact of conditions such as ADHD on these tasks and challenges is different from its impact on younger children and adults. Therefore, clinicians working with adolescents who may have ADHD need standards of care and suggestions for diagnosis and treatment which take the special nature of adolescence into account.

4. Research reviewed in Chapters 2 and 4 indicates that children with ADHD are at risk for developing serious comorbid conditions during adolescence, particularly Conduct Disorder, Mood Disorders, Substance Use Disorder, truancy, and school dropout. If not adequately addressed, these comorbidities significantly worsen the prognosis for adult functioning in such adolescents. We must be able to recognize and respond to these comorbidities to prevent them from incapacitating the adolescent and leading to a lifetime of subjective misery, relationship problems, psychiatric disorders, personality problems, unfulfilled educational and vocational potential, and lost productivity to society.

5. Not all adolescents with ADHD look or act alike. In fact, there is a tremendous heterogeneity in how teenagers with ADHD present, perhaps more so than with younger children. Only a volume that fully concentrates on the adolescent stage of life can hope to prepare practitioners to deal with this heterogeneity.

Through my personal clinical work and research with hundreds of adolescents and parents over the past two decades, I have come to realize the importance of these five points. Accordingly, this book reflects the life span perspective of ADHD as a condition originating in childhood that often continues into adolescence and adulthood, and blends developmental knowledge regarding adolescence with knowledge about ADHD, psychiatric diagnosis, comorbidity, parent–adolescent relationships, and psychosocial, medical, and educational interventions.

ORGANIZATION OF THE BOOK

The book is divided into three sections. Section I focuses on definitions, descriptions, and theoretical models. After an introduction using four case studies to acquaint the reader with the multifaceted nature of ADHD in adolescence, Chapter 1 critically reviews the current definition and diagnostic criteria of ADHD and presents reformulations of the disorder such as Barkley's (1997b) response inhibition theory and a temperament model. Chapter 2 summarizes the results of the major follow-up studies about what happens to children with ADHD as they move through adolescence, and then applies behavioral family systems theory and social learning coercion theory to adolescents with ADHD.

Section II focuses on assessment and diagnosis. After an introduction outlining the overall assessment process, this section addresses specific topics in assessment. Chapter 3 focuses on questionnaires and rating scales; Chapter 4 focuses on the clinical interview and differential diagnosis; Chapter 5 focuses on continuous performance tests, psychological testing, and behavioral observation; and Chapter 6 focuses on integration of diverse assessment results.

In Section III a comprehensive treatment plan for an intensive burst of short-term, multimodal intervention is presented. The philosophy, organization, and sequencing of this treatment is discussed in an introduction, followed by chapters devoted to each aspect of it. Educating families about ADHD and enhancing acceptance of ADHD are the topics of Chapter 7. Chapter 8 contains a comprehensive discussion of medical treatments for ADHD, while Chapter 9 focuses on educational interventions. Chapters 10 through 14 cover parenting issues, home-based interventions, conflict management, and family therapy, including two stories written by adolescents with ADHD. A brief epilogue closes the book.

FOR WHOM IS THIS BOOK WRITTEN?

I wrote this book for psychologists, physicians, social workers, educators, and other professionals who work with adolescents with behavioral and emotional problems. It is not written primarily for parents of adolescents or the adolescents themselves, although parents familiar with psychological constructs may benefit from it. I also wrote it for students and trainees preparing for careers working with adolescents in mental health and health care settings, and it is appropriate for use during both their formal academic training and their clinical internships.

To ensure effective implementation of the assessment and treatment methods described in this book, readers should already have received advanced professional training in the mental health field. Typically, psychologists, psychiatrists, behavioral and developmental pediatricians, clinical social workers, marital and family therapists, and licensed professional counselors have received such training. Although many of the ideas in this book will be extremely helpful to others (e.g., primary care physicians, nurses, teachers, and parents), I wish to caution that without explicit training in mental health assessment and intervention, success in using these techniques with a difficult population such as adolescents diagnosed as having ADHD may be hard to achieve.

Contents

———— ◯ ————

SECTION ONE

○

DEFINITIONS, DESCRIPTIONS, AND THEORY

Introduction

At the outset, it is important for the clinician to understand the scope of the clinical phenomena that go with the territory we call "ADHD." In this Introduction, I attempt to give the reader a clearer understanding of that territory by presenting four case examples of the many faces of ADHD in adolescents. Then, I discuss diagnostic issues and theoretical reformulations of the disorder in Section I.

FOUR CASE STUDIES

Michael

Michael Ginsberg's 16th birthday present to himself was the first report card with straight A's he had ever received, and he and his parents are beaming. Michael and his family had struggled long and hard to cope with ADHD. While he and his parents beam with pride and delight at his accomplishments, shadows of a darker past loom in the background. Michael can vividly recall his third grade teacher nagging at him to "pay attention, finish your work, try harder, concentrate," and the other students beginning to feel they could pick on him too. Once, after the teacher left the room, a group of boys pinned him to the floor, calling him terrible names and kicking and hitting him. Afterward the principal called the parents in and said that the school wanted to help him but since he wasn't "learning disabled," the only way they could give him any support was to label him "emotionally impaired!" His parents immediately yanked him out of that school, not knowing what to do next.

It was shortly after this horrible incident that Michael was diagnosed as having ADHD. There were not yet any plans to accommodate the needs of ADHD students through regular or special education in that district at that time. Michael was enrolled in private school for several years. When he returned to public school in sixth grade, his parents started asking for a

3

plan of accommodations in regular education under the guidelines of Section 504 of the Rehabilitation of the Handicapped Law, discussed in Chapter 5 of this volume. It took until ninth grade for such a plan to be developed, but fortunately for Michael, middle school went reasonably well due to the intervention of a very caring and supportive principal.

In time Michael has come to accept the need for religiously taking his Ritalin (methylphenidate), without which he cannot juggle advanced placement academic courses, a lot of homework, being an Eagle Scout and leading a large Boy Scout Troop, being a winning member and co-captain of the State Championship Varsity Swimming team, and having a social life.

When it turned out that the optimal time to take the second dose of Ritalin was during the middle of math class, Michael asked to step out for a moment and go to the water fountain; the teacher agreed. When I pointed out to Michael that it was very unusual for an ADHD adolescent to take medication in a way that was obvious to his peers, opening himself up to possible ridicule, Michael calmly responded, "ADD is a part of me and I'm proud of what I am." At age 16, Michael had achieved a degree of self-acceptance rare for ADHD adolescents.

It isn't only medication that helps Michael cope. Supportive parents who knew when to step in and advocate relentlessly for him and when to back off and let him do his own thing have been a crucial ingredient in his recipe for success. An understanding middle school principal also helped steer Michael through his sixth, seventh, and eighth grade years. Mr. and Mrs. Ginsburg, a business executive and a professional educator, fought to get their son a plan of accommodation in regular education under the Federal civil rights law known as Section 504 of the Rehabilitation Act of 1973. Starting in ninth grade, the school assigned a case manager to look after Michael's needs and insure that his teachers adhered to the Section 504 plan. His accommodations included timely administration of medication, extensive availability of computers even during examinations, organizational assistance, regular progress reports to parents, close in-school monitoring, careful selection of teachers, and several other features. Michael felt he would not have succeeded to the same degree without these accommodations. He still struggled with homework, and panicked the night before final exams, but it was the normal panic of a tenth-grader who had a fair chance of success, not the hopeless frenzy of an ADHD adolescent who had no idea how to cope or what to do first.

Michael was successfully coping with ADHD through medical and educational interventions, and with a great deal of emotional, intellectual, and financial support from his highly able professional parents. Fortunately, he did not have any serious comorbid conditions to complicate the picture. Through all his trials and tribulations, he had neither lashed out aggressively at others nor engaged in self-destructive behaviors or turned to illegal substances. In recent years, Michael began helping other, less fortunate ADHD teenagers by talking to them informally, giving lectures to their parents, participating in educational videotapes, and writing about his experiences. In the fall of 1996, he entered Stanford University, where he is continuing to do well and receiving accommodations for his ADHD. He wrote his own story, which appears in Chapter 14 of this volume and has permitted his actual name to be used here.

Adam

Adam Smith, age 14, is exploding with rage. He was just suspended from school for 5 days for cursing out another kid who dared him to fight, and for pushing the teacher who told him to watch his language; as usual, the other teenager did not get into any trouble. Three weeks ago, Mrs. Smith placed Adam in a local inpatient psychiatric unit for 1 week after he had an explosion of rage during which he kicked two large holes in the wall and chased his 12-year-old brother around the house, threatening to slice him up with a kitchen knife. Adam's tirade was set off by his brother's pulling out the plug on the Nintendo game as Adam got to the highest level. This was his fifth such short-term hospitalization in the past 2 years. Most of his life, Adam has had difficulty controlling his temper, channeling anger in productive directions, and tolerating criticism or frustration. To dissipate his anger, Adam gets physical, punches walls or trees, kicks doors, lifts weights, throws things, and so on. His mother gets out of his way until he calms down; there is no controlling him at such times.

Adam lives with his mother, 12-year-old brother, and pregnant 19-year-old sister. When Adam was 5, Mrs. Smith took the kids and left Adam's father, who was a violent alcoholic who beat her and their children indiscriminately. Mr. Smith moved to West Virginia, where he remarried and had two more children. Mrs. Smith works the day shift at a local auto assembly plant and rents a cramped, two-bedroom apartment, where she lives with her three children. She is a well-meaning person but is very overwhelmed by her life situation, Adam's problems, and tight finances. She has one or two female friends but has not had any significant male relationships since she left her husband. She is very isolated and has been depressed for many years. She is finding it increasingly difficult to deal with Adam, who often outwits her and gets around her rules. Her inability to get him to do what she wants gets her even more depressed so she spends most of her time at home watching TV.

Adam was first diagnosed as having ADHD in first grade. At the school's suggestion, Mrs. Smith took Adam to the pediatrician at CARE-FORME, the local health maintenance organization (HMO) to which she belongs. The pediatrician started Adam on 5 mg of Ritalin twice a day, which has gradually been increased over the years to 20 mg three times a day. Adam sees a different pediatrician each time he returns for a follow-up visit. Mrs. Smith got tired of telling her son's life story each time she needs a medication refill, so she wrote it down and now gives the paper to each new doctor. The HMO approves five sessions of therapy per year, which constitutes Adam's entire annual outpatient mental health benefit. The therapist attempts to help restore parental control and help Adam deal with his anger. To achieve this, the therapist asks Mrs. Smith to clarify the basic rules for living in the home and to negotiate behavioral contracts that specify privileges in return for following these rules, and punishments for failure to follow them. However, more than five sessions per year are needed to help Mrs. Smith effectively implement these contracts. By the beginning of each new year, all past progress is lost.

Adam's response to medication is like a "light switch." When the Ritalin is in his body, he is as sweet as can be; he rarely engages in aggressive behavior and is only moderately oppositional. When the Ritalin wears off or he has not taken it, he is moody, irritable, quick to flash into aggression, and so on. Mrs. Smith recalls that Adam has always been this way, just like his alcoholic father. Unfortunately, as Adam has moved into adolescence, he has increasingly refused to take his Ritalin and often spits it out when no one is looking or "forgets" to go to the office to get it (the school refuses to remind him, saying that he is old enough to take it on his own). This is a particular problem in the morning, as Mrs. Smith leaves for work at 5 A.M. and Adam rarely takes his medicine on his own.

Adam denies that anything is wrong with him. He claims that Ritalin does not help him and that his mother and teachers are too strict. He externalizes blame for all his misbehavior. He spends his free time playing Nintendo, his one passion in life. He has no goals for the future and talks about running away from home, but has no idea where he would go.

Adam has difficulty concentrating on schoolwork. When he knows what his homework is, he ignores it, and he usually does not write down the assignments. As a boy of average intellectual ability, without any learning disabilities, he just squeaks by, getting C's, D's, and an occasional failing grade. He has a difficult time with authoritarian teachers, and consistently gets into trouble in their classes.

In school, he does not ask for help with material he does not understand and is opposed to receiving any educational accommodation. Adam's school does not recognize that he is handicapped by ADHD, despite several attempts by his mother to prove it, and has not provided any extra help. The teachers view him as "bad and unmotivated," and many have virtually given up on him.

Adam has ADHD plus Oppositional Defiant Disorder (ODD), rapidly graduating to Conduct Disorder (CD). His moodiness also has a hypomanic quality to it. His impulsively explosive nature makes daily life a mine field of interpersonal disasters waiting to happen. He leaves a trial of damaged property, broken relationships, and hurt feelings; but most seriously, inside his hard veneer lies a fragile, hurting person, who may intellectually understand his handicap but emotionally fails to accept it. Even though Adam has poor impulse control and can be aggressively destructive, he never became involved in substances or committed any illegal acts in the community. Unfortunately, because the HMO to which Mrs. Smith belongs does not provide the necessary coverage to meet the Smiths' medical care needs, it ends up with frequent, costly inpatient hospitalizations when Adam gets violent and Mrs. Smith cannot tolerate it anymore.

Sarah

Fourteen-year-old Sarah Peterson is an attractive, highly social young adolescent with many friends. She gets along well with her parents and 8-year-old brother, whom she often babysits. Adults as well as adolescents find Sarah charming, and teachers often overlook her chronic tardiness with school assignments, accept her creative excuses for incomplete work, mistake her extroverted verbal style for high intellectual ability, and do not discipline her for socializing instead of doing written work. Although she had satisfactory grades in elementary school, the increasing demands for organization and long-term planning inherent in the middle school curriculum, overwhelm her limited ability to concentrate and organize. She often comes to her eighth-grade classes unprepared, with incomplete homework, and she often loses the work she has done before class or turns it in late. Recently, Sarah had to do a major paper in English and she felt lost; it was by accident that her mother discovered, the night before the paper was due, that Sarah even had that assignment. She worked hard, under her parents' close supervision for 3 nights, and turned in the paper late, receiving a failing grade. At midsemester, in her eighth-grade year, every academic teacher sent home progress reports indicating that many assignments were incomplete or poorly executed, and that Sarah could fail.

Her parents were surprised by these problems because Sarah had always done well in school. They acknowledged that she was a "total slob," an "air head," and disorganized at home, but they always viewed her as a capable student, just a bit "flighty." A comprehensive psychological evaluation revealed not only that Sarah had ADHD but also that her overall intellectual ability was in the low-average range, suggesting that even a little inattention might cause her to fall behind in school.

Sarah and her parents learned about ADHD and the methods for coping with it, and opted for medication and enrollment in short-term family and individual therapy. Sarah was prescribed Ritalin, which was titrated over 4 weeks to a daily dose schedule of 20 mg three times a day. Sarah reported that her mind was sharp as a whip in class and that she could complete her schoolwork more efficiently on Ritalin but that it changed her personality, making her less bubbly. Through therapy, she eventually understood that her "bubbly personality" was also, in part, a form of verbal impulsivity and hyperactivity. When the dose of Ritalin was adjusted Sarah accepted the compromise that allowed her to concentrate without curbing her impulsive nature too much. Chapter 8 describes the adjustments to Sarah's medication regimen in detail.

The preferred provider organization (PPO) through which Sarah was insured authorized 10 outpatient therapy sessions. Therapy focused on school and home issues. For example, in the school domain, the therapist collaborated with Sarah and her parents to analyze how she approaches homework and to develop a comprehensive homework plan. Sarah rarely wrote down her assignments, and thus did not consistently have the materials she needed to do or understand it. The therapist helped her use an assignment sheet to track her assignments and arranged for her school counselor to meet with her three times a week to go over the assignment sheet and help her track what she needed to do. Sarah never thought about which assignment to do first, or how to maximize concentration by timing Ritalin with homework. The therapist helped Sarah and her mother to begin brief, daily planning sessions to learn to prioritize homework. He also helped the family monitor the medication and talk with their physician about timing the homework dose. He gave the physician feedback about the effectiveness of the medication, helping to facilitate fine tuning.

Sarah and her parents were present at the sessions, although sometimes Sarah wanted to discuss peer problems so she saw the therapist individually. He arranged a school meeting with Sarah, her teachers, and her parents; the teachers agreed to send home weekly progress reports, monitor Sarah's on-task behavior in class, give her smaller assignments with several progress checks, and let her start her homework in school. Therapy ended after 10 sessions, but follow-ups authorized by the PPO were conducted every 3 months. In this case, therapy worked synergistically with stimulant medication and school-based interventions to improve the quality of Sarah's life.

Adolescent girls with pure ADHD and no comorbidity often present as Sarah did; her ADHD is moderate in intensity, without the angry impulsivity that characterized Adam. Her well-developed social skills, coupled with a strong history of positive relationships with her family, teachers, and peers, insulated her against the damage to self-esteem which occurred in differing but equally serious ways for Michael and Adam. In such cases, a short burst of intensive behavioral/psychological intervention is usually followed by long-term medical and educational interventions, with occasional follow-up bursts of psychological intervention when new crises emerge at significant transition points in life, such as entering high school or college.

Melissa

Melissa Bernstein presented as a depressed 19-year-old sophomore who recently dropped out of Michigan State University. She had been unable to turn around her poor academic record, which had caused her to be placed on academic probation the previous semester. Throughout elementary and middle school, she breezed through the academic curriculum, getting on the honor roll. In high school she had trouble with writing but nonetheless received outstanding grades. Her family and friends described her as a pleasant adolescent, who has a tendency to "zone out," to be "flighty," daydreamy, and disorganized, but who is not oppositional or rebellious. Her parents remembered as an adolescent, Melissa always had difficulty getting to places on time, and became easily overwhelmed when she had to make important decisions.

In the freedom of the college environment, Melissa was unable to structure her time, set priorities, organize her study, focus her attention, and balance her social life with her academic commitments. She spent her freshman year socializing and getting involved with marijuana and alcohol rather than studying. She discovered that with a little bit of marijuana, she could concentrate so she used it to socialize and to study. She had difficulty with writing assignments. During her sophomore year, Melissa tried to focus less on her socializing and concentrate more on her studies. Despite her best efforts, she soon realized that she could not concentrate in class or during study sessions and her note-taking skills were very poor. She could not study effectively in the dorms, where there were too many social temptations, or in the library, where she was distracted by every squeak or minor sound. In the middle of the first semester of her sophomore year, she was failing most of her courses and became frustrated and depressed and planned to take her own life, but her closest girlfriend stopped her. Feeling defeated, Melissa quit school and went home to live with her parents. She took a job helping out at a local day-care center. She loved kids and wanted to become a teacher but saw no hope of succeeding in college. Her parents took her for therapy. Shortly thereafter, her mother heard me give a talk on adolescent ADHD and thought that my case descriptions sounded just like Melissa. After talking to Melissa and her therapist, she arranged for me to evaluate her daughter.

I diagnosed Melissa as having ADHD, Combined subtype, along with Major Depressive and Substance Abuse Disorders. I found that Melissa had superior verbal but average performance IQ, with above-average to superior achievement in all areas except written expression, which was on the low side of average. By history and testing, she fit the profile of an adolescent with a learning disability in the written expression area. Throughout elementary, middle, and high school, she compensated effectively for her ADHD by using her superior memory and cognitive ability, and the structure of her family life helped keep her on track. However, faced with the need to produce her own structure in a stimulating, residential college environment, she fell apart. College work also required a great deal of writing ability, but her ADHD and the learning disability in written expression severely handicapped Melissa.

When Melissa's diagnosis was given to her, she heaved a big sigh of relief; she was glad to learn that there was a good reason for her seemingly hopeless struggle to do better in college. She asked if she could now go back to college and succeed if she started taking Ritalin. However, when I explained to her that medication such as Ritalin was not a "quick fix," and that she would have to quit marijuana before she could be treated medically for ADHD, she was disappointed. After I thoroughly discussed the treatment options with Melissa and her parents, she agreed with my recommendations to attend a local community college and live at home for several semesters, until she learned to cope more effectively with ADHD, depression, and substance abuse, and then transfer back to a residential college.

She agreed to continue regular individual therapy, to learn self-organization techniques, and to achieve a better balance in her life. In the therapy sessions, I asked Melissa to specify which major elements of her life needed better balance. Her list included school, part-time work, social life, health, and self-care/appearance. Together, we developed specific goals in these areas, and began to work toward achieving these goals. For example, Melissa wanted to study daily for her college courses and also to exercise and talk to her friends daily. Whatever she started first, she would keep doing, failing to prioritize and organize her time to achieve balance. We made a daily schedule, and she learned how to use a voice-activated personal organizer to remind her to adhere to her schedule. She was much happier when she divided her time between school, friends, and exercise than when she devoted too much time to any one area.

Melissa began to take Prozac, which helped her depression but not her concentration. Two months after she quit smoking marijuana, Melissa was also started on Ritalin; her dose was titrated up to 20 mg four times a day. Now, she is beginning to experience academic success in a local community college, she can concentrate much better with the Ritalin, and is working on her other issues in therapy. She has learned that coping with ADHD is a lot more than just taking a pill.

FOUR FACES OF ADHD IN ADOLESCENTS

These case studies represent four of the many faces of ADHD in adolescents. Michael, gifted and introspective, overcame a shaky start and, with a lot of family support and external treatment, is now doing well. Adam, faced with family adversity, denial of his disability, comorbid ODD with a violent temper, and a short-sighted HMO that did not authorize sufficient therapy, is headed down the path of disaster. The organizational demands of middle school caught up with bubbly Sarah's biological limits for attention, but she was able to quickly recover with help from her family and treating professionals. Brooding Melissa, unable to cope with college, fell apart, became depressed, withdrew from life, and turned to drugs until her disability was correctly diagnosed. Effective therapy coupled with medication helped her pull her life together.

Yet all four adolescents share common characteristics: (1) They do not naturally focus quickly, concentrate well, organize effectively, pay attention to details, or complete tasks requiring sustained mental effort and planning, such as schoolwork; (2) they have difficulty regulating their impulses and restlessness, cognitive, emotional, and/or behavioral problems; (3) their self-esteem suffered greatly from the increasing number of failures in life, leaving inner scars and suffering, or leading to lashing out at a world they perceive as hostile; (4) their ADHD symptoms have interfered with their accomplishment of the normal developmental tasks of adolescence; and (5) their functioning depends in part on their receptivity to and the availability and accessibility of medical, psychological, and educational interventions for coping with ADHD.

Four important, but interdependent factors, aside from innate biological/personality differences, differentiate between their various manifestations of ADHD and their abilities to benefit from coping interventions: (1) the stage of adolescent development, (2) the severity of ADHD, (3) the presence of comorbidity, and (4) the family environment. Early-to-mid-adolescents (11–14) typically deny any chronic illness or disability and have more difficulty coping with it, whereas middle to later adolescents (15–19) accept their disabilities and are willing to try coping techniques. Michael and Melissa fit into this latter category, but Adam is in early adolescence. Although Sarah is also an early adolescent, her ADHD was not as severe as the others, and other things were going positively in her life (e.g., her social life and her family life). Thus, the diagnosis of ADHD was not a big blow to her self-esteem, and she was able to accept the necessary interventions. In general, milder ADHD symptoms, coupled with partial success in non-academic life pursuits, make it easier for adolescents to accept and cope with ADHD.

Melissa and Adam also displayed comorbidities for other psychiatric conditions, whereas Michael and Sarah did not. Sometimes, these comorbidities appear to be secondary consequences of the cumulative impact of life failure on an ADHD teen, as in the case of depression and marijuana use for Melissa. Other times, family interactions and environmental conditions may exacerbate comorbidities, but the manifestations of these conditions have been there since birth; Adam had always been coercive and aggressive, as long as his mother could remember. Common comorbidities to ADHD in adolescence include ODD, CD, Mood Disorders, Anxiety Disorders, and Substance Abuse Disorders. Learning disabilities, and common educational comorbidities, further impede school performance but do not necessarily contribute to antisocial behavior or other negative psychiatric conditions. Michael's and Melissa's learning disabilities required specific educational interventions but did not spur negative family interactions or acting-out behavior.

Family adversity and parental psychopathology hindered their success, while a healthy family environment helped considerably. However, it cannot simply be asserted that ADHD teenagers with supportive, helpful parents do better than those with disrupted, dysfunctional families. Adam had more family adversity than Michael or Sarah, but Melissa's problems developed despite a positive family environment. In reality, family systems are both architects and victims of negative interactions, and severe ADHD with certain comorbidities contributes to the shaping and maintenance of coercive interactions, even in the most well-meaning families.

As this account of adolescent ADHD unfolds, the clinician is given specific techniques to recognize, assess, and treat these very different manifestations of ADHD, and these four cases are revisited to illustrate diverse approaches to diagnosis and intervention. The research evidence supporting the importance of the factors discussed here is critically reviewed, with suggestions for future research.

ORGANIZATION OF SECTION I

Chapters 1 and 2 comprehensively address diagnostic issues and theoretical models relevant to ADHD in adolescence. These chapters cover the following topics:

Chapter 1

- DSM-IV diagnostic criteria for ADHD
- Core features of ADHD
- Associated problems
- Critical review of DSM-IV with regard to age, gender, onset, subtypes
- Is the incidence of ADHD increasing?
- *Diagnostic and Statistical Manual for Primary Care, Child and Adolescent Version*
- Positive aspects of having ADHD
- ADHD and temperament
- Response Inhibition Theory of ADHD
- Argument that ADHD does not really exist

Chapter 2

- Follow-up and cross-sectional studies on adolescents with ADHD
- Behavioral Family Systems theory of parent–adolescent conflict
- Coercion theory for the development of oppositional behavior
- Integration of these two theories in explaining the nature of adolescent ADHD
- Implications of these theories for assessment and intervention

CHAPTER ONE

―――――――― O ――――――――

Definitions and Diagnostic Criteria

"Attention-deficit hyperactivity disorder is a heterogeneous disorder of un-known etiology." This is the opening line of a major review of the litera-ture on medication for treating ADHD by one of the leading child psychia-try research teams in the country (Spencer et al., 1996, p. 409). To this line, we could easily add the phrase "and of highly changeable definition." The name, definition, and prevailing diagnostic criteria for what we today call "ADHD" have changed at least five times in the past few decades, reflect-ing changes in our conceptualization of the disorder but creating confusion among practitioners and the public, and making the task of standardizing samples in research very difficult (see Barkley, 1990 for a complete histo-ry). Currently, ADHD is defined by the fourth edition of the *Diagnostic and Statistical Manual of Mental Disorders* (DSM-IV; American Psychi-atric Association, 1994) (see Table 1.1). There have also been redefinitions and reformulations of ADHD, as well as nihilistic attempts to negate the existence of the disorder, which the well-informed clinician should be aware of. Specifically, I address the following seven issues:

1. Manifestations of the "traditional" core symptoms of inattention, impulsivity, and hyperactivity in the second decade of life.
2. The associated problems commonly coinciding with these core symptoms in adolescents.
3. The positive and negative features of the DSM-IV approach to defining ADHD.
4. The possible assets, strengths, or positive attributes of the individ-ual with ADHD.
5. The relationship between temperament and ADHD.

13

TABLE 1.1. DSM-IV Criteria for ADHD

Definitions

The essential feature of Attention-Deficit/Hyperactivity Disorder is a persistent pattern of inattention and/or hyperactivity–impulsivity that is more frequent and severe than is typically observed in individuals at a comparable level of development. . . . Some hyperactive–impulsive or inattentive symptoms that cause impairment must have been present before age 7, although many individuals are diagnosed after the symptoms have been present for a number of years. . . . Some impairment from the symptoms must be present in at least two settings (e.g., at home and at school or work). . . . There must be clear evidence of interference with developmentally appropriate social, academic, or occupational functioning. . . . The disturbance does not occur exclusively during the course of a Pervasive Developmental Disorder, Schizophrenia, or other Psychotic Disorder, and is not better accounted for by another mental disorder (e.g., a Mood Disorder, Anxiety Disorder, Dissociative Disorder, or Personality Disorder). . . .

Two lists of nine symptoms

A. Either (1) or (2):

(1) six (or more) of the following symptoms of **inattention** have persisted for at least 6 months to a degree that is maladaptive and inconsistent with developmental level:

Inattention

  (a) often fails to give close attention to details or makes careless mistakes in schoolwork, work, or other activities
  (b) often has difficulty sustaining attention in tasks or play activities
  (c) often does not seem to listen when spoken to directly
  (d) often does not follow through on instructions and fails to finish schoolwork, chores, or duties in the workplace (not due to oppositional behavior or failure to understand instructions)
  (e) often has difficulty organizing tasks and activities
  (f) often avoids, dislikes, or is reluctant to engage in tasks that require sustained mental effort (such as schoolwork or homework)
  (g) often loses things necessary for tasks or activities (e.g., toys, school assignments, pencils, books, tools)
  (h) is often easily distracted by extraneous stimuli
  (i) is often forgetful in daily activities

(2) six (or more) of the following symptoms of hyperactivity–impulsivity have persisted for at least 6 months to a degree that is maladaptive and inconsistent with the developmental level:

Hyperactivity

  (a) often fidgets with hands or feet or squirms in seat
  (b) often leaves seat in classroom or in other situations in which remaining seated is expected
  (c) often runs about or climbs excessively in situations where it is inappropriate (in adolescents or adults, may be limited to subjective feelings of restlessness)
  (d) often has difficulty playing or engaging in leisure activities quietly

(continued)

TABLE 1.1. *(continued)*

(e) is often "on the go" or often acts as if driven by a motor
(f) often talks excessively

Impulsivity

(g) often blurts out answers before questions have been completed
(h) often has difficulty awaiting turn
(i) often interrupts or intrudes on others (e.g., butts into conversations or games)

Three subtypes

314.01 Attention-Deficit/Hyperactivity Disorder, Combined Type: if both Criteria A1 and A2 are met for the past 6 months
314.00 Attention-Deficit/Hyperactivity Disorder, Predominantly Inattentive Type: if Criterion A1 is met but Criterion A2 is not met for the past 6 months
314.01 Attention-Deficit/Hyperactivity Disorder, Predominantly Hyperactive–Impulsive Type: if Criterion A2 is met but Criterion A1 is not met for the past 6 months

Note. From the American Psychiatric Association (1994). Copyright 1994 by the American Psychiatric Association. Reprinted by permisson.

6. ADHD as a fundamental problem of impaired response inhibition rather than a problem of attention (Barkley, 1997b).
7. The arguments that have been made against the very existence of ADHD, and their validity.

CORE SYMPTOMS OF ADHD

Attention

In adolescence, the construct of "attention" encompasses a broad range of phenomena at various levels of molarity or molecularity, and teenagers may manifest difficulties in any one or more of these areas: (1) selecting and focusing on the relevant stimuli in the environment, coupled with starting or executing tasks; (2) maintaining concentration and resisting distraction; (3) consistently mobilizing effort in a task-oriented direction; (4) organization, forgetfulness, and recall of learned information; and (5) making transitions from one task to another. Brown (1996) in fact developed a questionnaire that assesses these various subcategories of attention.

Adolescents for whom it is difficult to select and focus on the relevant stimuli procrastinate on homework and chores. They go to their rooms, perhaps with the best intentions of doing their homework, but instead day dream, fiddle with things on their desks, look out the window, and do everything but start their homework. They socialize so much in class that they never start their independent classwork. They study for their examination at the last minute, or start the term paper the night before it is due. They say "Yes, in a few minutes," when mothers ask them to take out the trash or get ready for bed; in a few minutes, they have totally forgotten the request and are involved in television, video games, or a telephone call. They may seem indecisive when faced with choices, such as what to buy in a store or which video game to play first; that is, they are overwhelmed by a rich array of stimuli and can not get focused or make a selection. For example, when faced with a desk full of papers to sort, they may go to pick up one paper but notice five others, and go to pick up the next. Not being able to decide what to do first, they get emotionally overwhelmed and end up doing nothing. Some may have a sluggish cognitive tempo, a slow processing speed, and may even look hypoactive and spaced out. However, they do not have difficulty getting started on all tasks but only on tasks that require sustained mental effort, are not intrinsically interesting to them, and/or require dealing with a complex array of environmental stimuli. Barkley (1990) argued that deficits in focused attention are the primary attentional problem in ADD without Hyperactivity, known in DSM-IV as ADHD, Predominantly Inattentive subtype.

Maintaining concentration has been considered the main difficulty of ADHD, with distractibility as a byproduct. When classwork or chores begin, the youngster shifts gears to something else midway through and either leaves the original task incomplete or later completes it inefficiently. Poor sustained attention may represent a process of active distraction, where visual, auditory, or kinesthetic stimuli successfully compete for the adolescent's attention, as when a teenager says he or she cannot tune out the noises, sights, thoughts, fantasies, or feelings. Alternatively, Barkley recently argued that poor sustained attention may really represent a modified form of impaired behavioral inhibition, in that the adolescent's brain cannot delay the impulse, for neurochemical reasons, to switch attention to the next incoming sensory stimulus. It takes 3 hours to do a 10-minute assignment or a 1-hour examination because of frequent lapses of concentration or temporary shifts to other activities which momentarily capture the youngster's attention. This forces the adolescent to read the same paragraph over and over again. At a more molar level, the adolescent may sign up for many extracurricular activities but quit them after a short time. He or she may start hobbies or artistic endeavors but abandon them in midstream; one talented young artist had four splendidly half-painted walls in his room, an avant garde testimony to his poor sustained task performance.

Difficulty maintaining effort is closely aligned with difficulty maintaining concentration. This attention deficit can best be summarized in two words often uttered by ADHD teens: "I'm bored." They become easily bored with most mundane, repetitive, low-stimulation activities, especially schoolwork, chores, hobbies, and even peers, relationships, sports, or their lives in general. They often seek out new and exciting experiences to maintain their interest; such thrill seeking may lead them to perfectly innocent activities such as roller blading, dancing, video games, or bike racing, or to more risky behaviors such as drag racing, experimentation with alcohol or drugs, sexual promiscuity, shoplifting, or violence. Zentall (1985) called this trait an attentional bias toward novelty. ADHD teens cannot properly perform tasks that require sustained mental effort. When deep thought is required, they look for the easy way out, glossing over the details and giving incomplete answers. If forced to sustain their effort for a long time, they often complain of mental fatigue.

Difficulty with organization, forgetfulness, and recall of learned material leads to many of the educational handicaps encountered by ADHD adolescents. They come to class unprepared, turn in assignments late or not at all, do not have the necessary books or papers to do homework, fail to write down assignments, keep their rooms and lockers in messy condition, and do not track long-term commitments adequately. During an exam, they may blank out and forget everything they knew the night before. They do not manage time well and are unable to prioritize efficiently. They have a warped perception of how much time has passed, or of the amount of time a task will take, and they are chronically late.

Difficulty making transitions refers to becoming hyperfocused on one detail of a situation, to the exclusion of all the other relevant details, or rigidity (e.g., spending all one's time on math homework and ignoring English or history, or refusing to stop watching television or video games at bedtime).

Impulsivity

Adolescence is characterized by poor impulse control or impaired response inhibition, although ADHD teenagers display even more impulsivity than do other teenagers. I find it clinically useful to explain the symptoms to families in order to divide impulsivity into its behavioral, cognitive, and emotional components, even though this clinical conceptualization does not necessarily correspond to the latest research findings. *Behaviorally,* the impulsive teenager has to have things right now, and thus acts on a whim. He or she does whatever pops into mind, becoming a victim of the moment, blurting things out, opting for short-term pleasure despite long-term pain, and not considering the consequences of actions before taking them. It is difficult for them to regulate their behavior in accordance with external or internal standards or rules. *Cognitively,* the impulsive adolescent rushes through schoolwork, overlooking crucial details, making careless mistakes, and writing sloppily. He or she cannot slow down cognitive tempo. *Emotionally,* impulsive teenagers become easily frustrated, agitated, moody, and/or emotionally overactive, losing their temper, and having angry and/or violent outbursts which may be accompanied by aggressive physical and verbal responses, directed either at others or at oneself (e.g., suicidal behaviors). Life is a series of highs and lows for the adolescent with ADHD, but it is important that the clinician distinguish between the unpredictable moodiness of ADHD and the more protracted, episodic mood swings of the bipolar individual. In teenage girls with ADHD, I have observed clinically (although there is no research on this yet) that moodiness and hyperemotionality increase exponentially compared to their non-ADHD peers shortly before they menstruate (i.e., PMS). It is the impulse control aspect of ADHD that can get an adolescent into serious life difficulty and may even lower life expectancy (Barkley, 1996a), when the adolescent makes poor decisions about sexuality, substances, driving, and other high-risk situations.

Hyperactivity

Although we now know that hyperactivity and impulsivity are different expressions of impaired behavioral inhibition (i.e., failure to inhibit the impulse for motor movement), it may nonetheless be clinically useful to discuss hyperactivity separately. The classic motor overactivity of young children is often diminished or transformed by adolescence, and is either channeled in different directions or transformed into subjective feelings of restlessness. Although ADHD teens do not necessarily appear restless to the external observer, they often feel that way inside. They fidget or exhibit other signs of minor motor restlessness. They feel confined when in a classroom for a long time or if they have to sit at a desk and study for a long time. Nonstop talking (especially in girls) and badgering are two additional manifestations of hyperactivity. Those who channel high energy levels into many activities may be on the go day and night, wearing out their friends and family. They may only need 4 or 5 hours of sleep a night.

Clinicians will, however, encounter a relatively small number of adolescents who continue to exhibit the driven, nonstop on-the-go quality characteristic of the young hyperactive child. They constantly have to do something, otherwise they feel as if they will go crazy.

ASSOCIATED PROBLEMS

Children with ADHD may have a host of associated problems, including academic, behavioral, family, emotional, social, and developmental/medical difficulties, which are present to a greater degree in children with ADHD than in other children but are not intrinsic to the core symptoms of ADHD. Nor do such problems rule out the diagnosis when they are absent, so they cannot be considered defining features of ADHD. These problems often multiply exponentially as children become adolescents and the demands and expectations for performance increase. In some cases, these problems take the form of formal comorbid psychiatric syndromes; in other cases, they are equally significant difficulties but do not fall into any diagnostic category. In this section, I briefly survey the most common difficulties associated with ADHD, which are discussed in greater detail in later chapters on differential diagnosis and treatment.

Academics

Academic performance and learning problems are probably the most common associated difficulty that ADHD adolescents experience. The demands of the school environment increase dramatically upon entering middle and high school. The student has several teachers, a locker, and a variety of assignments and is expected to function more autonomously and master a lot more material and do long-term assignments more independently than in elementary school. The greatest academic difficulty for the average ADHD student is completing all of his or her homework and turning it in on time. These students gradually fall further behind, as their compromised organizational and executive abilities are overwhelmed. In some cases, they also have learning disabilities in reading, mathematics, written expression, or other areas. Some learning disabilities become impairments more in secondary education than in primary education, because high school students are expected to be able to put their thoughts into writing much more than are elementary school students. The ADHD student with a learning disability in written expression may run into problems with essays and term papers for the first time in high school. In other cases, deficits in memory, organization, or simply consistent follow-through rather than learning disabilities interfere with academic success.

Intellectual ability may become a factor in one of two ways. Students with ADHD and above-average ability were often able to coast through elementary school without much effort. They did not have to pay attention much of the time to be successful in the average public school. However, they can no longer get by on sheer brilliance in high school, college, and beyond. Now they must devote long hours to often tedious study and paper writing, which demand full concentration. This helps to explain why we often diagnose ADHD in gifted adolescents or young adults. Research (Barkley, 1990) suggests that for reasons we cannot explain, many ADHD youngsters score 7–10 points below others on standardized IQ tests; this may be a result of the impact of ADHD symptoms on test-taking behavior, or it may be a true neurobiological difference.

Conduct

Behavioral/conduct problems along with academic problems are the number one associated difficulty in adolescents with ADHD. In fact, many people mistakenly assume that oppositional and/or aggressive behavior is a core characteristic of ADHD. Such conduct problems frequently take the form of noncompliance to parents' requests, stubbornness, argumentativeness, back talk, rebellion, getting easily annoyed, and generally agitating siblings and others in provocative ways. The teenager often behaves in such a defiant manner to avoid completing effortful tasks such as household chores or homework. Agitating others and making a general nuisance out of oneself is sometimes an expression of hyperactivity in adolescents. Because a certain amount of rebelliousness is normal as young teenagers individuate from their parents (Robin & Foster, 1989), it is often difficult for parents to determine whether a given adolescent's defiance is a natural developmental phenomenon or an associated feature of ADHD. When argumentative, defiant behavior reaches clinical proportions, we often diagnose ODD as a comorbid condition to ADHD. ODD occurs in 59% to 73% of adolescents with ADHD (Barkley, Fischer, Edelbrock, & Smallish, 1990; Biederman, Faraone, Milberger, Guite, et al., 1996).

A smaller number of adolescents with ADHD display more serious conduct problems, including lying, stealing, truancy, and physical aggression. Such adolescents are often diagnosed as having CD. Research reviewed in Chapter 2 suggests that 28% to 43% of adolescents with ADHD meet the criteria for CD (Barkley, Fischer, et al., 1990; Biederman, Faraone, Milberger, Guite, et al., 1996). This subgroup of adolescents with ADHD and CD has been found to be at serious risk for substance abuse, although ADHD itself has not been found to be a risk factor for substance abuse (Grilo et al., 1995; Martin, Earleywine, Blackson, & Vanyukov, 1994).

Family Conflict

Academic and conduct problems inevitably promote family conflict. Families of normal adolescents experience a period of increased conflict at the onset of puberty, but this period is usually more intense for families with ADHD adolescents. These conflicts are characterized by negative communication (mutual accusations, defensiveness, interruptions, poor eye contact, not listening, lecturing, etc.) and inadequate problem solving (power assertion, failure to negotiate). Parents sometimes lose control over their adolescents, who often outwit them to avoid effort and responsibility and get their way. Such unpleasant conflicts separate family members, creating disengagement, rattling the parents' marriage, and often bringing out the worst in everybody. These conflicts can be particularly severe and debilitating in families with ADHD adolescents who are dealing with parental separation, divorce, and/or remarriage.

Emotions

Common emotional disturbances in adolescents with ADHD include various forms of depression, anxiety, and low self-esteem. The cumulatively increasing life failure experiences, which often occur as children with ADHD move into adolescence, take their toll on self-esteem and induce periods of depression in most adolescents. This is especially true for adolescents who are diagnosed for the first time in their late teenage years. They had no explanation for their troubles and often were blamed for being stupid, lazy, and unmotivated, which most come to believe over time. Low mood and low self-esteem set in, just as with Melissa, the 19-year-old we met earlier.

In most cases, the depression may be phenomenologically significant but may not meet the full diagnostic criteria for Dysthymia or Major Depressive Disorder. The clinician may find that the adolescent's mood disturbance meets the criteria for the cluster of a Sadness Problem, a subclinical variety of Major Depressive Disorder, according to the *Diagnostic and Statistical Manual for Primary Care (DSM-PC), Child and Adolescent Version* (American Academy of Pediatrics, 1996). By adulthood, more ADHD adults than adolescents meet the formal criteria for a Mood Disorder. Biederman, Faraone, Milberger, Guite, et al. (1996) reported that 45% of the teenagers in his follow-up study met criteria for Major Depressive Disorder. One may speculate that there would be an increased risk for suicide caused by depression, among adolescents with ADHD, but further research is needed in this matter.

The clinician should not underestimate the tremendous negative impact of low self-esteem and sadness resulting from life failure experiences caused by ADHD. Even though the sadness may not meet clinical criteria, the clinician needs to help the adolescent with these problems.

Clinically, most adolescents with ADHD are not particularly anxious individuals, and many could benefit from some facilitative anxiety about the consequences of not pulling it together in school and at home. Adults often report high levels of anxiety in ADHD youngsters, but upon further investigation, the clinician typically learns that it is a form of nervousness that is really an example of restlessness and hyperactivity but not true anxiety. Nonetheless, clinicians will find selected symptoms of anxiety in some ADHD adolescents, particularly performance anxiety. Those who try to cope but have difficulty may exhibit performance anxiety. Michael and Melissa often had periods when they felt overwhelmed and anxious. When faced with an unexpected crisis, the ADHD individual may more readily overreact emotionally than do non-ADHD individuals, displaying temporary panic and anxiety symptoms.

Some adolescents with ADHD meet formal criteria for comorbid Anxiety Disorders. Biederman studies the frequency of multiple Anxiety Disorders in his follow-up sample of adolescents, finding it to be 35% compared to 9% in a non-ADHD control group.

Developmental/Medical Problems

Younger children with ADHD exhibit elevated rates of developmental difficulties such as enuresis, speech and language delays, and "soft" neurological signs (Barkley, 1990). They also exhibit elevated rates of minor physical anomalies and medical problems such as an index finger longer than the middle finger, adherent ear lobes, maternal health and perinatal complications, recurring respiratory infection, allergies, sleep difficulties, and asthma. These children are also considerably more likely to have accidents than are normal children (Barkley, 1990).

No particular medical syndromes are known to be specifically associated with ADHD in adolescents. However, the poor choices that impulsive adolescents make in terms of life style issues (e.g., having unprotected sexual relations, failing to wear a seat belt, drinking and driving, and engaging in other high-risk behaviors) may in fact shorten life expectancy of ADHD individuals (Barkley, 1996a). Future follow-up studies will need to examine these possibilities. No data yet compare life expectancy in ADHD versus non-ADHD individuals. However, one large, longitudinal investigation (Friedman et al., 1995) found that impulsivity in childhood often predicts reduced life expectancy by all causes of death.

Adolescents are often brought to clinicians because of these associated features of ADHD (poor academic performance, family conflict, substance abuse, depression, anxiety, or even bulimia nervosa). Males are more likely to present with conduct problems and females with depression or internalizing problems. Through the careful process of evaluation and differential diagnosis described in Section 2, the clinician uncovers what is really going on and plans a course of intervention.

EVALUATION OF THE DSM-IV APPROACH TO ADHD

To understand the core and associated features of ADHD in adolescence, we need to critically examine the adequacy of the DSM-IV categorical approach to defining ADHD: Either you have it or you do not. Compared to DSM-III-R, DSM-IV advances our ability to conceptualize ADHD by adding and/or rewording many of the attention items, making them more relevant to adolescents and adults. Items such as "fails to pay close attention to detail," "has difficulty organizing tasks or activities," and "often avoids, dislikes, or fails to engage in tasks which require sustained mental effort" broaden the formal definition of inattention to include most of the attentional deficits discussed earlier in the chapter. Explicitly requiring clinically significant impairment across two or more settings, recognizes the cross-situational nature of ADHD. Requiring that the symptoms not only to be present but also be interfering with or impairing an individual's life helps to differentiate between normal variations in temperament and a disorder. Unfortunately, DSM-IV does not provide any guidelines defining "clinically significant impairment," leaving this open to subjective interpretation. In future chapters, the issue of significant impairment becomes especially important when considering the need for educational interventions. In addition, the requirement for pervasiveness across situations may be a problem in some cases as research has repeatedly demonstrated that parents and teachers typically agree only modestly (.30 to .50) on the presence of ADHD symptoms (Barkley, 1995a). Important issues related to age, gender, onset, and subtypes remain unsettled in DSM-IV (Barkley, 1995a).

Age

The requirement that the symptoms be more severe than is typically observed in individuals of a comparable level of development emphasizes the importance of taking age and level of development into account, yet the number of symptoms required to make a diagnosis is not adjusted for different ages. The subjects in DSM-IV field trials were primarily ages 4 to 16. It is well established that the base rate of ADHD symptoms in the population declines with increasing age (Murphy & Barkley, 1996a). Applying the same diagnostic threshold across all ages may result in diagnosing a larger than expected percentage of preschoolers and a smaller than expected percentage of older adolescents and adults. The appropriateness of the item set for capturing the core features of the disorder may also be different at different ages. Inattention items have a wide applicability across the life span, but hyperactivity/impulsivity items may be more limited to age-related appropriateness. Hyperactivity in adolescents and adults is less overt than are most of DSM-IV items. There is an insufficient number or variety of impulsivity items; they fail to tap domains of functioning such as decisions about high-risk behaviors (sexuality, substances, driving), which are relevant for older adolescents and adults, for example.

Gender

The complicated question is whether there ought to be separate diagnostic thresholds for males and females. Research on ADHD and related characteristics generally suggests that males display greater frequencies and higher intensities of these characteristics than do females in the general population (Achenbach & Edelbrock, 1983; DuPaul, 1991). If so, applying the same symptom cutoff to males and females will result in females having to meet a higher threshold relative to other females to be diagnosed as ADHD than do males relative to other males; that is, more severe cases will be identified in females than males, and milder cases will more often go unidentified in females than in males (Barkley, 1995a, 1995b). Barkley (1995a) suggested that the 95th percentile of deviance be applied to each gender equally, resulting in a lower absolute symptom threshold for females than for males, meaning that equal numbers of girls and boys would be identified as having ADHD.

Gordon (1996) objected to Barkley's suggestion and argued that more boys than girls are identified because males naturally display more inattention and hyperactivity/impulsivity symptoms than do females (i.e., ADHD is more of a "guy thing"). He noted that other problems such as Anorexia Nervosa and depression occur more often in females than males, so why couldn't ADHD occur more often in males than females? If we adjusted the diagnostic criteria to have equal numbers of boys and girls diagnosed as having ADHD, Gordon further argued that the girls so identified would have lower levels of impairment than the boys, and we would be offering clinical services to children with milder symptoms. He considers this problematic, both on philosophical grounds (i.e., labeling a less impaired population as having a psychiatric disorder), and on economic grounds, (because of limited availability of treatment resources in our managed care era). Gordon points out that the argument about identifying children with less impairment rests on the assumption that a greater number of symptoms correlates with a greater degree of impairment, and that the evidence supporting this assumption is mixed, at best. Finally, he cautions us that if we adjust diagnostic criteria for ADHD based on sex, we might be opening the door to adjusting criteria for many other diagnoses based on a variety of factors such as gender, race, ethnicity, and so on. Where would we draw the line?

Barkley (1996b) rebutted Gordon's arguments against adjusting ADHD diagnostic criteria on the basis of sex. First, he pointed out that we currently use rating scales as part of our diagnostic practice, and that most rating scales have been normed separately for males and females. Therefore, we are already implicitly using separate thresholds for deviance on rating scales as part of our diagnostic criteria, so why not make this practice explicit? Furthermore, he disagreed with Gordon's reasoning that ADHD may be more of "a guy thing." He pointed out that DSM-IV ADHD criteria were developed empirically, using a large sample of children, mostly boys. Therefore, the symptom lists are based primarily on manifestations of inattention and hyperactivity/impulsivity in boys. So it explains why symptoms derived from research primarily on males result in the identification of more males than females as having ADHD. If more girls were studied in subsequent revisions of DSM-IV, perhaps a more balanced symptom list would be developed, providing equal results.

Barkley also strongly seconded Gordon's concern that the evidence for the link between the number of symptoms and the degree of impairment is shaky. Furthermore, there is no evidence that shows that the types of impairments caused by ADHD are comparable in males and females. Perhaps the clinical problems caused by ADHD in females are different than those caused by ADHD in males. Solden (1995) vividly documented at the clinical level the many ways that women with ADHD suffer from a variety of emotional and self-esteem problems, compounded by different cultural expectations from women than from men. Arcia and Conners (1998) supported Solden's (1995) contention in a comparison of male and female children and adults with ADHD. They found no gender diferences in cognitive or neuropsychological functioning, but adult women ADHD had significantly more negative self-perceptions than adult men with ADHD. Barkley concluded by calling for more research on the nature of the impairments in women with ADHD, to help us decide whether we ought to have different diagnostic thresholds.

Where does this debate leave the practitioner? Clearly, we currently have to apply the same DSM-IV symptoms thresholds to males and females for the sake of standardization, but I agree with Barkley that we should make explicit our current practice of implicitly using rating scales with different norms for males and females. Clinically, I agree with Solden that there may be very different pictures of impairment in men and women with ADHD, as the case studies in this chapter and the research by Arcia and Conners (1998) have already begun to illustrate. Clinicians need to be sensitive to the different clinical presentations and types of impairments and to gear their treatments to them while researchers begin to investigate the possible differences in the degree and types of impairments in males versus females with ADHD.

Onset

Requiring an age of onset of 7 may be too restrictive. DSM-IV field trials did not show any differences in degree of ADHD and degree of impairment between those meeting and not meeting the criterion of age 7 for onset (Barkley, 1995b). It may be wiser to stipulate some time during childhood for age of onset. Research suggests that many young children's hyperactivity lasts six months but does not later become a disorder; thus 12 months' persistence may be more reasonable.

Subtypes

The presentation of the three subtypes as part of a unitary disorder goes against current research, which Spencer et al. (1996) aptly summarized with the phrase "ADHD is a heterogeneous disorder of unknown etiology." A preponderance of research suggests that the Predominantly Inattentive subtype is fundamentally a separate disorder (Barkley, DuPaul, & McMurray, 1990; Lahey & Carlson, 1992), while family genetic research suggests that ADHD plus certain comorbidities such as CD are better considered subtypes of ADHD than independent disorders (Biederman, Faraone, & Lapey, 1992). Recent reconceptualizations of ADHD have suggested that it may be primarily a disorder of executive function based on a wide-umbrella cognitive model with either inattention (Brown, 1996) or behavioral disinhibition as the central organizing construct (Barkley, 1994, 1997b). It isn't clear whether the Hyperactive–

Impulsive subtype is truly a separate subtype or an earlier developmental stage of ADHD, Combined subtype. In the field trials, the Hyperactive–Impulsive subtype was found primarily in preschoolers. By school age, these same youngsters develop inattention symptoms, and as Barkley (1994, 1997a) has recently argued, inattention may not be the central construct in ADHD, Combined type.

Research on the validity of the DSM-IV subtypes is just beginning to appear. Paternite, Loney, and Roberts (1996) conducted a preliminary test of the criterion-related validity of DSM-IV ADHD subtypes. Using 132 6- to 12-year-old boys, they approximated DSM-IV ADHD diagnoses with DSM-III versions of structured psychiatric interviews and selected rating scale items. Their sample divided into 28 children with the Inattentive subtype (ADHD INATT), nine with the Hyperactive–Impulsive subtype (ADHD HI), 59 with the Combined subtype (COMB), and 18 non-ADHD residual cases. The remainder of the sample, which did not clearly fall in any one group, was discarded from the analysis. They compared the INATT, HI, COMB, and residual groups on a comprehensive set of measures of the extent of problem identification, impairment, cognitive–attentional variables, family factors, and disruptive and nondisruptive behavior.

All the subtypes differed from the residual group, and there were consistent differences between the three subtypes on problem identification, extent of impairment, parent and teacher ratings of disruptive behavior, and playroom observations of behavior. However, there were no differences on IQ, academic achievement, and cognitive measures of attention such as continuous performance tests (CPTs). The COMB and HI subtypes generally exhibited more impairment at home and more disruptive behavior on parent and teacher ratings scales than did the INATT subtype but did not differ from each other. Although all three subtypes exhibited more learning and attention problems than did the residual group, few differences were found between the HI and the COMB groups. For example, the COMB group showed more learning and attention problems than did the HI group, while the HI group exhibited less delinquent behavior than the COMB group.

These results supported the criterion-related validity of the Inattentive and Combined subtypes of ADHD, but only provided limited evidence for the criterion-related validity of the Hyperactive–Impulsive subtype as a separate subtype of ADHD. Of course, this study was limited by the small sample size of the hyperactive–impulsive group, the use of DSM-III diagnostic approximations to the full DSM-IV criteria, and the exclusion of females. Nonetheless, the results support the clinical impression that the validity of ADHD, Hyperactive–Impulsive subtype is questionable. In addition, the fact that differences were found between the Inattentive and the Combined subtype on disruptive behavior and impairment does not provide evidence for or against the hypothesis that the Inattentive subtype may be a fundamentally different disorder.

Incidence

With the addition of a new subtype and a broadening of the diagnostic criteria, the concern arises as to whether the application of DSM-IV will result in diagnosing more individuals as having ADHD. In fact, the rate of diagnosis of ADHD in the United States has increased tremendously in the past few years, fueling criticisms concerning overdiagnosis (Armstrong, 1995). Baumgaertel, Wolraich, and Dietrich (1995) conducted three studies addressing this concern, comparing DSM-III, DSM-III-R, and DSM-IV criteria within a population of 1,000 German elementary school children in five rural and five urban public schools. They found that the prevalence of ADHD increased from 9.6% with DSM-III criteria to 17.8% with DSM-IV criteria, with most of the additional cases falling in the Inattentive and Hyperactive–Impulsive subtypes. The Inattentive subtype was more strongly associated with academic problems, whereas the Hyperactive–Impulsive subtype was more strongly associated with behavioral problems. The Combined subtype showed academic and behavioral problems. Interestingly, Baumgartel et al. (1995) also found the Inattentive Type to be more prevalent in the urban children and comorbid ODD to be more prevalent in the rural children.

More recently, Wolraich and Baumgaertel (1996) reported two additional studies of the change in prevalence rates using DSM-III-R compared to DSM-IV ADHD criteria. Subjects consisted of all the children in kindergarten through fifth grade in a middle Tennessee county during 1993–1994 in the first study, and during 1994–1995 in the second study. These included 398 teachers and 8,258 children during the first year and 214 teachers and 4,323 children during the second year. The teachers completed a comprehensive checklist of the DSM-IV ADHD and ODD characteristics, as well as seven depression and anxiety items. They also rated academic and behavioral impairments in the students, whether the student was formally diagnosed as having ADHD, and whether the student was being treated with stimulant medication. In the first study, the overall prevalence rate of ADHD increased from 7.3% under DSM-III-R criteria to 11.4% under DSM-IV criteria. The prevalence rates for the various DSM-IV subtypes were as follows: Inattentive subtype, 5.4%; Hyperactive–Impulsive subtype, 2.4%; and Combined subtype, 3.6%. In the second study, the prevalence rates were 16.1% for all subtypes of ADHD, broken down as follows: Inattentive subtype, 8.8%; Hyperactive–Impulsive subtype, 2.6%; Combined subtype, 4.7%. When the presence of impairment was also added as a criterion in the second study, the prevalence rates decreased to a total of 12.4%, with 6.6% Inattentive, 0.9% Hyperactive–Impulsive, and 4.9% Combined subtypes. A subset of 243 children had been rated in a similar study by their teachers the previous year, so that it was possible to examine the reliability of ratings meeting the ADHD criteria. Only 52% met the ADHD criteria for any subtype 2 years in a row.

These three studies suggest that application of the DSM-IV criteria may result in an increase in the number of children identified as having ADHD, which explains why more individuals are being diagnosed as having ADHD now than a decade ago. However, these studies relied on only one source of information—teacher ratings of the presence of sufficient inclusionary criteria for an ADHD diagnosis—and did not examine differential diagnostic factors. Clinicians need to study full diagnostic evaluations that also focus on adolescents before we can reach definitive conclusions about whether DSM-IV increases the number of children identified as having ADHD.

In addition to broader diagnostic criteria, other factors may be fueling the increase in diagnoses of ADHD in contemporary American society. First, the fast-paced, 15-second sound bite mentality of our culture tends to encourage ADHD-like behavior (Hallowell & Ratey, 1994). Second, the pressure in many middle-class circles for high achievement and the keen competition for good jobs may cause parents to look to diagnoses such as ADHD and treatments such as medication as ways to quickly help their children climb the social and economic ladder. Third, the recognition that ADHD is indeed a life span disorder has increased the number of adolescents and adults seeking evaluations. Further research is needed to determine the relative influence of each of these factors, together with the broader criteria of DSM-IV, in causing changes in the rate of diagnosis of ADHD.

DSM-PC, Child and Adolescent Version

One of the problems with DSM-IV is that it is a categorical diagnostic system. It has become more evident that disorders such as ADHD really reflect dimensions of functioning and temperament rather than discrete categories, and that the disorder is one end point of a continuum. Adolescents may exhibit the entire continuum of difficulties with attention and behavioral inhibition. We often encounter subclinical problems that create some impairment for the adolescent but do not meet the DSM-IV criteria. Primary care physicians in particular often face this dilemma. In response to this issue, a new diagnostic manual has been written and designed to bridge the gap between normality and disorders and to recognize that environmental situations are important contributors to children's mental health. The *Diagnostic and Statistical Manual for Primary Care (DSM-PC), Child and Adolescent Version* (American Academy of Pediatrics, 1996) is a collaborative effort of the American Academy of Pediatrics and the American Psychiatric Association. It consists of two major sections: (1) the child's environment, and (2) the child's responses to that environment. Section One recognizes that a child's environment has an important impact on his or her mental health and includes a detailed listing of over 30 environmental factors ranging from death of a parent, divorce, physical and sexual abuse, to acculturation, religious crisis, poverty, illiteracy, and homelessness. Each of the major factors includes a definition and a discussion of those factors that either put a child at risk or protect the child from the impact of the environmental situation. It is particularly noteworthy that factors that protect a child against the impact of a disorder are discussed along with risk factors, as characteristics such as a short attention span may not always be negative.

Section Two organizes children's responses into 29 clusters, which correspond roughly to DSM-IV Axis I disorders. Each cluster starts with common presenting complaints, definition and symptoms, and epidemiological information. Most important, this taxonomy recognizes that children's behavioral/emotional problems fall on a continuum by dividing each cluster into three levels: (1) *developmental variations* that may cause parents to be concerned but are actually normal variations, (2) *problems* that are severe enough to require intervention but are not severe enough to be diagnosed as a disorder, and (3) *disorders* that meet DSM-IV criteria. Readers are given detailed examples of common presentations of each level of the clusters in infancy, early childhood, middle childhood, and adolescence, along with differential diagnosis guidelines based on general medical conditions, substances and drugs, and other mental disorders.

Five clusters touch on ADHD and disruptive behavior disorders (1) Hyperactive–Impulsive behaviors; (2) Inattentive behaviors; (3) Negative emotional behaviors; (4) Aggressive/Oppositional behaviors; and (5) Secretive Antisocial behaviors. In the Hyperactive–Impulsive cluster, for example, a developmental variation is defined as a high level of restlessness or impulsivity which does not impair functioning, such as an adolescent engaging in active social pursuits for long periods (e.g., dancing) without any negative outcomes. A problem is defined as restlessness or impusivity that becomes intense enough to begin to impair functioning but does not consist of sufficient symptoms of ADHD to diagnose a disorder. An adolescent who meets four of the nine DSM-IV ADHD hyperactivity–impulsivity criteria might also be classified as having a Hyperactive–Impulsive behavioral problem.

The utility and psychometric characteristics of the DSM-PC await empirical evaluation through field trials and controlled investigations. Meanwhile, this primary care–oriented approach to mental health classification serves as a model for how the clinician who works with ADHD adolescents can better view the core characteristics of ADHD from a dimensional/developmental perspective rather than a dichotomous distinction. Clinically, I have found it useful to portray difficulties with concentration and inhibitory control to parents as falling on a continuum, with the DSM-IV diagnosis of ADHD being beyond a certain point toward the extreme end of the continuum. Adolescents may fall anywhere on that continuum, and DSM-PC is a way to classify milder forms of ADHD symptoms.

Assets and Positive Features of ADHD

As noted previously, the DSM-PC classified protective factors as well as risk factors related to childhood behavior and emotions. The emphasis on impairment, which is intrinsic to making a DSM-IV diagnosis, may obscure the individual's strengths. Individuals with ADHD may have unique strengths in addition to impairments caused by their symptoms, although this must be based on clinical experience because there is little research on this topic. Highly distractible individuals may not remain depressed or distraught for a long time because they are easily distracted. These individuals are frequently scanning the environment and are likely to notice things others overlook. Although they may forget where they put their own keys, wallet, or purse, they may often find things that others lost. They may notice defects in products or work situations, dangerous situations, or other details the highly focused individual may overlook.

Impulsive individuals may excel in situations that require quick thinking and immediate responses, such as emergencies. Hartmann (1993) argues that ADHD may have served an adaptive function at one time in the history of humankind, and that these characteristics may be useful in certain environments today. He points out that in ancient times when man was primarily a hunter, ADHD characteristics may have been an asset. Skilled hunters must notice their prey by constantly scanning the environment, and they must respond quickly with high bursts of energy; thus distractibility, impulsivity, and hyperactivity would serve a hunter well. Similarly, in today's world, ADHD individuals may also excel in situations in which brainstorming a variety of divergent, innovative ideas is required (e.g., think tanks and entrepreneurial business situations such as starting new companies). Situations in which high energy levels are adaptive may also be particularly suited to ADHD individuals. In sales, for example, many ADHD individuals excel because they keep on going when their non-ADHD colleagues have given up in fatigue. In addition, those ADHD individuals whose hyperactivity manifests as a high degree of talkativeness often become social butterflies who have many friends and are very well liked. Ironically, the hypersensitivity of many individuals with ADHD, which results from a lifetime of being criticized, may heighten their sense of empathy toward others, making them excellent helpers in times of distress.

Clearly, more research is needed concerning the strengths and assets of having ADHD. Perhaps researchers can start by examining the positive characteristics of adolescents and adults with ADHD who are succeeding socially, academically, interpersonally, and vocationally.

The DSM-IV Approach: Conclusion

For descriptive and standardization purposes, the practitioner who deals with adolescents everyday needs to proceed by using the DSM-IV definition as the primary basis for diagnosis and treatment, while understanding and explaining to adolescents and their families that our conceptualizations of ADHD are evolving. The DSM-PC criteria may also be used for subclinical cases. It would be a mistake for the practitioner to adhere to other, less standardized definitions of ADHD, as this impedes research and reduces the reliability of treatments. An analogy to the disease of cancer may prove useful in explaining this to families. Fifty years ago, when a physician diagnosed a patient as having cancer, the general term "cancer" was a meaningful diagnosis because the tremendous heterogeneity of the disease was not well understood and subtyped. In addition, we did not have a wide variety of treatments for various types of cancer; most resulted in the same outcome—death. Today, the diagnosis of "cancer" without more detail is a virtually meaningless diagnosis which communicates very little about prognosis and treatment, because we have a much finer-grained understanding of the various types of cancer, their different treatments, and their very different prognoses. Some are completely curable, and others still result in a nearly certain death. Diagnosing an adolescent as having ADHD today is like diagnosing cancer 50 years ago because we have only a broad understanding of ADHD and its subtypes today. Our treatments are crude in the absolute scheme of things; we use a general stimulant to stimulate specific parts of the central nervous system, like using an elephant to kill an ant. The elephant gets the job done but has a lot of other effects too. In 50 years we will have more precise definitions and diagnostic criteria for ADHD, based on neurobiological and genetic subtyping.

THE RELATIONSHIP BETWEEN TEMPERAMENT AND ADHD

If we agree that a pure categorical model of mental illness is a gross oversimplification of the continuum of human functioning, is ADHD simply a type of temperament? "Temperament" refers to an individual's behavioral style or characteristic way he or she experiences and reacts to the environment, and it is generally thought to be a lifelong aspect of personality that is based on a combination of genetic, biological, and environmental factors.

One popular model (Thomas & Chess, 1977) defines nine basic dimensions of temperament: activity, rhythmicity, approach/avoidance, adaptability, intensity, mood, persistence/attention span, distractibility, and sensory threshold. Within this model, certain combinations of temperaments have been found to be risk factors for negative outcomes when the child's temperament does not fit with the demands and expectations of the environment. The temperament clusters that predict poor school adjustment and poor school performance include (1) low task orientation—low persistence/attention span, high distractibility, and high activity; (2) low flexibility—low approach and low adaptability, and negative mood; and (3) high reactivity—low sensory threshold, high intensity, and negative mood.

Historically, the temperament model of human behavior and the biological psychiatry model of disorders have developed in a parallel fashion but with little communication between the proponents of each (Carey & McDevitt, 1995). As a result, clinicians and researchers who study and work with the concept of temperament have pointed out that we may be mistakenly labeling extreme variations in temperament as an attention disorder (Carey & McDevitt, 1995). Carey and McDevitt (1995) argue that the definition of ADHD as it is commonly used in the United States refers to

> an oversimplified grouping of a complex and variable set of normal but incompatible temperament variations, disabilities in cognition, problems in school function and behavior, and sometimes neurological immaturities. We believe that many different conditions are being called by this one name. We propose that many of the children now being given this diagnosis of brain dysfunction or disorder simply have normal temperament variations that do not fit at school and that nothing at all is wrong with their brains. (p. 147)

The low-task-orientation temperament cluster is seen as predisposing a child to ADHD but not as the disorder itself. Because of certain environmental demands and expectations such as a traditional school system, the low-task-orientation temperament cluster may result in behavior that is a poor fit with the environment; clinicians then diagnose these children as having ADHD. Carey and McDevitt (1995) believe that it is wrong to diagnose a child as having a disorder when, in fact, he or she is at the extremes of certain normal temperament characteristics and therefore does not have a good fit with certain traditional societal environments (e.g., public school classrooms).

On this basis, Carey and McDevitt (1995) criticize the construct of ADHD as it is defined in DSM-IV:

1. ADHD is not a coherent syndrome because there is neither sufficient concurrence of its elements nor sufficient differentiation between them and other phenomena.
2. The behavioral components of ADHD are not clearly distinguishable from what is normal; that is, there is no clear-cut point at which normal activity level or normal attention span becomes abnormal.
3. Many children who are inattentive, distractible, and active do not develop clinical problems but do well in school and other settings.
4. The behaviors thought to constitute the disorder instead really con-

stitute risk factors for a disorder in some individuals, given a bad fit to their environments.

5. Low adaptability and inflexibility may be more prevalent among ADHD children than the supposed core symptoms of the syndrome.
6. ADHD in DSM-IV fails to take an evolutionary view, that is, that these characteristics may have been useful in the past.

Carey and McDevitt's (1995) solution is to maintain the concept of attention deficits but not to consider them a standard syndrome as readily as we do under DSM-IV. Instead, they suggest that we acknowledge multiple causes of attention deficits, ranging from cognitive dysfunction to extremes of the temperament characteristics of low persistence to other problems such as depression, anxiety, or even physical illness. They urge practitioners to adopt a more comprehensive diagnostic formulation, including the following factors: (1) general physical status, including growth, (2) neurological status, (3) information processing abilities, (4) cognitive and psychomotor maturation, (5) temperament or behavioral style, particularly the low task persistence characteristics, and (6) psychosocial adjustment, including social competence, task performance, self-assurance, and other mental and physical functions. They suggest that a profile of each child be constructed along these dimensions, and that if abnormalities in any area are identified, the person identifying them should be specified, and the "bad fit" between the child and that person should be specified in detail.

They urge researchers not to confuse extremes of normal temperament with a brain dysfunction, and to reserve the term "ADHD" for a small number of children who have an objectively demonstrable brain dysfunction. They also ask researchers to continue to conduct biologically based research to define the boundaries of the smaller group of individuals with a true neurobiologically based attention-deficit disorder.

Essentially, Carey and McDevitt are arguing that by confusing temperament extremes with a disorder, many individuals are diagnosed and treated as ADHD even though they do not have a disorder but, rather, a bad fit between their temperament and the environments with which they are compelled to cope. Furthermore, the true ADHD group with a genuine brain disorder is probably a much smaller number of children than are diagnosed using DSM-IV criteria.

Many of Carey and McDevitt's concerns parallel those expressed earlier in this chapter about DSM-IV—its categorical nature when, in reality, there are continua of behavioral phenomena; the lack of specification of how to assess impairment, which is really the same as a "bad fit" between the child and the environment; and the premature reification of subtypes in the absence of sufficient empirical knowledge, given that ADHD is a heterogeneous disorder of unknown etiologies. Whether the basic dimensions of functioning relevant to ADHD are to be considered constructs such as behavioral disinhibition or combinations of the nine temperament factors is a matter partly of semantics and partly of research outcomes. Research is needed, for example, to determine whether the low-task-persistence characteristics accurately characterize ADHD individuals across the life span, and whether useful treatment prescriptions follow from this conceptual model. Now that Carey and McDevitt (1995) and their colleagues have developed a psychometrically sound series of temperament rating scales, investigators should be able to conduct such research in the near future.

A BEHAVIORAL INHIBITION-BASED EXECUTIVE FUNCTIONING THEORY OF ADHD

We now recognize that impulsivity and hyperactivity are really two facets of a single dimension: behavioral disinhibition. Barkley (1997a, 1997b) has taken this line of reasoning one step further and reviewed the research indicating that impaired behavioral inhibition, not inattention, is the primary dimension underlying all the ADHD symptoms. He has constructed a hybrid model of executive functions based on a synthesis of Bronowski's (1977) theory of the uniqueness of language in human beings and Fuster's (1989, 1995) theory of the functioning of the frontal cortex, and he has grounded his theory in our current neurobiological and neuropsychological understanding of brain functioning in normal and ADHD individuals. He has eloquently described how this theory accounts for the myriad clinical symptoms and phenomena we call ADHD and has reviewed the emerging research support for it (Barkley, 1997b). I describe this theory in some detail and show how it applies to ADHD because of its importance to the field and its commonsense clinical utility in understanding the adolescents we treat. It is important to note that this theory applies to those individuals who have ADHD, Combined or Hyperactive–Impulsive types, not to those with ADHD, Inattentive type.

Figure 1.1 outlines the six components of Barkley's hybrid model of executive functions. The first component is behavioral inhibition—the foundation on which four other executive functions are dependent. These four executive functions include (1) nonverbal working memory (also known in earlier versions of his theory as prolongation), (2) verbal working memory or internalization, (3) self-regulation of affect/motivation/arousal, and (4) reconstitution. Barkley considers these four executive functions to be covert, self-directed forms of behavior which yield information that is internally represented and exerts a controlling influence over the sixth component of the model—the motor control and execution system. Barkley indicates that although he has heuristically chosen to depict these executive functions in neuropsychological terms, he could just have easily described them in the language of applied behavior analysis.

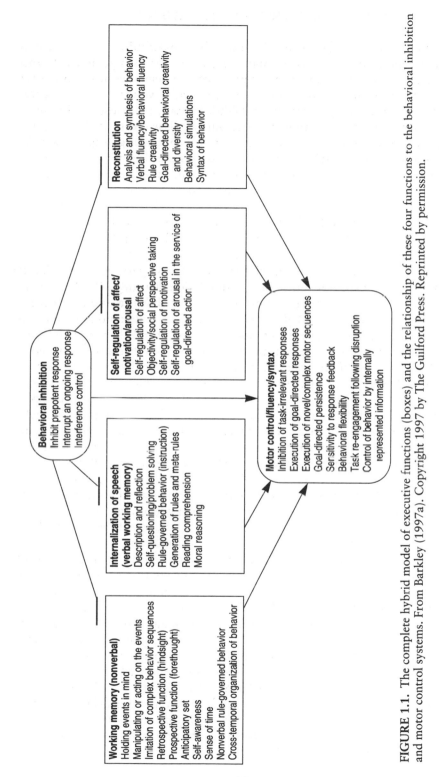

Behavioral inhibition
Inhibit prepotent response
Interrupt an ongoing response
Interference control

Working memory (nonverbal)
Holding events in mind
Manipulating or acting on the events
Imitation of complex behavior sequences
Retrospective function (hindsight)
Prospective function (forethought)
Anticipatory set
Self-awareness
Sense of time
Nonverbal rule-governed behavior
Cross-temporal organization of behavior

Internalization of speech (verbal working memory)
Description and reflection
Self-questioning/problem solving
Rule-governed behavior (instruction)
Generation of rules and meta-rules
Reading comprehension
Moral reasoning

Self-regulation of affect/ motivation/arousal
Self-regulation of affect
Objectivity/social perspective taking
Self-regulation of motivation
Self-regulation of arousal in the service of goal-directed action

Reconstitution
Analysis and synthesis of behavior
Verbal fluency/behavioral fluency
Rule creativity
Goal-directed behavioral creativity and diversity
Behavioral simulations
Syntax of behavior

Motor control/fluency/syntax
Inhibition of task-irrelevant responses
Execution of goal-directed responses
Execution of novel/complex motor sequences
Goal-directed persistence
Sensitivity to response feedback
Behavioral flexibility
Task re-engagement following disruption
Control of behavior by internally represented information

FIGURE 1.1. The complete hybrid model of executive functions (boxes) and the relationship of these four functions to the behavioral inhibition and motor control systems. From Barkley (1997a). Copyright 1997 by The Guilford Press. Reprinted by permission.

Behavioral inhibition includes three interrelated processes: (1) inhibition of an initial prepotent response to an event; (2) stopping of ongoing responses, which thereby delays the decision to respond; and (3) interference control—protection of the period of the delay and the self-directed responses that occur within it from disruption by competing events and responses. Inhibition of an initial prepotent response creates a delay during which the other four executive functions can operate, guiding motor responding; thus, these four executive functions are dependent for their effectiveness on effective behavioral inhibition. Stopping ongoing responses and interference control are also essential to protect the operation of the four executive functions from being overwhelmed by impulsive response tendencies and distractions.

Good behavioral inhibition in all three of these domains sets the stage for effective self-regulation by permitting the individual to delay his or her response to an incoming environmental stimulus long enough to engage in self-regulated behavior rather than to respond reflexively, as most animals do. Barkley defines self-regulation, in cognitive-behavioral terms as any response that alters the probability of an individual's subsequent response to an event and, in doing so, functions to alter the probability of a later consequence related to that event; for example, doing something less pleasant now to achieve a more desired outcome later. Self-regulatory behavior may be public or private (e.g., cognitive events). The following types of executive functions are examples of self-regulatory behaviors: (1) self-directed actions, (2) self-directed speech, (3) organization of behavioral contingencies across time, (4) delayed gratification, and (5) goal-directed, future-oriented, purposive, intentional actions.

Let's consider the next four executive functions in more detail.

1. *Nonverbal working memory/prolongation* represents a covert sensing to the self of visual (seeing to oneself) and auditory (hearing to oneself) information, or in more commonsense terms, the retention and reactivation of prior visual and auditory sensory representations; that is, the capacity to hold or prolong visual or auditory stimuli in mind to use them to control a subsequent response. Nonverbal working memory give us the ability to refer backward and forward in time and to exchange messages with others who propose action in the future; it requires retaining the event in working memory during the delay in responding and later fixing it in some symbolic form that can be retrieved for comparison with other stimuli and construction of hypothetical-situation courses of action, anticipating and planning future actions. This form of memory gives us our sense of time and imagination, as well as hindsight and forethought. The referencing of the past to regulate present behavior and aim it toward future events makes possible our sense of self-awareness, permits us to develop an anticipatory set or anticipation of hypothetical futures, and governs the cross-temporal organization of our behavior.

2. *Internalization of speech or verbal working memory* refers to self-directed, covert speech. It provides a means for the individual to describe and reflect on the nature of an event or situation before responding to it. Through internalization, individuals direct themselves, ask themselves questions, solve problems, and generate rules. It is therefore central to the development of rule-governed behavior, which makes possible functions such as reading comprehension and moral reasoning. Barkley outlines how this is consistent with a behavioral/developmental theory of the stimulus control of behavior by language, going through three stages: (a) the control of behavior by the language of others, (b) the control of behavior by self-directed public speech which eventually becomes subvocal or private speech, and (c) problem solving or the novel creation of new rules.

Rule-governed behavior has several consequences: (a) the variability of responses to a task is much less when it is in effect than when behavior is contingency shaped, (b) it is less affected by immediate contingencies in the situation, (c) it can be inflexible, and (d) it can continue even in the absence of immediate environmental consequences to maintain it.

3. *Self-regulation of affect/motivation/arousal* involves distinguishing between the emotional and informational content of a message and regulating one's emotional response by one's self-directed, executive reasoning abilities; that is, not reacting based purely on emotion but evaluating events objectively and rationally, then reacting. This involves self-regulation of emotion by reason, as when a person acts calm despite feeling angry. Barkley adds to this ability the self-generation of drive or motivational and arousal states that facilitate goal-directed actions and persistence toward the goal. Examples of this latter ability would be staying home from an enjoyable party to study for a chemistry exam (i.e., giving up an immediate gratification and mustering the self-motivation to work toward a long-term goal). The delay in emotional responses inherent in self-regulation of affect permits us to take various perspectives other than our own on an issue, making possible a sense of objectivity. To the extent that we can be objective and take other's perspectives, we do not have to be self-centered or egocentric. Thus, this executive function enables us to develop a sense of empathy for others and become nurturant of others' needs in addition to our own.

4. *Reconstitution* refers to (a) the analysis of a signal, now prolonged in working memory, into its component parts, and (b) the synthesis of these dissembled parts into entirely new messages, recombining them in innovative, creative ways. Reconstitution endows humans with tremendous problem-solving abilities and creativity.

Enabled to work efficiently through effective behavioral inhibition, the four executive functions discussed previously guide the individual's motor behavior in reasoned, intentional, and goal-oriented directions.

Impaired Behavioral Inhibition, Executive Functions, and ADHD

Barkley argues that impaired behavioral inhibition is the core difficulty of individuals with ADHD. This inhibitory deficit disrupts the control of goal-directed motor behavior by its detrimental effects on the four executive functions and the internally represented information they normally generate. ADHD delays the internalization of behavior that is central to executive functions and consequently delays the self-regulation that the executive functions afford to the individual. ADHD individuals do not as readily or efficiently engage these capacities in daily adaptive living compared to non-ADHD individuals. As a result, information will not feed forward as well in the brains of ADHD individuals compared to others, resulting in the performance problems with which we all are so familiar.

Deficits in Nonverbal Working Memory

Barkley's theory predicts that ADHD adolescents will show deficits in all forms of nonverbal working memory, including covert visual imagery and covert audition, as well as representational activities for taste, smell, and touch. Their behavior should be more influenced by context (i.e., living for the moment) and less influenced by internally represented information than that of non-ADHD peers. They should have more limited hindsight or a sense of the past, more limited foresight or a sense of the future, more distorted time perception, and more limited control of their ongoing behavior by past events and constructions of hypothetical future consequences. The rampant difficulties with procrastination, meeting deadlines, making the same mistakes repeatedly despite negative consequences for the past behavior, and the inability to plan meaningfully for a future are certainly consistent with a deficit in nonverbal working memory. Barkley also argues that difficulties with nonverbal working memory could help us understand why many ADHD adolescents have trouble with mental arithmetic: Restriction of working memory may make it difficult to hold the relevant information long enough to manipulate it and achieve the correct answer.

Deficits in Working Verbal Memory or Internalization

Concomitantly, poor internalization of language results in poor self-directed speech, with a clear negative impact on the regulation of the ongoing stream of daily adaptive behavior. As outlined earlier, the second stage of internalization is the increasing power of such speech to control behavior; this theory predicts that individuals with ADHD will have deficits in using self-directed speech to guide their behavior. This helps us to explain the why ADHD adolescents do not consistently follow rules. Clinically,

ADHD adolescents are victims of the moment, failing to recall or adhere to an internalized rule structure; they do poorly in situations involving delayed consequences and show great variability in performance. More globally, because moral development depends on internalization of societal standards, poor internalization could help explain the socialization and social skill difficulties of many ADHD adolescents.

Deficits in Self-Regulation of Affect/Motivation/Arousal

Barkley has pointed out that an integral part of private, self-directed sensing and speech is its associations with affective, motivational, and even arousal states. Because individuals with ADHD are less capable of mentally representing and sustaining internal information about prior contingencies, they are less able to reawaken their associated affective and motivational states. As a result, individuals with ADHD are less able to motivate themselves without external contingencies. Common complaints about adolescents with ADHD are that they display deficits in self-motivation and also learn less from environmental contingencies. They are less able to postpone immediate gratification for long-term gratification because of the self-motivational and arousal deficiency.

The difficulties inhibiting prepotent responses to events and delaying their response to those events diminishes the capacity to inhibit emotional prepotent responses. For example, adolescents with ADHD blow up, lose their temper, and have emotional outbursts more than non-ADHD adolescents. The greater emotional overreactivity, thin-skinned nature, and poor frustration tolerance characteristic of ADHD adolescents are consistent with this deficit in self-regulation of affect, for example. More important, the difficulty that ADHD adolescents have remaining objective in social situations, rather than responding to affective cues, would also be predicted to follow from poor self-regulation of affect. Clinical descriptions of ADHD teens are replete with factors such as a reduced likelihood of distinguishing personal meaning from objective information being communicated in a social exchange which might also lead to a greater display of self-centered, selfish behavior, and poor social perspective taking.

Deficits in Reconstitution

The reconstitution deficits in ADHD adolescents would be expected to manifest themselves as deficiencies in dissembling signals, messages, and events into their components and recombining such components into new responses (e.g., problem solving and creativity). Clinically and in research, it has been found that ADHD adolescents often act on the first solution to a problem that comes to mind, failing to generate a variety of alternatives and to evaluate their relative advantages versus disadvantages. They have a very difficult time with taking another's perspective, particularly in the case of emotionally charged issues.

Developmental Course and Instinctual Nature of Executive Functions

The normal development course of the appearance and maturation of these four executive functions is unclear. Barkley points out the capacity for delayed responding is known to begin to emerge by 12 months of age, and he suggests that self-regulation of affect/motivation/arousal might emerge next and that reconstitution probably matures last but does not yet have a clear hypothesis about the overall developmental course of these abilities. He does suggest, however, that the development of these four capacities is probably delayed in ADHD children, compared to normal children, in addition to being less efficiently utilized after development. Clearly, such a developmental trajectory is crucial to our application of this theory to ADHD adolescents.

Barkley hypothesizes that the development of self-control through the functioning of the executive functions is instinctual, with a strong genetic basis rather than learned from environmental experience. In other words, he believes that humans do not so much acquire self-control through formal social indoctrination or education but develop it largely as a result of the unfolding maturation of the neural structures of the prefrontal cortex, which he believes subserve it. Environmental conditions may facilitate or hinder this natural maturational process but do not account completely for it.

Because behavioral inhibition is the central construct, this theory explains that the role of inattention in ADHD represents an impairment in goal-directed persistence arising out of poor inhibition and resulting in negative impact on self-regulation. The adolescent cannot inhibit the impulse to respond to the next stimulus and is therefore frequently task shifting, not persisting with any one stimulus or response for any length of time. Therefore, the adolescent appears "inattentive" to the external observer. This theory accounts for the failure to find a true neuropsychological attention deficit in ADHD while nonetheless finding factors that represent perceptions of inattention on rating scales.

Research and Implications

Barkley (1997b) points out that to date, relatively little research directly addresses the many aspects of his theory, but the research that exists supports the theory, particularly regarding the central role of behavioral inhibition in ADHD, the role of working memory, poor self-regulation of motivation, and motor control and sequencing. Readers interested in a review of the research supporting this theory along with a detailed account of it should consult Barkley (1997b). Certainly, many clinical examples of difficulties with the four executive functions arise with adolescents. Readers can expect to see a great deal of research in the coming years, testing the many new hypotheses that follow from this theory.

Barkley's theory has clear-cut implications for treatment. If ADHD represents a neurobiologically based impairment in inhibitory control affecting key executive functions, then treatments that directly target the underlying neurobiological difficulty are most likely to be helpful. Medication is the only real example of such an intervention available today. Behavioral and educational interventions are likely to be helpful to the extent that they help the individual become aware of and work around the neurobiological deficit. Because the difficulty is not a lack of knowledge, skills training interventions would not be predicted to be that helpful. Rather, interventions that target the point of performance (e.g., behavior modification) would be predicted to be more helpful. To date, the treatment outcome data are consistent with this prediction.

DOES ADHD REALLY EXIST?

The most radical reformulation of ADHD has been to deny its validity. Is ADHD a valid syndrome or entity, or is it somehow an invention of self-interested professionals, support groups, lobbyists, or businesses that stand to benefit from its existence? This question surfaces regularly in the media in the United States. Every practitioner should be prepared to address it in a convincing manner. *The Myth of the ADD Child* (Armstrong, 1995) is the most sophisticated exposition of the nihilistic position about ADHD in print, written by a respected author and frequent presenter to educational audiences, who has credibility in the educational community because of his previous work, particularly on multiple intelligence.

According to Armstrong (1995) "ADD exists only because of a unique coming together of frustrated activist parents, the drug industry, a new cognitive research paradigm, a growth industry in new educational products, and a group of professionals eager to introduce them to each other—all of this taking place under a climate of benevolent government agencies" (p. 10). In other words, rather than being a true scientific entity, "ADD" is a construct invented by several groups of people for economic, political, cultural, and perhaps emotional reasons. These groups include the organized mental health community, pharmaceutical firms, support groups such as Children and Adults with Attention Deficit Disorder (CH.A.D.D.), and selected government agencies.

The following are a few of the reasons Dr. Armstrong gives for why he believes ADD is an invented construct rather than a real clinical syndrome.

Following each argument are my responses to his concerns ("Counterpoint").

1. *ADD is the disorder that goes "poof."* By stating that ADD is a medical disorder, experts are placing the source of the problem inside the child. Yet, unlike other medical disorders, ADD pops up in one setting, only to disappear in another. If ADD really existed, like diabetes or pneumonia, it would always be present.

Counterpoint: The fact that a person does not display the symptoms of a disorder all the time in all settings has nothing to do with the existence of the disorder. People with allergies only show symptoms in certain settings. People with ulcers only show symptoms at certain times. People with Bipolar Disorder only are manic some of the time; this is intrinsic to the definition of Bipolar Disorder, just as situational variability is intrinsic to the definitions of ADHD. Would we dispute the existence of allergies, ulcers, or Bipolar Disorder on this basis? Furthermore, by saying that ADD is a medical disorder, we are not placing the source of the problem completely within the child. Many medical disorders are reactive to environmental factors. Asthma is aggravated by smoking. Lead-based paints can lead to organic brain damage. Would we say asthma does not exist when the individual is not in the presence of smoke, or that organic brain damage does not exist because a child has not ingested lead chips?

2. *Diagnostic methods for ADD are poor.* The wide range of incidence figures for ADD cited in the literature calls into question the assessment methods used to make this diagnosis. If the diagnostic tools were valid, we would have a clear-cut figure for the incidence of ADD. There are also problems with all the common methods used to diagnose ADD. Ratings scales are merely subjective opinions, biased because many teachers and parents want their children to get diagnosed and medicated. Continuous performance tests bear little resemblance to what children do in the real world and are pitiful assessment techniques. In fact, all the measures used to assess ADD are fatally flawed because they were originally validated by comparing ADHD diagnosed children with control groups. Because there is no infallible, gold standard for ADD, there is no accurate way to form the comparison group to validate the measures.

Counterpoint: Any one assessment tool for ADD or any other disorder is fallible. That is why knowledgeable professionals rely on a battery of interview, parent rating, teacher rating, and testing data. That is why it takes 4–5 hours to conduct a thorough evaluation. Each of the major tools such as rating scales have undergone rigorous validation using generally accepted methodological standards in the social sciences. If we followed Armstrong's logic, we would have to stop all social science research. Many advances have been made through these research methods, and although they are not perfect, there is no compelling scientific reason to reject them.

3. *There is no attention deficit in ADD.* Research has failed to find

any real attention deficit in ADD, and Armstrong implies that reconceptu-alizations of ADHD in terms of deficits in rule-governed behavior (Barkley, 1990), and subsequent reasoning that we need to encourage better rule-governed behavior, will encourage the kind of blind obedience that oc-curred in Nazi Germany. We are already making our children obey too much. What they need is more inner-oriented self-actualizing experiences, not more obedience.

Counterpoint: Science advances by studying phenomena and changing one's conceptualizations of them. It is perfectly natural to expect that as we study ADD, we will learn that our earlier conceptualizations (i.e., first that hyperactivity was the central construct and then that attention was the cen-tral construct) are incorrect, and we will search for a better understanding. Premature reification would be dangerous. It is a travesty and totally ridiculous to liken the emphasis on increasing rule-governed behavior to societies such as Nazi Germany where too much compliance was a prob-lem. As anyone who has ever spent a few hours with an ADHD/ODD child knows, the issue is certainly not too much compliance but, rather, any compliance at all.

4. *Biological research is inconclusive.* The evidence for a neurobiolog-ical cause of ADD is incomplete. In particular, Armstrong points to Zimetkin's two published PET scan studies (Zimetkin et al., 1990), and to the fact that the second study only partially replicated the first.

Counterpoint: It is the convergence of many different types of evi-dence—PET scan research, family genetic research, biochemical assays, MRI structural research, etc.—that points to a neurobiological origin for many cases of ADD. Of course, not every study unequivocally supports the neurobiological etiology of ADD, because ADD is very heterogeneous. It represents a logical error of selective abstraction and magnification to pick on two studies and because one does not replicate the other, conclude that the ADD does not exist or have a neurobiological basis.

Next, Armstrong goes on to argue that ADD really is a simplistic an-swer to a complex problem. Perhaps society has invented ADD because it needed a simple explanation for the breakdown of the Protestant work eth-ic in the late 20th century. Perhaps ADD is a result of our 15-second sound-bite culture, which caters to short attention spans. Perhaps ADD is the response of children to boring classrooms, or a reflection of normal gender differences whereas boys are more active than girls. Perhaps ADD is a parent's excuse for a temperament mismatch between parent and child, or perhaps it is simply a different way of learning. If parents would parent and teachers would teach, we would not need to blame our children's fail-ures on ADD. In fact, Armstrong would agree with our earlier discussion of the possible assets of having ADHD, but he would argue that we are pe-nalizing individuals with these characteristics by giving them a diagnostic label at all.

Armstrong's Solution

Dr. Armstrong suggests that we should not diagnose children with problems as having any disorder but, rather, focus on their individual strengths. He certainly does not suggest that we use either stimulant medication or behavior modification. He believes that we are drugging our children into compliance (although interestingly he does say that in severe cases of hyperactivity, and when nothing else works, Ritalin should be tried) and we are killing their creative spirit through externally controlled behavior modification systems. Instead, he indicates that we should internally empower children to respect, listen, collaborate, and problem-solve with adults. In the second half of his book, he gives us 50 techniques to achieve this, although he does not give us any systematic approach for deciding which techniques to use with which children because he is against any kind of diagnosis.

Many of Armstrong's specific techniques are in fact common behavior modification techniques or classroom accommodations. Examples include (1) teach self-talk skills, (2) use color to highlight information, (3) find the child's best time of alertness, (4) give instructions in attention-grabbing ways, (5) provide positive role models, (6) help your child with organizational techniques, and (7) establish consistent rules, routines, and transitions. Most of his suggestions make a great deal of sense and are commonly used by parents and teachers of ADD children, as well as by therapists.

There is always a place for lively debate and checks and balances in science and society. Armstrong's book certainly reminds us to avoid the excesses of sloppy diagnosis, overdiagnosis, and shooting from the hip with a prescription pad. Unfortunately, there are sufficient half-truths, distortions, and inaccuracies in this book which, if seriously adhered to, would hurt the plight of many youngsters who continue to need lifelong interventions for ADHD. It is also truly unfortunate that such a useful compendium of intervention techniques resides in a volume that tears down the prevailing paradigm for understanding ADHD and offers nothing constructive in its place.

MOVING ON

This first chapter has illustrated how the core symptoms of inattention and poor response inhibition can vary widely as a function of many other factors such as IQ, family situation, sex, associated features, stage of adolescent development, and so on. ADHD truly is a heterogeneous disorder, and I have discussed how our current diagnostic system, for better or worse, has tried to grapple with this heterogeneity. I have presented Barkley's new theory of ADHD as a disorder of response inhibition involving four aspects of executive functioning, a discussion of temperament and ADHD, and ideally I have prepared the reader to deal with attempts to deny the existence of ADHD. With this foundation in place, we now move onto the research on the many different faces of ADHD in adolescence.

CHAPTER TWO

———————— ○ ————————

Follow-Up Studies and Theoretical Models

The Introduction to Section I and Chapter 1 introduced us to Michael, Adam, Sarah, and Melissa. From meeting them and reviewing the clinical characteristics of ADHD and its associated features, we learned about the different facets of ADHD in adolescents. Now we must turn our attention to the research data on the many faces of ADHD in adolescents and the theoretical models postulated to explain the data. What, in fact, are the outcomes of ADHD in adolescence? How does growing up with this neurobiological disorder mold the developing personality?

Research suggests that three different outcomes can generally be detected (Hechtman, 1992):

1. A small group of children function fairly well in adolescence and are not significantly different from matched normal control group (i.e., these adolescents "outgrow" ADHD or are remitters).
2. The majority of children continue to have significant concentration and behavioral disinhibition symptoms which increasingly impair their functioning in school and in their families, and negatively affect their self-esteem and the achievement of the developmental tasks of adolescence.
3. A minority of children develop severe antisocial behavior patterns and/or substance abuse in addition to persistent ADHD by adolescence.

At this point, little is known about exactly how growing up with ADHD molds a person's personality. We do know, however, that even though ADHD is typically neurobiologically based, environment makes a huge difference in how such children turn out as adolescents and adults. Given two 6-year-old children with similar constellations of ADHD symptoms, how their parents discipline, nurture, and rear them, together with their school

46

experiences, can result in one ending up in juvenile detention by age 16 and the other becoming an honor roll student. We cannot always translate this knowledge into effective interventions, but we can generally write prescriptions for success or failure.

FOLLOW-UP AND CROSS-SECTIONAL STUDIES

Two types of research are relevant: (1) follow-up studies of ADHD children into adolescence and (2) cross-sectional studies comparing ADHD adolescents to demographically comparable control groups. These studies provide some answers to specific questions:

1. What percentage of ADHD children continue to have ADHD as adolescents?
2. What factors predict the persistence of ADHD into adolescence and beyond?
3. How are ADHD adolescents doing in school?
4. What other psychiatric disorders do these adolescents have, and how do these comorbid conditions influence outcomes?
5. How does having ADHD all these years affect their self-esteem?
6. How do ADHD adolescents get along with their families?
7. What kind of drivers are ADHD adolescents?

The follow-up studies to date vary considerably in their methodological rigor. Prospective follow-up studies generally provide more methodologically clear-cut answers to these questions than do retrospective studies. In the typical prospective study, a group of ADHD children and a matched control group are selected at time 1 in childhood, and their functioning is measured. Then, the investigators wait a number of years and measure their functioning as adolescents. In typical retrospective studies, the investigator locates a group of adolescents with ADHD, then retrospectively studies how they were as children and relates their childhood characteristics to their adolescent outcomes. Retrospective studies suffer from a variety of sampling biases which limit their generalizability compared to prospective studies. Early prospective studies were hampered by lack of clear-cut diagnostic criteria and reliable diagnostic instruments for ADHD (called Minimal Brain Dysfunction or Childhood Hyperactivity at the time these studies began) (Thorley, 1984; Weiss & Hechtman, 1993). The work of Russell Barkley (Barkley, Fischer, et al., 1990), Joseph Biederman (Biederman, Faraone, Milberger, Guite, et al., 1996), and Ben Lahey (Hart, Lahey, Loeber, Applegate, & Frick, 1995) provides examples of more recent studies which relied on clearer definitions with more objective measurement techniques. Barkley, Fischer, et al. (1990) initially selected 158 hyperactive and 81 normal children between ages 4 and 12, based on clear-cut research criteria, administered a wide battery of measures, and followed them up prospectively 8 years later—locating 71% of the hyperactive children and 81% of the controls. Biederman, Faraone, Milberger, Guite, et al. (1996) used a systematic three-step ascertainment procedure—including rigorous structured psychiatric interviews, based on the revised third edition of the *Diagnostic and Statistical Manual of Mental Disorders* (DSM-III-R; American Psychiatric Association, 1987)—to recruit 140 children with ADHD along with 454 first-degree relatives, and 120 controls along with 368 first-degree relatives. The sample population was assessed at baseline, 1-year follow-up, and 4-year follow-up, when 91% of the original sample was retained for assessment. Hart et al. (1995) recruited 177 boys ages 7 to 12 based on DSM-III-R ADHD criteria and, after a baseline assessment, reassessed them annually for 4 years.

In this chapter, I try to provide answers to the questions outlined earlier based on composite pictures gleaned from the soundest follow-up and cross-sectional studies on ADHD adolescents done to date.

What Predicts Persistence of ADHD into Adolescence?

Using DSM-III-R criteria, the three prospective follow-up studies (Barkley, Fischer, et al., 1990; Biederman, Faraone, Milberger, Guite, et al., 1996; Hart et al., 1995) found that a mean of 77.9% of the ADHD children compared to 3% of the controls continued to have ADHD in adolescence (71.5%, 85%, and 77.4%, respectively). By comparing three age cohorts within their sample, Hart et al. (1995) showed that the number of inattention symptoms declined over four years, independent of the age of the children, but the number of hyperactivity–impulsivity symptoms declined over 4 years with increasing age, especially in early adolescence. The rate of age-related decline in hyperactivity–impulsivity symptoms was also independent of any pharmacological or inpatient psychiatric treatment the patients received, although it was related to outpatient psychotherapy in an inverse direction (less improvement with more psychotherapy). Three factors predicted persistent ADHD: (1) familiarity of the ADHD, (2) family adversity, and (3) presence of psychiatric comorbidity (Biederman, Faraone, Milberger, Curtis, et al., 1996). Children who had more ADHD in their families (e.g., parents and siblings), had greater exposure to paternal mental illness and more conflict in their families, and had comorbid Conduct, Mood, or Anxiety Disorders were more likely to persist with ADHD in adolescence than those who did not have these factors present. Barkley, Fischer, et al. (1990) found that the baseline prevalence of ADHD symptoms in the normal control group decreased from childhood to adolescence, and that the diagnostic criteria do not provide any developmental adjustment for such changes; therefore, the cutoffs for adolescents are more stringent than the cutoffs for children, perhaps artificially lowering the number of cases identified. Barkley showed that if he kept the criterion of 2 standard deviations above the normative mean constant from childhood to adolescence, the percentage of persistent ADHD in his sample would go up from 71.5% to 83.3%.

How Are ADHD Adolescents Doing in School?

All the follow-up studies concur that children whose ADHD persists into adolescence are having more and more difficulty succeeding academically in school. Barkley, Fischer, et al. (1990) found that by early adolescence, one to three times as many ADHD as control youngsters had failed a grade, been suspended, or expelled. Specifically, 29.3% of the ADHD teens had been retained in a grade compared to 10.6% of the controls; 46.3% had been suspended, compared to 15.2% of the controls, and 10% had dropped out of school compared to none of the controls. The ADHD group had significantly lower reading, spelling, and arithmetic scores on the Wide Range Achievement Test, and displayed more off-task behavior when observed in an analogue academic task setting. Biederman, Faraone, Milberger, Guite, et al. (1996) found that from baseline to follow-up, the ADHD adolescent cohort showed an increase in academic impairment, lower IQ and mathematics achievement scores, and more learning disabilities compared to the control group. Other follow-up studies reached similar conclusions (Mannuzza et al., 1991, 1993; Weiss & Hechtman, 1993; Wilson & Marcotte, 1996).

What Other Psychiatric Problems Do ADHD Adolescents Have?

Early follow-up studies suggested that by adolescence, a relatively high percentage of ADHD individuals display comorbid antisocial behavior problems (Weiss & Hechtman, 1993; Mannuzza et al., 1991) but low rates of mood or anxiety disorders. The more recent studies have broadened the picture on comorbidities. Barkley, Fischer, et al. (1990) found that at follow-up, 59% of adolescents with ADHD had ODD, compared to 11% of the controls; 43% had CD compared to 1.6% of the controls.

Biederman, Faraone, Milberger, Guite, et al. (1996) reported the most detailed analysis of comorbidities, based on reliably administered structured psychiatric interviews conducted at baseline and follow-up. At baseline, the ADHD group displayed a fair amount of comorbidity not only for CD (22% vs. 3% for controls) and ODD (65% vs. 9% for controls) but also for Major Depressive Disorder (29% vs. 2% for controls), Bipolar Disorder (11% vs. 0% for controls), multiple Anxiety Disorders (27% vs. 5% for controls), Tic Disorders (17% vs. 4% for controls), and Enuresis (30% vs. 14% for controls). Four years later, the lifetime diagnosis rates for all of these conditions had increased, in most cases significantly. The control group increased only for ODD and substance use disorder. Relatively higher rates of Mood and Anxiety Disorders were found here for the first time in such research, and these results need to be replicated by independent investigators working in other states. If replicated, such high rates of mood and anxiety disorders will paint a much broader picture of the range of comorbidities to ADHD than was previously thought to be the case.

Comorbidity clearly complicates the ADHD picture at follow-up. When two disorders co-occur, the outcomes of one disorder might be erroneously attributed to the other. Early outcome studies consistently reported that antisocial personality, delinquency, and substance abuse were outcomes of ADHD in adolescence and adulthood (Thorley, 1984; Weiss & Hechtman, 1993). Are these outcomes the result of ADHD, or its common comorbidities such as CD and Major Depressive Disorder? Barkley, Fischer, et al. (1990) found that in adolescence, the subgroup of ADHD patients with CD account for the elevated use of substances and antisocial behavior; however, he did not assess the presence of comorbid conditions to ADHD at baseline. Biederman, Faraone, Milberger, Guite, et al. (1996) addressed this question by examining the impact of comorbidity at baseline on outcome at 4-year follow-up. Relative to noncomorbid ADHD cases, baseline comorbid CD significantly increased the risk for CD and ODD, Bipolar Disorder, and alcohol and drug dependence at follow-up. Comorbid major depression at baseline increased the risk for ODD, Major Depressive Disorder, Bipolar Disorder, and Agoraphobia at follow-up. Multiple Anxiety Disorders at baseline increased the risk for Anxiety Disorders. Those youngsters with noncomorbid ADHD had an increased risk for ODD, Tic Disorder, and language disorders compared to the controls at follow-up.

Baseline comorbid CD, Major Depressive Disorder, or multiple Anxiety Disorders also predicted more impaired psychosocial functioning in adolescence on a global assessment measure relative to pure ADHD youngsters. However, the pure ADHD youngsters and the ADHD youngsters with various comorbid conditions at baseline had comparably increased degrees of impairment in school and family conflict at follow-up relative to normal controls.

The fact that comorbidity at baseline predicted outcomes with regard to psychiatric status but not cognitive and family functioning suggested to Biederman, Faraone, Milberger, Guite, et al. (1996) that the cognitive and family problems in adolescence are a result of the ADHD but that the other psychiatric problems in adolescence are a result of the comorbidity to the ADHD. Although this may be true for the cognitive problems, as shown when we discuss family interaction research, other factors in addition to ADHD symptoms account for the development of significant family interaction problems by adolescence.

How Does Having ADHD Affect Self-Esteem?

The clearest data on the relationship among ADHD, self-esteem, and outcome in adolescence and beyond come from the Mannuzza and Klein follow-up studies. Slomkowski, Klein, and Mannuzza (1995) examined whether ADHD children suffer from low self-esteem as adolescents, whether low self-esteem is associated with poor functioning in adolescence, and whether poor self-esteem is associated with poor functioning in adulthood. Sixty ADHD males and 60 comparable controls were followed up at a mean age of 18 and then again at a mean age of 26. An 11-item self-esteem questionnaire developed by Weiss and Hechtman (1993) for their follow-up studies was administered along with structured psychiatric interviews, ADHD symptoms questionnaires, and overall ratings of psychosocial adjustment. Occupational attainment and educational achievement were also measured at the adult follow-up. Compared to controls, the ADHD individuals displayed lower self-esteem and psychosocial adjustment by adolescence and lower educational achievement and occupational status in adulthood. Self-esteem in adolescence was correlated with eventual occupational status and educational achievement in adulthood for both the ADHD and control subjects, albeit modestly (.26 to .32). Adolescents who had better self-esteem achieved higher educational and occupational status.

The ADHD and control groups were subdivided into those who had any psychiatric diagnosis in adolescence and those who did not. Even the ADHD subgroup with no psychiatric diagnosis in adolescence had lower self-esteem than the comparable control group, which suggests that lowered self-esteem is part of the longitudinal outcome of ADHD in childhood even when ADHD is no longer a diagnosable mental condition in adolescence. Poor self-esteem is also one of the factors Weiss and Hechtman (1993) found to predict long-term outcome for adults in their classic follow-up study.

How Are ADHD Adolescents Getting Along with Their Families?

As children with ADHD mature into adolescents, ADHD and its comorbid conditions take their toll on family relations. We are now beginning to understand exactly what this toll is, based in great part on the work of Barkley, who provided the most thorough information regarding parent–teen relations in families with ADHD adolescents from both his longitudinal follow-up study (Barkley, Fischer, et al., 1990) and a cross-sectional study (Barkley, Anastopoulos, Guevremont, & Fletcher, 1992). In the follow-up study, 100 ADHD adolescents and their mothers were compared to 60 matched controls; comparisons were made between the entire ADHD group and the controls, as well as between the controls and subgroups of ADHD adolescents with ODD versus ADHD without ODD. In the cross-sectional study, 56 ADHD/ODD adolescents and their mothers were compared to 27 ADHD without ODD adolescents and their mothers and to 77 demographically comparable control families without any psychiatric conditions. Barkley also mentioned that because all the ADHD adolescents with CD were also diagnosed as having ODD in his research, he lumped them together for analysis of family interaction data. The majority of the participating adolescents were male in both studies. Dr. Barkley found no differences in family relations between the males and females, although the small number of females limited the power to detect such differences.

Common to the two studies were a number of family interaction measures that I developed and discuss in more detail in Chapter 3 (in this volume):

1. The Conflict Behavior Questionnaire—a 20-item true–false self-report questionnaire where parents and adolescents independently report on communication and conflict in their relationship.
2. The Issues Checklist—a 44-item self-report checklist of specific issues parents and adolescents encounter, where the parent and the adolescent independently report the frequency and anger intensity of discussions regarding these issues.
3. Videotaped observations of discussions of a neutral and a conflictual topic later coded with the Parent–Adolescent Interaction Coding Systems (PAICS), which yields frequencies of six maternal and six adolescent behaviors: put-downs/commands, defends/complains, defines/evaluates, problem solves, facilitates, and talks.

In the cross-sectional study, the mothers and adolescents also filled out the Family Beliefs Inventory (FBI), a self-report inventory of cognitive distortions and unreasonable beliefs about parent–teen relationships. The FBI yields scores for six parental beliefs (ruination, obedience, perfectionism, approval, self-blame, and malicious intent) and four adolescent beliefs (ruination, autonomy, unfairness, and approval). These beliefs are derived from the cognitive component of a behavioral family systems model of parent–adolescent relations, discussed later in this chapter. Measures of parental psychopathology were also collected. Mothers in both studies rated themselves on the Symptom Checklist 90—Revised, Beck Depression Inventory, and Locke–Wallace Marital Adjustment Test.

In many respects, the results of the two studies were very similar and complemented each other. Table 2.1 summarizes the patterns of significant effects on the dependent measures common to the two studies. Generally, the ADHD/ODD adolescents had the most conflict, with the ADHD alone group in between the ADHD/ODD and control groups. In some cases in the follow-up study, the combined ADHD group was also different from

TABLE 2.1. Significant Effects in Barkley's Family Interaction Studies with ADHD Teens

Measure—agent	Follow-up study	Cross-sectional study
CBQ—Mothers	Comb. ADHD > Control ADHD/ODD > Control ADHD/ODD > ADHD	ADHD/ODD > ADHD > Control
CBQ—Adolescents	None	ADHD/ODD > Control ADHD/ODD > ADHD
IC—Mothers		
Number of conflicts	Comb. ADHD > Control ADHD/ODD > Control ADHD/ODD > ADHD	ADHD/ODD > Control ADHD > Control
Mean intensity	Comb. ADHD > Control ADHD/ODD > Control ADHD/ODD > ADHD	ADHD/ODD > Control ADHD > Control
IC—Adolescents		
Number of conflicts	Nothing	ADHD/ODD > Control
Mean intensity	Nothing	ADHD/ODD > Control
PAICS, Neutral Discussion—Mothers		
Put-down/command	ADHD/ODD > Control ADHD/ODD > ADHD	ADHD/ODD > Control
Problem solves	Nothing	ADHD/ODD < Control
PAICS, Neutral Discussion—Adolescents		
Put-down/command	Comb. ADHD > Control ADHD/ODD > Control ADHD/ODD > ADHD	ADHD/ODD > Control
Defends/complains	Nothing	ADHD/ODD > Control
Facilitates	Nothing	ADHD/ODD < Control
Talks	Comb. ADHD < Control	Nothing
PAICS, Conflict Discussion—Mothers		
Put-down/command	Comb. ADHD > Control ADHD/ODD > Control ADHD/ODD > ADHD	Nothing
Defends/complains	Comb. ADHD > Control ADHD/ODD > Control	Nothing
Talk	Comb. ADHD < Control ADHD/ODD < Control	Nothing
PAICS, Conflict Discussion—Adolescents		

(continued)

TABLE 2.1. *(continued)*

Measure—agent	Follow-up study	Cross-sectional study
Talk	Comb. ADHD < Control ADHD/ODD < Control	Nothing
MAT—Mothers	ADHD/ODD < Control ADHD/ODD < ADHD	ADHD/ODD > Control ADHD/ODD > ADHD
BDI—Mothers	ADHD/ODD > Control ADHD/ODD > ADHD	ADHD/ODD > Control
SCL-90-R		
Obsessive–compulsive	ADHD/ODD > Control ADHD/ODD > ADHD	ADHD/ODD > Control
Hostile	Comb. ADHD > Control ADHD/ODD > Control ADHD/ODD > ADHD	ADHD/ODD > Control
Anxious	Nothing	ADHD/ODD > Control
Depression	ADHD/ODD > Control ADHD/ODD > ADHD	Nothing
Somatization	ADHD/ODD > Control ADHD/ODD > ADHD	Nothing
Interpersonal sensitivity	ADHD/ODD > Control ADHD/ODD > ADHD	Nothing
Phobic anxiety	ADHD/ODD > Control ADHD/ODD > ADHD	Nothing

Note. CBQ, Conflict Behavior Questionnaire; IC, Issues Checklist; PAICS, Parent Adolescent Interaction Coding System; Comb. ADHD, combined ADHD group; BDI, Beck Depression Inventory; SCL-90-R, Symptom Checklist 90—Revised; MAT, Locke–Wallace Marital Assessment Test. Data from Barkley, Fischer, Edelbrock, & Smallish (1991) and Barkley, Anastopoulous, Guevremont, & Fletcher (1992).

the controls, but subgroup analyses usually revealed that the ADHD/ODD families accounted for the significant differences. On the Conflict Behavior Questionnaire for both studies, mothers in the ADHD/ODD group and the ADHD group reported more conflict and negative communication than did mothers in the control group. ADHD/ODD mothers also reported more conflict than ADHD mothers. The results for adolescents differed across the two studies. In the follow-up study, ADHD adolescents did not perceive more conflict or negative communication than control adolescents, but in the cross-sectional study, ADHD/ODD adolescents did report more conflict than controls or ADHD alone adolescents. Analogously, on the Issues Checklist, mothers of ADHD/ODD adolescents and ADHD alone adolescents in both studies reported more frequent and more intensely anger-producing disputes with their adolescents than did mothers of control adolescents. In the follow-up study, mothers of ADHD/ODD adolescents also reported more frequent and intense disputes with their teenagers than did mothers of the pure ADHD group. For adolescents, there were no group differences in the follow-up study. By contrast, ADHD/ODD adolescents in the cross-sectional study reported more frequent and intense conflict than did control adolescents.

It is not clear why the results varied across studies for the adolescents. Barkley, Fischer, et al. (1990) speculated that the adolescents in the follow-up study may have been less self-aware of conflict or underreporting it. Perhaps they had habituated to the chronic state of conflict with their parents in which they lived, so it did not seem unusual to them, whereas their parents, who have a more external frame of reference, did find it unusual. Robin and Foster (1989) found that adolescents generally report lower scores than do parents on these measures in previous research. In any case, these speculations do not account for the fact that the ADHD/ODD adolescents in the cross-sectional study reported more conflict than did the control adolescents. Perhaps more of the adolescents in the cross-sectional study were diagnosed as ADHD for the first time in adolescence, and their perceptions of family relations may have differed from a group diagnosed for the first time in childhood. More information is needed about the impact of age of diagnosis on perceived family interactions.

On the videotaped observations in the neutral topic discussion, mothers of ADHD/ODD adolescents exhibited more put-downs/commands compared to controls in both studies and compared to the ADHD alone group in the follow-up study. Mothers of ADHD/ODD adolescents also exhibited fewer problem-solving suggestions than did controls in the cross-sectional study. Adolescents with ADHD/ODD exhibited more put-downs/commands than did controls in both studies and more put-downs/commands than the ADHD alone group in the follow-up study. Adolescents in the cross-sectional study exhibited more defends/complaints and less facilitative remarks in the ADHD/ODD group than did the control group. ADHD adolescents in the follow-up study exhibited a lower frequency of talk than did control group adolescents.

Surprisingly, the videotaped observations in the conflict topic discussion revealed a major difference between the results of the two studies. No effects were obtained in the cross-sectional study, with all three groups exhibiting equally high rates of negative interaction. The follow-up study obtained a variety of effects: the combined ADHD group and the ADHD/ODD subgroup exhibited more negative and less positive behavior than did the controls. Specifically, mothers of ADHD/ODD adolescents emitted higher rates of put-down/command and defend/complain than mothers of either control adolescents or ADHD alone adolescents. Mothers and adolescents in the ADHD/ODD group emitted lower rates of talk than did those in the control group. Barkley, Anastopoulous, et al. (1992) speculated that the task in the conflict situation elicited high rates of negative interactions in both groups, overriding other factors, but it is not clear why this did not occur in the follow-up study, where there were differences between groups using identical tasks on the categories of put-down/command, defend/complain, and talk. As with the self-report results, perhaps differences between the two samples of subjects accounted for the different results.

For the parental psychopathology measures, virtually all significant differences were between the ADHD/ODD and the control groups in the two studies. This group reported greater marital conflict, more depression, greater hostility, obsessive–compulsive tendencies, anxiety, and several other domains of pathology. Parents of pure ADHD adolescents did not report any more marital or personal problems than did parents of control adolescents.

Analysis of the FBI in the cross-sectional study revealed significant differences between the ADHD/ODD and control groups for parents on rumination and for adolescents on rumination and autonomy. Parents of the ADHD/ODD group also displayed more malicious attributions about their adolescents' actions than did parents of the ADHD without comorbidity group.

Finally, in the follow-up study, Barkley was able to correlate parent–child interactions at baseline with PAICS scores at follow-up. During the initial evaluation of the children at baseline, they interacted with their mothers in a free-play and a structured-playroom setting. The interactions were coded with the Response Matrix System, which yields summary scores for such variables as mother interaction, mother command, mother negative, mother facilitates, mother praises, child compliance, child play, child off task, and so on. Despite differences in coding systems, Barkley, Fischer, Edelbrock, and Smallish (1991) found significant relationships between parent–child interactions over the 8-year follow-up period. Positive parent–child interactions at entry into the study predicted continued positive interactions and diminished negative interactions in adolescence. Negative parent–child interactions at entry into the study predicted continuing conflicts in adolescence and fewer positive interactions. The magnitude of the correlations was modest (.20 to .30) but significant.

I (Robin, Kraus, Koepke, & Robin, 1987) also conducted an investigation comparing the mother–adolescent relationships of 63 ADHD adolescents (mean age 14) to a demographically comparable nondistressed group of 65 control mothers and adolescents. We selected the ADHD subjects based on clinical diagnosis and elevations on the Conners Parent Hyperactivity Questionnaire; the resulting sample would, in DSM-IV terms, have ADHD, Combined Type, most with ODD. The mothers and adolescents independently completed a multidimensional family assessment questionnaire, the Parent–Adolescent Relationship Questionnaire (PARQ), which includes true–false items sampling skill deficit–overt conflict, cognitive distortions, and family structure (Robin, Koepke, & Moye, 1990). The skill deficit/overt conflict scales include global distress, communication, problem solving, warmth/hostility, school-related conflict, and sibling-related conflict. For parents, the cognitive distortion scales tap ruination, obedience, perfectionism, malicious intent, and self-blame; for adolescents they tap ruination, autonomy, unfairness, perfectionism, and love/approval. The family structure scales included cohesion, coalitions, and triangulation. Chapter 3 discusses the PARQ in more detail.

Mothers and adolescents with ADHD reported significantly higher scores than did the control group on all of the skill deficit/overt conflict scales, including global distress, communication, problem solving, warmth hostility, school-related conflict, and sibling-related conflict. These findings replicate Barkley's finding on the Issues Checklist and the Conflict Behavior Questionnaire. Mothers of ADHD adolescents also reported significantly stronger adherence to unreasonable beliefs than did mothers of control adolescents concerning ruination, obedience, and malicious intent. However, there were no differences between groups for the adolescent belief scales. These results partially replicate the effects obtained on the FBI in the Barkley, Anastopoulous, et al. (1992) study.

Significantly more disengagement was reported on the Cohesion scale by the ADHD adolescents and their mothers compared to the controls. Although there were no differences on coalitions, the ADHD adolescents reported less triangulation than did the controls. There was a trend toward a similar difference on triangulation for mothers. These findings represent the first evidence of differences in perceptions of family structure between families with ADHD adolescents and control families.

Taken together, these studies indicate that parent–adolescent relationships between ADHD teenagers and their parents are generally characterized by increased conflict, negative communication, distorted beliefs, and more disengagement, but these effects are typically attributable to those families in which the adolescents are diagnosed with ODD in addition to ADHD. Pure ADHD families often have more conflict than controls but usually not significantly more. The outstanding exception to this rule was on the mother's self-reports of negative communication and disputes; mothers of the pure ADHD adolescents also reported more negative interactions than the control mothers. Later in this chapter in the section on coercion theory and entrenched oppositional behavior, I further explore the worsening family relations of ADHD/ODD adolescents.

We need to consider the results of the research on family relations between ADHD adolescents and their parents in light of the comorbidity data collected by Biederman, Faraone, Milberger, Guite, et al. (1996). Barkley did not assess comorbidity to ADHD when he first enrolled his subjects in the follow-up study as children, and he only assessed comorbidity for ODD and CD at follow-up. We do not know whether the outcomes for family relations would differ as a function of various other comorbidities at baseline (depression, anxiety, bipolar disorder, etc.). Further research is needed to study this issue.

What Kind of Drivers Are ADHD Adolescents?

Although a number of studies have examined the driving behavior of older adolescents and adults with ADHD, Barkley and his colleagues conducted the most thorough analyses in two studies. Barkley, Guevremont, Anastopoulous, DuPaul, and Shelton (1993) reassessed 3–5 years later the sample of ADHD and control adolescents who participated in the Barkley, Anastopoulous, et al. (1992) family interaction study discussed earlier. At the time of the follow-up, the adolescents/young adults ranged in age from 16 to 22, with mean ages of 19.1 and 18.6 in the ADHD and control groups. The investigators mailed a comprehensive survey of driving behavior, driving-related risks, and outcomes to the mothers of these adolescents and young adults. Fifty-four percent of the ADHD and 61% of the control mothers returned the questionnaires (no differences between those who returned and those who did not return surveys), and after eliminating those whose adolescents did not have licenses, 35 ADHD adolescents were compared to 36 control adolescents.

Mothers of the ADHD group rated their teenagers as using significantly less sound driving habits than mothers of non-ADHD teenagers, and this deficiency was associated with a variety of negative driving outcomes. ADHD adolescents were more likely than control adolescents to have driven without a license or had their licenses revoked, to have had auto crashes, to have had more such crashes, and to be at fault for more crashes than control subjects. They were also more likely to have received traffic citations and received more such citations than did control subjects, particularly for speeding and failing to stop.

The contribution of ODD and CD to driving risk and outcomes was assessed through multiple regression with the combined ADHD and control groups. The number of ADHD, ODD, and CD symptoms were entered as predictors in a series of multiple regressions predicting driving outcomes. The combination of ODD and CD symptoms significantly predicted maternal ratings of driving behavior, driving without a license, license suspensions and revocations, crashes, bodily injuries, crashes with subjects at fault, and traffic citations. The number of ADHD symptoms only made a unique contribution to predicting driving without a license. However, the frequency of ODD and ADHD symptoms was so highly correlated (.91) that even though we can conclude that the presence of more ODD/CD symptoms predicts greater driving risk in ADHD adolescents, we cannot completely separate the contribution of the ODD and ADHD symptoms based on this study alone.

This study suffered from two methodological limitations: (1) the data were based exclusively on surveys completed by parents rather than official government records or direct measures of driving behavior; and (2) the study could not tell us whether the subjects' driving difficulties were due to impaired knowledge of driving rules or poor driving performance itself. In a second study, Barkley, Murphy, and Kwasnik (1996) corrected these deficiencies by comparing 25 young adults with ADHD (mean age = 22.5) to 23 demographically comparable controls (mean age = 22.0) on a structured interview of driving behavior, driving behavior ratings by self and others, a video test of driving knowledge, a computer-simulated driving test, and official motor vehicle records.

The results of this second study corroborated and extended the results of the first survey study. Official motor vehicle records indicated that ADHD young adults received more citations for speeding, were more likely to have had their licenses suspended or revoked, had more such suspensions/revocations than did controls, and showed a trend toward being more likely to have had a crash and a greater number of accidents than controls. Comparable results were found based on the interviews with the young adults. In addition, the ADHD young adults and their significant others rated their driving behavior as significantly worse than the control group. Interestingly, although there was no difference between the two groups on the test of driving knowledge, the ADHD young adults performed more poorly than did the controls on the computer-simulated driving performance test, particularly with regard to steering control and crashes and scrapes. These results strongly suggest that the poor driving records of the ADHD young adults were due to performance problems rather than lack of knowledge of driving procedures and regulations.

Clinically, we often see that ADHD individuals who take their stimulant medication while driving exercise better judgment and have fewer infractions than those who do not, although this effect remains to be demonstrated in a research study. The question arises as to whether the young adults in the Barkley et al. (1993, 1996) studies were taking medication at the time of their participation in the study; the answer is that none of the young adults in the first study were taking medication, and five of the ADHD subjects in the second study were taking medication (four taking stimulants, one taking antidepressants). The four who took stimulants were asked to refrain from taking their medication during the time of the study, and we have no information to indicate whether these four subjects generally took their medication while driving. Thus, the results of Barkley's studies should be viewed as representing primarily the driving behavior of ADHD individuals without medication.

In summary, Barkley et al's two studies (1993, 1996) demonstrated that ADHD individuals off medication have worse driving habits and more negative driving-related outcomes than do non-ADHD controls, and that these outcomes are primarily performance rather than knowledge problems. Symptoms of antisocial behavior made a significant contribution to most of these outcomes in the first study. In helping our clients understand the results of this study, it is important to remind them that these poor driving behaviors were obtained in an unmedicated sample and do not necessarily generalize to individuals who take medication while driving.

Summary of Follow-Up Studies

The aggregate data from all the follow-up and cross-sectional studies discussed here generally support Hechtman's earlier statement about three common outcomes for ADHD children in adolescence. A small number of ADHD children, probably around 15–20%, have a remission of ADHD symptoms and are indistinguishable from controls by adolescence on measures of psychiatric status, school functioning, and psychosocial functioning, although they may have suffered some damage to their self-esteem. These adolescents typically had milder forms of ADHD and little or no comorbidity for other psychiatric disorders and were raised in families with more less family history of ADHD or other major mental disorders and in more benign family environments.

The majority of youngsters with ADHD in childhood continue to meet the full criteria for ADHD and have significant impairments in school and some family difficulties, with comorbid ODD at times. If these youngsters are raised by parents without severe marital problems, depression, or other major psychopathology in a relatively benign home environment, they will grow up to be productive citizens but will have some emotional scars and will have to continue to use compensatory strategies to cope with ADHD symptoms and their sequelae throughout their adult years. A significant minority, who already were showing severe psychiatric comorbidities in childhood, or who are raised by disturbed parents in malignant family environments, go on to develop serious problems with continued comorbidity, antisocial behavior, and substance problems in adolescence.

These conclusions apply primarily to males and to those who have ADHD, Combined Subtype. There are no follow-up studies on the outcomes in adolescence or adulthood of those who have ADHD, Inattentive Subtype, and the numbers of females in the existing follow-up studies have been too small to provide the statistical power to determine how the outcomes may differ for women with ADHD.

As my focus is primarily adolescence, I do not review in detail the follow-up studies on the adult outcomes of ADHD children. Suffice it to say that many adolescents with ADHD persist in having the symptoms into adulthood, and that the picture of ADHD in adults is highly varied. As in adolescence, the most powerful predictors of positive versus negative outcomes are not the core symptoms of ADHD themselves but rather the associated factors such as comorbid CD and mood disorders, IQ, socioeconomic status, the mental health of other family members, and a variety of other family-related factors. Readers interested in a review of this literature might consult Goldstein (1997) or Weiss and Hechtman (1993).

EXPLAINING DEVELOPMENTAL TRAJECTORIES IN ADHD FAMILIES

How do the kinds of family and environmental variables identified in the follow-up studies exert their influence over time to set the developmental trajectories of ADHD children going into adolescence? Through what processes do these variable operate? Although little is known for sure about these processes, the available data are at least partially supported by several promising theoretical models. I will review and apply my own behavioral family systems model of the development of parent–adolescent conflict (Robin & Foster, 1989) and Barkley's adaptation of Patterson's (1982) social learning model for the development of aggressive behavior to help answer three questions:

1. What factors determine the degree of conflict which arises between parents and teenagers?
2. How does the presence of ADHD symptoms heighten such family conflict?
3. How do entrenched repertoires of severe oppositional behavior develop alongside ADHD in such adolescents?

What Factors Determine Parent–Adolescent Conflict?

A comprehensive behavioral family systems model is helpful in understanding the factors that determine the degree of conflict and/or harmony experienced by the family with an ADHD adolescent (Robin & Foster, 1989). Within such a model, families are viewed as social systems of members, held together by bonds of affection, who exercise mutual control over each other's actions. A family has a definite structure or pecking order which permits it to accomplish goals within a developmental time frame. In Western civilization, parents are generally in charge of children, even adolescent children. Individual members of families have repertoires of skills and beliefs relevant to family life, which both determine and in part are determined by their interactions with other members. The family takes as its implicit goal the preservation, growth, and nurturance of its members. Over time, families develop systems of checks and balances (or "homeostatic patterns") to regulate the behaviors of their members within definite limits or boundaries. Sometimes, these systems may be explicitly stated, as when a parent says to a child, "You will obey your mother." Other times, they may be implicit to everyone, such as natural barriers against incest.

Adolescence is a time of exponential physiological, cognitive, emotional, and behavioral change. A complex constellation of biological changes known as puberty set in motion an equally complex set of reverberating psychosocial changes within the individual and the family. In addition, physically and socially imposed changes occur. Teenagers' physical size increases relative to their parents. School tasks require more independent organization and problem solving. Teenagers naturally spend less time with adults. As these changes occur, teenagers are expected to accomplish five major developmental tasks during the second decade of life: (1) individuate from their parents, (2) adjust to sexual maturation, (3) develop new and deeper peer relationships, (4) form a self-identify, and (5) plan for a career. Individuating from parents underlies all of the other developmental tasks.

These changes associated with adolescence pose challenges to the pre-existing homeostatic patterns of interaction families have developed prior to the adolescence of their children. For example, to become independent, a teenager must push away from his or her parents. Pushing away inevitably involves a certain amount of rebellion against parental authority and conflict over rules regulating freedom and independence. Parents naturally react by trying to maintain authority as they adjust to having a more independent adolescent in their midst. Thus, a period of normally increased perturbation occurs in early adolescence. How the parents react to this natural period of increased rebellion determines, in great part, whether it subsides or escalates to clinical proportions. "Clinical proportions" means, in DSM-IV terminology, Oppositional Defiant Disorder. Unfortunately, DSM-IV totally fails to capture the fact that ODD is really an interfactional problem of a family system, not a disorder that simply resides inside an adolescent. It would be more accurate to say that a family rather than an individual has ODD.

A behavioral family systems model postulates that three dimensions of family functioning determine the degree of clinically significant conflict that results as teenagers individuate from their parents: (1) problem-solving/communication skills, (2) cognitive distortions, and (3) family structure. Difficulties in one or more of these dimensions propels a family toward clinical distress. Strengths in these areas helps the family reestablish a new homeostatic pattern which gives the adolescent gradually increasing freedom in return for demonstrations of responsibility.

Problem-Solving/Communication Skills

Problem-solving/communication skills refer to the way parents and adolescents handle specific disputes within the context of the developmental task of independence seeking. Simply dictating to adolescents without discussion does not work because adolescents typically have the ability to circumvent parental rules, and because dictating does not prepare adolescents for resolving conflicts in an adult world. Negotiating mutually acceptable solutions to disagreements is much more consistent with the developmental task of individuation. Problem solving is a cognitive-behavioral process whereby one or more individuals follow a set of steps to reach a mutually acceptable agreement to a problem (D'Zurilla & Goldfried, 1971; Spivack, Platt, & Shure, 1976).

Problem solving typically involves (1) problem finding, recognizing the presence of an interpersonal problem; (2) problem definition, formulating the problem in clear-cut terms and communicating that formulation to others; (3) generation of solutions, creative brainstorming of a wide variety of potential solutions to the problem; (4) evaluation, projecting and weighing the advantages and the disadvantages of each solution for solving the problem; (5) decision making, negotiating a solution or combination of solutions that maximizes the advantages and minimizes the disadvantages for everyone involved in the problem; (6) implementation planning, working out the details necessary for effective implementation of the selected solution; and (7) verification, after implementation, evaluating the extent to which the solution solved the original problem and, if not, recycling through the steps of problem solving to find a better solution.

Communication refers to the verbal and nonverbal components of how parents and adolescents communicate with each other. Family members need to express their opinions and feelings to each other assertively but unoffensively, to listen to each other attentively, and to decode messages accurately. Accusations, denials, threats, commands, excessive interruptions, sarcasm, poor eye contact, and a host of other negative communication habits impede effective expression of feelings and listening to others. Nonaccusatory "I statements," paraphrases, reflections, empathetic remarks, signaling when one needs to talk, good eye contact, and appropriate posture all facilitate problem solving. Family members become so enraged by negative communication that they get sidetracked from problem solving and stuck in reciprocally negative communication loops (e.g., "No I didn't," "Yes, you did").

Cognitive Distortions

Family members' beliefs, expectations, and attributions concerning parenting, growing up, and family life are habitual cognitive responses learned from life experiences and from families of origin. Following the cognitive and rational-emotive models of human behavior (Beck, 1976; Ellis & Grieger, 1977), I believe these cognitions mediate affectual and behavioral responses to common conflictual situations that arise between parents and adolescents, and if the cognitions are unrealistic or distorted, the responses to the situation may be overreactive or inappropriate. A father, for example, may believe that if his ADHD son fails to complete his chores, the boy will grow up to be an worthless, aimless, unemployed welfare case; such extreme thinking would be an example of ruination. If a disagreement over the chores arose, it might be very difficult for the father to remain calm and negotiate a mutually acceptable compromise because of his extreme belief.

The son may believe that teenagers should have as much freedom as they wish, and that any parental restrictions will ruin their teenager years. In the conflict with his father over chores, this son may also have a difficult time remaining flexible and open to compromise solutions because of his extreme beliefs. We have found that the following belief themes commonly arise and get in the way in parent–adolescent relationships:

Parents

1. *Ruination.* Parents believe that giving adolescents too much freedom will end up in disaster.
2. *Obedience.* Parents believe that adolescents should always comply with their requests willingly and without question.
3. *Perfectionism.* Parents expect their adolescent to behave in a flawless manner at all times.
4. *Malicious intent.* Parents believe that adolescents misbehave on purpose to anger the parents or to get even with them for perceptions of having been wronged by them.
5. *Self-blame.* It is the parent's fault if the adolescent make mistakes.
6. *Love/appreciation.* Parents believe that their adolescents should always approve of their actions, and it is terrible if they disapprove.

Adolescents

1. *Ruination.* Teenagers believe that parental restrictions on their freedom will ruin their lives.
2. *Unfairness.* Teenagers have a keen sense of injustice and believe that it is unfair for their parents to put restrictions on them, especially restrictions that may be more stringent than those put on their peers and/or siblings.
3. *Autonomy.* Teenagers believe that they should have as much freedom as they desire, and that they can handle such freedom effectively.
4. *Love/appreciation.* Teenagers believe that their parents really do not care about them, love them, or respect their opinions, and if they did, they would give them more freedom.

All parents and teenagers adhere to these beliefs to a certain degree. It is blind, rigid adherence to these beliefs in the face of clearly conflicting evidence that impedes effective problem solving and conflict resolution. As mentioned earlier, both the FBI (Vincent-Roehling & Robin, 1986) and the PARQ (Robin et al., 1990) have been validated as self-report measures of the beliefs discussed here. These two studies found that families with oppositional youth (regardless of whether or not ADHD was also present) exhibit greater adherence to beliefs concerning ruination, obedience, perfectionism, malicious intent, autonomy, and unfairness (but not self-blame or

love/approval) than do families in a normative population and families selected because their youth did not have any clinical distress.

Family Structure

Family structure also contributes to parent–adolescent conflict. Cohesion,
hierarchy, and the distribution of power in families are the molecules of
family structure, which combine to form the elements of parenting style.

Cohesion is a dimension of connectedness which goes from enmeshment or overinvolvement to disengagement or lack of involvement. A balanced or moderate degree of cohesion is optimal. The instrumental aspect
of cohesion is monitoring (e.g., the extent to which a parent keeps track of
what an adolescent is doing). Too little monitoring may lead to adolescents
getting into trouble. Too much monitoring represents an invasion of privacy, fueling conflict. The affectual aspect of cohesion is how close family
members feel to each other. Too little closeness leads to feelings of alien-
ation and lack of development of self-confidence. Too much closeness sti-
fles individuation. Lack of adequate parental monitoring is associated with
increased risk for a variety of antisocial behaviors (Forgatch & Patterson,
1989; Snyder, Dishion, & Patterson, 1986; Steinberg, Fletcher, & Darling,
1994).

Difficulties in the hierarchy typically involve alignment or taking sides
(e.g., coalitions and triangulation). Coalitions refers to two people consistently taking sides against a third, in a three-person system. If a parent
sides with an adolescent against another parent (e.g., a cross-generational
coalition), problems are likely to arise because parental discipline is diluted
and adolescent misbehavior may go unchecked. When two parents work
consistently as a team (e.g., a within-generational coalition), discipline is
more effective. Triangulation occurs when two family members put the
third in the middle, and the third vacillates between allegiance to one or
the other. Like cross-generational coalitions, frequent triangulation can impede effective parental discipline and limit setting. Triangulation often occurs when the father comes home and finds that the mother and ADHD
son have had a major battle earlier that afternoon. Each appeals to him for
support, placing him in the middle.

The degree of cohesion and the nature of the hierarchy or power
structure contribute to parenting style. Child development researchers have
identified and extensively studied four parenting styles: (1) authoritative,
(2) authoritarian, (3) indulgent, and (4) neglectful. These four styles represent combinations of two basic dimensions: (1) acceptance/involvement
and (2) strictness/supervision. Authoritative parenting is characterized by
high acceptance/involvement and moderately high strictness/supervision,
including parental warmth, inductive discipline, consistency, and nonpuni-
tive punishment. Authoritarian parenting is characterized by low accep-
tance/involvement and very high strictness/supervision; indulgent parent-

ing by high acceptance/involvement and low strictness/supervision; and neglectful parenting by low acceptance/involvement and low strictness/supervision. Researchers found many differences in outcomes among adolescents parented in authoritative, authoritarian, indulgent, or neglectful styles. In general, adolescents from authoritative environments score highest, and adolescents from neglectful parenting environments score lowest on measures of adjustment; adolescents from either authoritarian or indulgent environments show a mixed picture of positive and negative adjustment outcomes (Steinberg, Lamborn, Darling, Mounts, & Dornbusch, 1994). With regard to conflict, authoritarian and authoritative environments are likely to produce more frequent conflict than are indulgent and neglectful environments, where parents are not monitoring their adolescents closely. Authoritarian environments are likely to produce more conflict than are authoritative environments, where parents reason and negotiate with their adolescents.

In summary, parental style and structural problems may contribute to parent–adolescent conflict and outcomes by virtue of the importance of parental monitoring and consistency. Families characterized by triangulation and cross-generational coalitions create "divide and conquer" situations in which the adolescent can continue to engage in some inappropriate behavior because the parents are not able to work well as an executive team, setting and enforcing limits.

How Do ADHD Symptoms Heighten Family Conflict?

To these three factors of skill deficits, cognitive distortions, and family structure problems we must add the core symptoms of ADHD. Adolescent ADHD symptoms function like a catalyst in the chemical reaction which fuels early adolescent individuation-related conflict. Inattention spurs increased conflict by making it difficulty for the ADHD adolescent to stay on task when resolving conflicts during family discussions; to carry out agreements with parents; and to complete schoolwork, chores, or other responsibilities. Behavioral disinhibition leads adolescents to "lose it" in conversations with their parents; they say things that really upset their parents and sidetrack the discussion and they impulsively do something other than carrying out their part of agreements made with their parents. Such adolescent expressions of impulsivity as poor frustration tolerance, wide mood swings, and failure to consider the consequences of an action lead to frequent, angry confrontations with parents. The hyperactivity side of behavioral disinhibition makes it possible for adolescents to keep badgering their parents when all others would have given up, often resulting in their parents giving in, thereby negatively reinforcing the badgering behavior.

Because adolescents with ADHD do and say unpredictable and at times irresponsible things, it is easy for parents to "throw out the baby with the bath water" and overgeneralize in a negative direction, adhering to distorted beliefs. It is easy for parents to attribute failure to complete a task to malicious motives, to suspect that giving their adolescents a little freedom will have ruinous consequences, or to conclude that the adolescent is not meeting parental expectations. It is easy to misinterpret restlessness as "disrespect." It is very difficult for parents to maintain perspective and say to themselves, "This ruinous-looking behavior is just another example of ADHD in action; I need to provide some consequences, but not reach catastrophic conclusions."

Imagine the added complications of having a parent and/or a sibling with ADHD, which is the case in many families. The ADHD parent is likely to have a difficult time utilizing whatever effective problem-solving/communication skills are in his or her repertoire when provoked by his or her ADHD adolescent. Maintaining good communication between an ADHD parent and an ADHD teenager can be a real challenge. The parent and the adolescent are only really listening to a fraction of each others' conversation, and probably not even the same fraction! The potential for misunderstanding is immense. Simply organizing one's daily life to find the time for a problem-solving discussion may be a major challenge for the family with an ADHD adolescent and an ADHD parent. It is easy to understand why Biederman, Faraone, Milberger, Curtis, et al. (1996) found that a family history of ADHD was one of the predictors of persistence of ADHD symptoms into adolescence.

How Does Entrenched Oppositional Behavior Develop Alongside ADHD?

Barkley (1990) integrated three research streams to formulate a theoretical model to explain how severely oppositional and/or aggressive behavior develops over time in children with ADHD as they move from childhood into adolescence. These three streams are (1) the literature on the shaping of aggressive behavior in deviant youth (Patterson, 1982), (2) Barkley's own research on parent–child relations in families with ADHD children, and (3) the literature on the relationship between parental psychiatric disturbances and child behavioral problems. To this material, I add comments integrating elements of the previously discussed behavioral family systems theory of parent–adolescent conflict.

The first part of this model follows from the cognitive-behavioral conceptualizations of Beck and Ellis discussed earlier about how extreme thinking induces negative mood, which then skews subsequent thinking and behavior in a negatively constricted direction. According to Barkley's model, parental psychiatric symptoms such as depression or marital conflict have a negative impact on parental mood. I would add substance abuse, personality disorders, and parental ADHD to Barkley's short list and note that really any parental psychiatric or emotional problem is likely to affect parental mood and skew thinking in absolutistic, negative directions. Over time, these problems induce parents to be in a chronically and consistently negative mood. Depending on the parents' form of psychopathology, this mood may be depressed, hostile, paranoid, and/or anxious. This chronic negative emotional state and distorted cognitions regarding their children's behavior decreases parents' tolerance for ADHD-related misbehaviors. Parents come to view the behavioral patterns of admittedly challenging ADHD children as more deviant than they really are, for example, they all too readily think the worst of their children and attribute malicious motives to their typically nonthinking, impulsive behavior. Parents are likely to engage in the kinds of distorted thinking discussed earlier (e.g., erroneously expecting ruination, making inappropriate demands for obedience or perfection, and incorrectly making malicious attributions about their adolescent's behavior). The ADHD children are in fact challenging, posing many situations that demand immediate parental action. Thus, there are many opportunities for negative mood and distorted cognitions to color a parent's reaction to the ADHD child.

The homeostatic balance of the family system has already been disrupted by the adolescent's natural striving for autonomy, the changes in relative physical size of teenagers and their parents, and the other developmental challenges of adolescence, taxing problem-solving communication skills and family structure. Now the additional family adversity of parental psychiatric problems further unbalances the system. Parents dealing with own problems are even less likely to use effective problem-solving or positive communication than are healthy parents, and problems such as marital conflict are even more likely to spur triangulation, disengagement, and cross-generational coalitions.

As a result of this chronic negative mood state and high rate of distorted thinking, the parents reduce their rate of social reinforcement and general interaction with their children. The children, in return, comply less with their parents and engage more in negative attention-getting behaviors, at first minor ones, but later major ones, if they do not obtain a parental reaction to the more minor misbehaviors. As the children become less positive and more negative, the parents spend even less time interacting with their children. Negative behavior "works" to capture the parent's attention because it cannot be easily ignored by the depressed or angry parent.

At this point in the model, Barkley invokes Patterson's concept of coercive parent–child interactions. Patterson (1982) found that parents of aggressive/noncompliant children are more likely to respond to their children with aggressive behavior, indiscriminant aversiveness, and/or eventual submissiveness to their children during management encounters. The children make demands or disobey a rule; the parent comes on like "gangbusters." The child's negative behavior may be temporarily suppressed, but the child finds a way to up the ante by escalating the pattern of misbehavior. Eventually, the parent caves in. The child gets his or her way, removing the threat of parental action. Behaviorally, the child escapes or avoids punishment; demanding, coercive behavior is reinforced. The child's misbehavior toward the parent ceases when the parent caves in; parental cave-in is negatively reinforced by the removal of an aversive stimulus. Patterson called this pattern of parent–child interaction "coercion."

Because parental pathology, negative parental mood, distorted parental thinking, and structural problems predispose parents to cave in easily, they set the stage for parents to fall into a coercion trap with their ADHD children. Family interaction becomes characterized by frequent, unpleasant coercive exchanges. Through the negative reinforcement and shaping that is intrinsic to coercive exchanges, the children with ADHD in such families learn that they can avoid their parents' wrath and escape from having to comply with their parents' demands if they keep escalating their defiant behavior to increasingly more extreme proportions. Over the years from childhood to adolescence, thousands of such negative interactions occur, and slowly the child solidifies a repertoire of hostile, defiant, and antisocial behavior.

By the adolescent years, the parents find that they have run out of effective disciplinary procedures and eventually reach a state of "learned helplessness." They give up and withdraw or may disengage from their adolescents. They may ignore their adolescents, who now can do whatever they like with impunity. With a strong repertoire of coercive behavior and little or no monitoring of their actions or whereabouts by parents, it is then very easy for adolescents to become involved in criminality, antisocial behavior, promiscuity, and even substance abuse. Of course, they do little schoolwork and fail academically.

Summary of Theoretical Model of ADHD and Family Interaction

Figure 2.1 summarizes this model of ADHD and family interaction, integrating behavioral family systems and coercion/performance theories. Three antecedent factors disrupt the homeostatic balance of the family system and promote increased conflict between ADHD adolescents and their parents, rebellious behavior, and coercive interchanges: (1) parental pathology such as depression, marital conflict, substance abuse, or ADHD; (2) the developmental challenges of adolescence, particularly teenager's natural striving for independence; and (3) adolescent ADHD symptoms, along with any comorbid conditions such as mood or anxiety disorders. The reaction of the parents to this disruption of homeostatic functioning in great part determines whether coercive parent–teen interchanges remain occasional events which are effectively dealt with or whether they become an entrenched pattern permeating all aspects of family life. Coercive interactions come to permeate family life when parents react with (1) poor problem-solving skills; (2) negative communication; (3) a negatively skewed, distorted view of the adolescent's behavior characterized by ru-

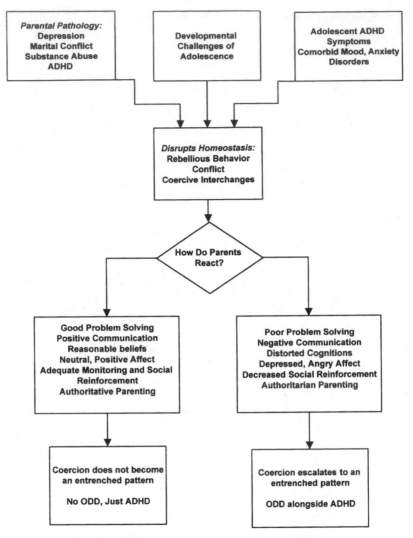

FIGURE 2.1. Integrative model of ADHD and family interaction.

inous thinking and malicious motives; (4) excessively depressed or hostile affect; (5) decreased social reinforcement; and (6) authoritarian parenting styles. Adolescents escalate their negative attention-getting behavior and coercive interactions, spurring further negative parental reactions, and over time formidable repertoires of oppositional behavior develop. Parents may then feel helpless, give up on their adolescents, and monitor their actions less closely. Then, adolescents become more involved with deviant peer groups and antisocial behaviors.

Research Support for the Model

Although no studies of the overall integrative model presented here have yet been conducted, researchers have separately studied (1) the behavioral family systems model of parent adolescent conflict, (2) the relationship of maternal depression and marital conflict to family interactions between ADHD adolescents and their parents; and (3) the general impact of family adversity on the outcomes of ADHD children.

Robin and Foster (1989) extensively reviewed the research supporting the behavioral family systems model of parent–adolescent conflict in non-ADHD families. In summary, this research strongly supports the role of deficits in problem-solving communication skills and cognitive distortions as contributors to parent–adolescent conflict and provides preliminary evidence for the role of family structural problems in such conflicts. With regard to ADHD adolescents, Barkley's family interaction studies with ADHD adolescents and their parents (Barkley, Anastopoulous, et al., 1992; Barkley, Fischer, et al., 1990), as well as my own study (Robin et al., 1987), reviewed earlier, also provide support for selected aspects of the model. The differences between the ADHD and control groups on the Issues Checklist, Conflict Behavior Questionnaire, and the PARQ confirm that the ADHD adolescents and their parents in fact have more frequent and intense conflicts than do the demographically comparable controls. The group differences on selected categories of the PAICS are consistent with the hypotheses that families in conflict will have specific deficits in problem-solving communication skills; the differences on FBI and the PARQ Belief scales provide preliminary evidence for increased cognitive distortions in ADHD families relative to controls.

Barkley (1990) extensively reviewed research on the relationship of maternal depression, marital conflict, and family interactions involving ADHD children. He found a clear-cut association of marital conflict and maternal depression with aggressive behavior in preadolescent children with ADHD. In further analysis of the family interaction data discussed earlier from his follow-up study, he also found significant correlations between the maternal Beck Depression Inventory and the maternal Locke–Wallace Marital Adjustment Test and observed maternal behavior during the analog parent–adolescent interactions. Mothers with higher depression scores used more put-downs/commands, and less general talk behavior; mothers with higher marital conflict scores used more put-downs/commands, more defends/complains, and less facilitative behavior with their adolescents. Similar relationships were found between maternal hostility and paranoia and observed maternal interactions with their ADHD adolescents.

Biederman and his colleagues examined the role of family adversity as a risk factor for the presence of ADHD and its comorbid conditions in children. They used Rutter's index of six factors within the family environment that were previously found to correlate significantly with child mental disturbances: (1) severe marital discord, (2) low social class, (3) large family size, (4) paternal criminality, (5) maternal mental disorder, and (6) foster placement. As part of a large-scale investigation of the familial transmission of ADHD, Biederman, Milberger, Faraone, Kiely, Guite, Mick, Ablon, Warburton, and Reed (1995a) operationalized the first five variables and compared 140 ADHD children to 120 normal controls based on them (none of his subjects had been placed in foster care). The families of ADHD children had higher conflict, lower socioeconomic status, and a greater rate of maternal psychiatric diagnosis than the controls, but no differences on paternal criminality and family size. The odds ratio for the presence of ADHD increased significantly with each increase in the number of Rutter's adversity indicators that were present (1 indicator = 7.4 odds ratio; 2 indicators = 9.5 odds ratio; 3 indicators = 34.6 odds ratio; 4 indicators = 41.7 odds ratio). There also were positive associations between the number of risk factors and the presence of conduct disorders, depression, anxiety, and learning disabilities, but these associations occurred similarly for both the ADHD and the control groups.

In a second analysis of data from the same sample of ADHD and control children, Biederman, Milberger, Faraone, Kiely, Guite, Mick, Ablon, Warburton, Reed, and Davis (1995) carefully operationalized exposure to parental psychopathology and exposure to parental conflict as indicators of family adversity and assessed their impact on ADHD and ADHD-related psychopathology and dysfunction. The ADHD group displayed significantly greater levels than did the control group of exposure to parental conflict, diminished family cohesion, number of parents psychiatrically ill during the child's lifetime, and the proportion of the child's life exposed to maternal psychopathology. Using regression analyses, there was a significant association between exposure to family conflict and measures of the child's relationships with peers, siblings, and parents, as well as internalizing and externalizing behavioral problems on the Child Behavior Checklist. However, exposure to parental psychopathology was only related to externalizing behavior problems and the child's use of leisure time. No associations were found between the indices of family conflict or exposure to parental psychopathology and Conduct Disorder, Major Depressive Disorder, or Anxiety Disorders.

Taken together, these three independent streams of research lend support to portions of the integrative model of ADHD and family interaction presented here. Biederman and Barkley's work clearly demonstrate the relationship between parental pathology and ADHD outcomes and family conflict. My own previous research and Barkley's family interaction work demonstrate the role of problem-solving/communication skills and cognitive distortions in mediating conflict between parents and ADHD adolescents. Careful longitudinal research is needed to study the development of entrenched coercive interchanges over time and their role in leading to the presence of comorbid ODD and CD in adolescents with ADHD.

CONCLUSION

The follow-up studies and theoretical model discussed in this chapter provide a number of practical implications for the clinician assessing and treating adolescents with ADHD:

1. *Consider the nature–nurture interaction.* The severity of the clinical presentation of ADHD and its associated problems is in great part an interaction of nature and nurture. For example, environmental factors such as family adversity, parental pathology, problem-solving skills, distorted cognitions, and family structure are as important as basic temperament and genetic predispositions in determining ultimate clinical problems.
2. *Cast a wide assessment net.* The clinician needs to cast a wide net when assessing adolescent ADHD and look at all the relevant family and environmental variables.
3. *Select broad intervention targets.* Intervention strategies must target not only ADHD symptoms but also family interaction, parental pathology, and issues in the family system.
4. *Remember adolescent development.* The clinician must keep in mind the adolescent's developmental stage at the time of assessment and intervention to plan effective strategies for helping the adolescent understand and accept ADHD and to motivate the adolescent to collaborate with the therapist in a meaningful intervention process.

With this background in place, we now turn to the practical issues of diagnosing ADHD in adolescents.

SECTION TWO

———— ◯ ————

EVALUATION
AND DIAGNOSIS

Introduction

To make an accurate differential diagnosis of ADHD and its associated conditions in adolescence, a clinician must thoroughly understand the DSM-IV criteria for these disorders as well as the limitations of the DSM diagnostic model, develop familiarity with the different presentations of ADHD and common ADHD look-alikes in adolescents, collect information from multiple informants, and become familiar with a wide variety of assessment methods. Above all, clinicians must take the time needed to collect, sift through, analyze, and interpret the assessment data. Because clinicians in any one discipline may be expert at some but not all of the assessment issues and methods, they often need to involve multiple disciplines on a consultative basis. To enlist the cooperation of the adolescent, the family, and the school, and to maximize the chances of acceptance of the diagnosis and compliance with the treatment recommendations, it is important for clinicians to demystify the diagnostic process. I explain what I am doing and why from the very first moment of the evaluation, and I actively solicit feedback about the assessment process and my explanations.

WHAT DO WE ASSESS?

Six primary areas constitute the content of the evaluation:

- Medical status
- Inclusionary criteria for ADHD
- Comorbidity
- Differential diagnosis
- Cognitive functioning
- Family functioning

We need to know the *medical status* of the adolescent. Is the adolescent in good health? Are vision and hearing normal or corrected to nor-

77

mal? Does the adolescent have any chronic diseases or neurological conditions which might contribute to ADHD-like symptoms, or are any of the medications being taken by the adolescent leading to such symptoms?

The *inclusionary criteria for ADHD* refer to the DSM-IV diagnostic criteria, supplemented by dimensional measures such as rating scales, designed to give the practitioner information about four essential points:

1. *Core symptoms* of inattention, impulsivity, and hyperactivity.
2. *Chronicity* of these symptoms over the course of time; that is, have they been present since childhood even if they were never diagnosed before?
3. *Pervasiveness* of these symptoms across situations and settings. ADHD must cause problems in a variety of situations with a variety of people, even though it may not cause problems in every situation.
4. *Impairment* in daily living or the extent to which these symptoms interfere with functioning in school, at home, and in the community. Some individuals may exhibit symptoms of inattention, impulsivity, or hyperactivity, but these symptoms may not be getting in the way of their functioning. We would not diagnose a disorder in such cases. Even if an adolescent meets the inclusionary criteria for ADHD, he or she may not truly have this disorder. We need to conduct a *differential diagnosis,* that is, rule out alternative conditions that may look like ADHD, including oppositional behavior problems, mood disorders, anxiety disorders, and chaotic environments leading to adjustment problems. In the course of ruling out these alternatives, we often find that they may be occurring in addition to ADHD rather than instead of it; that is, they are *comorbid conditions.*

One of the most common comorbidities or differential diagnoses to ADHD is a learning disability. Even when no learning disability is present, adolescents with ADHD typically present with academic underachievement. To assess patterns of underachievement and learning disabilities, we need to know the adolescent's *cognitive functioning,* that is, his or her intellectual ability and skill level in such academic areas as reading, written expression, and mathematics. Knowing intellectual ability also helps us understand the chronicity and pervasiveness of the youngster's impairments, because high intellectual ability may be a "protective" factor against early impairment. The bright youngster only needs to pay attention part of the time in the average public school classroom to obtain passing grades, but it becomes increasingly more difficult to do so as youngsters move up the educational ladder.

Although evidence is mounting that ADHD often has its roots in neurobiology, I described in Chapter 2 how the clinical expression of the disorder is indeed an interaction of nature and nurture. Therefore, we also need to assess patterns of *family functioning*. Not only do we need to assess how the adolescent and his or her parents get along, we also need to assess parental depression and marital conflict—the types of parental pathology noted in Chapter 2 to be most predictive of negative outcomes for adolescents with ADHD.

HOW DO WE ASSESS?

There is no single test for ADHD. We collect information about these five areas from the teenagers themselves, their parents, their teachers, and any other adults with whom they are closely involved. We rely on physical examinations and laboratory tests, clinical interviews, standardized rating scales, psychological tests, educational tests, behavioral observations, and reviews of archival records such as report cards and schoolwork samples, as methods to tap these five content domains. Any single method or informant might be fallible; it is the convergence of multiple methods and informants that helps us solve the diagnostic puzzle.

In addition, clinicians need to keep in mind that because ADHD has an onset during early childhood, it is essential to acquire a reliable history of past behavioral difficulties as well as present concerns. Parental recall of children's early life events, particularly in families with several siblings and ADHD parents, may not be accurate. Clinicians should routinely request "reliability checks" (e.g., report cards, school records, and medical records) for parental verbal reports. Unlike younger children, adolescents can provide valuable information concerning their ADHD symptoms as well as their perceptions of peer, family, and school difficulties, and the clinician should routinely seek their input.

WHAT IS THE "GAME PLAN" FOR SEQUENCING EVALUATION?

My "game plan" for evaluating adolescents for possible ADHD has nine steps, listed in the order in which I carry them out:

1. Collect, score the rating scales.
2. Orient the family to the evaluation.
3. Interview the adolescent.
4. Administer the IQ, achievement, and continuous performance tests.
5. Conduct direct observations.
6. Interview the parents.
7. Conduct medical evaluation.
8. Integrate all of the data.
9. Give feedback and recommendations.

Step 1. Collect, Score the Rating Scales

To increase my efficiency, I want to know as much as I can before I spend any time interviewing or testing the adolescent and the family. Therefore, following the telephone intake, verification of payment information, and scheduling of the appointment, I mail all the questionnaires and rating scales to the family, in a packet with sections clearly marked for the mother, father, adolescent, and teachers. I give the parents responsibility for having the teacher questionnaires completed, although when teachers prefer to communicate directly with me, I enclose stamped, addressed return envelopes for them. I ask parents to return all the questionnaires, along with copies of any past testing reports, report cards, Individual Educational Placement Conference (IEPC) reports, or other records, to me 1 week in advance of the appointment; I point out that if they are unable to return the completed forms to me before the evaluation, I spend the first 30 minutes of the appointment reviewing this information, while they sit in the waiting room. Most parents comply with the request. Often, the teenagers balk at completing their ratings scales or need to be prompted to work on them for short periods on multiple occasions. This becomes useful diagnostic information.

It takes me approximately 30 minutes to score and review my typical battery of rating scales and questionnaires. I compute all the quantitative scores, review the qualitative comments, and ask myself what I know about the six basic content areas to be assessed, in how much detail do I need to assess each area, and what the probable diagnostic outcomes are. In essence, I construct a mental profile of the adolescent and the family.

Step 2. Orient the Family to the Evaluation

During the first 15 minutes of the evaluation, the adolescent and the parents are briefly seen together to clarify the questions that will be addressed and explain the methods that will be used. Usually, the reason for such referrals is poor school performance and/or home-based conflict, with a suspicion of possible ADHD or learning disabilities. Each family member is encouraged to list specific questions they wish to address. Teenagers are particularly encouraged to raise questions, even if they differ dramatically from their parents' concerns (questions raised by teenagers are treated seriously). The following overview statement helps demystify the assessment process:

> "You are telling me that Sally is doing poorly at school and not getting along with you at home. There are generally four reasons that account for 99% of school problems with adolescents: (1) insufficient intellectual ability to do the schoolwork, (2) specific learning disabilities, (3) attention-deficit/hyperactivity disorder, and/or (4) other emotional/behavioral problems. We are going to figure out which one or more of these reasons applies to you, Sally. In a few moments, I will talk to you

and administer some IQ, achievement, and attentional tests. You have already filled out a bunch of questionnaires. After the testing is done, I will talk extensively with the two of you, Mr. and Mrs. Jones, using our conversation, the questionnaires, and the test results to address these four reasons. Any questions?"

The family is also given the DSM-IV definition of ADHD (see Chapter 1) and a traditional educational definition of a specific learning disability as an IQ/achievement discrepancy.

Steps 3–4. Interview the Adolescent and Administer the IQ, Achievement, and Continuous Performance Tests

Next, I conduct the part of the evaluation that directly involves the adolescent. I used to interview the parents before I talked to and tested the adolescent, but over the years I have changed the sequence of activities for several reasons. First, adolescents who sit in the waiting room for a long time while clinicians interview their parents are likely to become bored and to be less cooperative during their portion of the evaluation. Second, it is helpful to have completed and scored the formal testing before talking to the parents; then I have a clear idea of the adolescent's intellectual ability and whether he or she has any learning disabilities before I make a definitive judgment about the presence of ADHD symptoms. Third, I have a hands-on feel for the adolescent's response style and a better understanding of what the parents are dealing with on a day-to-day basis.

In the interview with the adolescent, I first establish rapport, then review the DSM-IV symptoms, possible comorbidities, school, and family functioning. This interview typically takes 30 minutes. Next, I administer IQ, achievement, and continuous performance tests (CPT). This testing typically takes 120 to 150 minutes. Next, I score the testing, which takes me, an experienced examiner, 15 to 20 minutes (often, I can complete the scoring of the IQ and achievement tests while the adolescent is taking the CPT).

Step 5. Conduct Direct Observations

Next I administer family interaction or analogue academic observational tasks, if being employed. Administration of a family interaction task typically takes 10 minutes, and administration of an analogue academic task typically takes 10 minutes.

Step 6. Interview the Parents

By the time I interview the parents, I have a good idea of what is going on, from a combination of the rating scales, the adolescent interview, the testing, and the direct observational tasks. This knowledge permits me to avoid redundancy and to organize my interview in an efficient manner. I review the

DSM-IV criteria for ADHD exhaustively using a semistructured interview; carefully probe for comorbid conditions or differential diagnoses; take a medical, developmental, and school history; and briefly explore the parents' personal and marital issues. This interview ranges in length from 60 to 90 minutes, depending on the complexity of the situation.

Step 7. Conduct Medical Evaluation

The medical evaluation, conducted by the youngster's physician, can be completed at any convenient time before I integrate the data and reach a conclusion. In cases referred by physicians, the medical evaluation has typically been conducted before I begin my evaluation. It is placed here simply to remind clinicians that medical problems should be assessed before they make a diagnosis.

Step 8. Integrate All of the Data

As an experienced clinician, I have learned to integrate all the data as I collect it, and complete the final integration as I interview the parents. This is the point at which I benefit from having scored all of the rating scales before beginning the evaluation. Thus, when time allows, I can go directly from the parental interview to the feedback and recommendations stage. Many clinicians may prefer to take some time to integrate the data and think through their conclusions after the interviewing the parents. Thus, they may schedule the feedback for a later time.

Step 9. Give Feedback and Recommendations

The age and maturity level of the adolescent determines how I format the feedback and recommendations. In the case of 12- to 15-year-old youngsters, I typically give the parents detailed feedback and recommendations, then bring the adolescent into the session for brief feedback. With adolescents ages 16 and older, I typically conduct the entire feedback and recommendation session with them and their parents at the same time. The younger adolescents do not listen to or benefit from the detailed feedback, whereas older adolescents do. The feedback and recommendation session takes approximately 30 minutes.

HOW LONG DOES IT TAKE TO CARRY OUT THE GAME PLAN?

Table II.1 summarizes the times needed to complete each step of the game plan. It is important to realize that the actual time it takes the practitioner to complete each phase of the evaluation depends on the complexity of the case and the level of experience of the assessor. Adolescents with pure

TABLE II.1. Time to Complete the Game Plan for Evaluation

1. Score the rating scales—30 minutes.
2. Orient the family to the evaluation—15 minutes.
3. Interview the adolescent—30 minutes.
4. Administer the IQ, achievement, and CPT tests—120 to 150 minutes.
5. Conduct direct observations—20 minutes.
6. Interview the parents—60 to 90 minutes.
7. Conduct medical evaluation—depends on physician.
8. Integrate all of the data—depends on experience level of clinician.
9. Give feedback and recommendations—30 minutes.
10. Write report—60 to 90 minutes.

Total time: 365 to 455 minutes; 6 to 7½ hours

ADHD and no learning disabilities can be assessed in much less time than oppositional, depressed adolescents from highly dysfunctional families with multiple learning disabilities. Bright adolescents take less time to test than do adolescents with cognitive difficulties or slow processing speeds. Experienced clinicians develop strategies that shorten many of these steps. I have included in this summary the time it takes to write a report of the evaluation.

If all the steps were carefully followed and a report were written, the clinician might spend from 6 to 7½ hours on the evaluation, not counting "thinking time" to integrate the data.

In this age of managed care and preauthorization, questions arise about the practicality of devoting so much time to a thorough evaluation (Gordon & Irwin, 1997). Few managed care organizations will authorize 6 hours of time for an ADHD evaluation, and many do not even consider the diagnosis of ADHD to be a covered benefit. Few insurance companies will pay the clinician for the time taken to score rating scales, integrate data, or write a report. For those readers who work in managed care settings, however, at least one managed care group has advocated allocating 4 hours for an ADHD evaluation (Gephart, 1997).

What, then, are the absolute essentials, and what shortcuts can the practitioner take? First, let me say that the reason I prefer to conduct the entire evaluation is to be absolutely certain of the diagnosis and not to miss any possibilities. In many clinical situations the practitioner is able to take the necessary time to complete the entire game plan, and many families recognize that it is worthwhile to pay for a comprehensive evaluation. Of course, life is a series of compromises and clinicians often must take shortcuts, but they do bring with them the risk of overlooking something. When shortcuts are necessary, consider the following suggestions:

1. Eliminate the direct observations; these are most expendable be- cause family interactions can often be assessed during the inter-

views, and behavior in academic settings can be inferred from teacher reports.

2. Arrange to have the adolescent's school conduct the IQ and achievement testing. Theoretically, if a parent makes a written request for a special education evaluation, schools are supposed to conduct such an evaluation within 30 days from the time of the written request, but in reality it often takes much longer. If the school does not conduct the testing, administer a short form of the IQ and achievement tests or eliminate the testing completely. Of course, this prevents the practitioner from ruling out a learning disability, but in some cases he or she may not have any choice.

3. Do not write a report as part of the evaluation. Write a brief letter. If the patient wants a report, the clinician may require that the patient pay out of pocket.

4. Eliminate the CPT. It is a helpful corroborative tool, but when time or resources are limited, the practitioner can make diagnostic decisions based on interviews and rating scales.

5. Use fewer rating scales to cut down on scoring time.

6. Do not cut down the practitioner interview. A thorough interview is essential to making a correct diagnosis.

Following these steps may cut the evaluation down to approximately 2 to 2½ hours.

WHERE TO FIND THINGS IN SECTION II

Section II of this book is organized according to the "game plan" outlined here. Chapter 3 discusses the medical assessment and the use of rating scales and questionnaires. Chapter 4 discusses clinical interviewing, differential diagnosis, and family assessment. Chapter 5 discusses the use of continuous performance tests, direct observation procedures, and psychological testing to assess intellectual ability, achievement, and learning disabilities; the determination of educational impairment due to ADHD; and the legal obligations of the schools to service youngsters with such impairments. Chapter 6 concludes with examples of how to integrate all the assessment data and present feedback to the family.

CHAPTER THREE

○

Medical Evaluation and Rating Scales

This chapter describes the medical evaluation and the use of standardized rating scales in the overall diagnostic process. These two essential but very different tools are part of the evaluation. A medical assessment may be conducted at various points throughout the overall evaluation process. Physicians evaluating adolescents might conveniently conduct the medical assessment along with the clinical interviews of the adolescent. Psychologists typically request that parents arrange for a thorough physical examination before or after the other parts of the assessment. In a managed care environment, the medical evaluation might best take place after the assessment. Thus, if the physician makes a positive diagnosis, a discussion of stimulant medication can take place during a single medical visit.

Standardized rating scales are an important tool for corroborating clinical impressions concerning behavioral/psychological problems. The clinician can compare ratings of a particular youngster to normative ratings of many similar youngsters; they supplement the artificially limiting categorical approach of the DSM-IV model with information based on a dimensional model of psychopathology. In contrast to the medical assessment, which can be completed at any time, the rating scales are best administered very early in the overall evaluation, so that the clinician can have the results available during the later clinical interviews.

MEDICAL ASSESSMENT

The medical interview may overlap somewhat with the psychological history but focuses much more on the child's disease and health history, genetic background, pre- and perinatal events, current health, nutritional status, and gross sensory/motor functioning. It is designed to provide a differential diagnosis of ADHD from other medical conditions. The physician will carefully assess whether ADHD symptoms are secondary to factors such as significant head or central nervous system (CNS) injury, CNS infection, cerebrovascular disease (e.g., strokes), sleep disorder, endocrine disorder, lead or other metal poisoning, or environmental toxins. It is important to evaluate medical conditions that may be comorbid to ADHD and may influence the medical management of ADHD (allergies, seizures, asthma, etc.) as well as medical contraindications to the prescription of stimulant medication (e.g., high blood pressure and cardiac difficulties).

The complete physical examination should begin with a height, weight, and head circumference. Next, the physician should conduct a general inspection to assess nutritional status and minor physical anomalies (short palpebral fissures, epicanthal folds, thin upper lip of fetal alcohol syndrome, clinodactyly, wide-set eyes, etc.). The physician should also check the ears, eyes, and throat for otitis and thyroid enlargement; perform a sexual maturity rating; and check testicular size in males. Large testes are associated with fragile-X syndrome, whereas small testes are associated with Klinefelter's syndrome. If indicated, the physician may conduct a neurological screening to evaluate the cranial nerves, muscle strength and tone, gait, coordination, reflexes, and sensory organs and to assess for tics or involuntary movements. Some physicians investigate the presence of "soft" signs such as reflex asymmetry, strabismus, coordination difficulty, motor overflow and mirror movements, and extinction to double simultaneous tactile stimulation.

Audiometric and visual acuity testing should accompany the physical examination. However, there is no evidence for the utility of blood tests, urinalysis, chromosome studies, PET (positron emission tomography) scans, CAT (computed axial tomography) scans, MRIs (magnetic resonance images), regular or enhanced EEGs (electroencephalograms), or any other similar tests in routine clinical assessment. Some of these tests are clearly useful in research, but none has proven valid for routine clinical screening.

Baseline liver function tests are necessary for those youngsters who are going to start on pemoline, and those who are going to start on a tricyclic antidepressant medication need a baseline EKG (electrocardiogram). In the case of sexually active female adolescents not using birth control, it is prudent to conduct a pregnancy test before starting any psychoactive medication.

RATING SCALES

The minimum, acceptable battery of rating scales should include a DSM-IV ADHD symptom checklist and at least one parent, one teacher, and one adolescent rating scale. Because there are numerous specific rating scales to choose from, I selectively review a small number of them here, but as long as psychometrically valid measures are used, the reader might also select from many others (See Barkley, 1990, for a review). Table 3.1 lists the rating scales I commonly administer, organized by parent, adolescent, and teacher respondents.

Parents, adolescents, and teachers each complete three types of rating scales:

1. *ADHD symptom-specific measures*—for example, the DSM-IV ADHD Behavior Checklist, ADHD School History Grid, Brown Attention Deficit Disorder Scales, and the TRF Attention Problems Scale.
2. *ADHD symptom and general psychopathology/classroom performance*—for example, the Child Behavior Checklist, the Behavior Assessment System for Children, Conners–Wells Adolescent Self-Report Scale, and the Classroom Performance Survey.
3. *Family functioning measures*—for example, the Conflict Behavior Questionnaire, Issues Checklist, Parent–Adolescent Relationship Questionnaire, and Marital Satisfaction Inventory.

The majority of the measures meet appropriate psychometric criteria, as discussed later, but I use several adjunctively, despite lack of good evidence for their reliability and validity, because they tap domains not adequately assessed by any validated measures.

Keeping in mind that ADHD runs in families, I also include a basic screening of the adolescent's parents by asking them to rate themselves at the present time and as children on the DSM-IV ADHD Behavior Checklist.

When interpreting even the reliable and valid rating scales on a case-by-case basis, the practitioner should keep in mind the following points: (1) the rating scales are based on subjective impressions of individuals who do sometimes have a vested interest in the outcome (e.g., parents and teachers searching for a positive ADHD diagnosis or adolescents who deny the presence of any problems); (2) secondary education teachers typically have not had the opportunity to get to know a student as well as elementary education teachers; (3) many of the manifestations of ADHD in adolescents are not overtly observable (e.g., mental restlessness), and can only be ascertained by adolescent self-report; and (4) the normative data are not always applicable throughout the entire age range of adolescence. As discussed in Chapter 1, the practitioner should be prepared to respond to the attacks of extremists who reject the existence of ADHD, in part based on the fact that subjective rating scales are part of the diagnostic procedures (Armstrong, 1995). Practitioners should never use rating scales as the primary criteria for diagnosing an individual with any disorder such as ADHD.

TABLE 3.1. My Standard Battery of Rating Scales

Name	Target	Availability
	Parent	
1. DSM-IV Behavior Checklists	ADHD symptoms	This chapter
2. ADHD School History Grid	ADHD symptom history	This chapter
Administer 3a, 3b, or 3c		
3a. Conners Parent Rating Scale—Revised	ADHD symptoms, pathology	Conners (1997)
3b. Child Behavior Checklist	Psychopathology	Achenbach (1991)
3c. BASC Parent Rating Scale	Psychopathology	Reynolds & Kamphaus (1992)
Administer 4a or 4b		
4a. Parent–Adolescent Relationship Questionnaire	Family conflict	Available from Robin
4b. Conflict Behavior Questionnaire	Family conflict	Barkley (1991a)
5. Issues Checklist	Specific disputes	Barkley (1991a)
6. Marital Satisfaction Inventory	Parents' marriage	Snyder (1997)
7. Beck Depression Inventory	Depression	Beck (1976)
8. SCL-90-R	Parental psychopathology	Derogatis (1983)
9. Demographic Data Form	History information	Barkley (1991a) Gordon (1995a)
	Adolescent	
1. DSM-IV Behavior Checklist	ADHD symptoms	This chapter
2. Brown Attention Deficit Disorder Scales	Attention problems	Brown (1996)
3. Conners–Wells Adolescent Self-Report Scale	Psychopathology	Conners & Wells (1997)
4. Conflict Behavior Questionnaire	Communication/ conflict	Barkley (1991a)
5. Issues Checklist	Specific disputes	Barkley (1991a)
	Teachers	
1. Classroom Performance Survey	School tasks	This chapter
Administer 2a, 2b, 2c, or 2d		
2a. Teacher Report Form Attention Problems	ADHD symptoms	Achenbach (1996)
2b. Child Attention Profile	ADHD symptoms	Barkley (1991a)
2c. Teacher Report Form	Psychopathology	Achenbach (1991)
2d. BASC Teacher Rating Scale	Psychopathology	Reynolds & Kamphaus (1992)

Parent Rating Scales

DSM-IV ADHD Behavior Checklist

It is helpful to have parents and adolescents complete a checklist of the 18 DSM-IV ADHD symptoms. I also used to administer this checklist to all the adolescent's teachers, but I found that because secondary education teachers may not directly observe behaviors relevant to many of the items, this checklist proves less useful than validated teacher rating scales, so I stopped administering it to the teachers. Table 3.2 contains the version of the DSM-IV ADHD Behavior Checklist completed by the parents rating the adolescent (Murphy & Barkley, 1995). With a change of initial instructions, the adolescent completes the same checklist. The odd-numbered items tap inattention; the even-numbered items tap hyperactivity/impulsivity. By tradition, any item endorsed "pretty much" (2) or "very much" (3) is considered significantly present. I review the completed checklists and highlight all the items endorsed as 2 or 3. I highlight the odd- and even-numbered items in different colors to expedite quick visual scanning for the core symptoms of various subtypes of ADHD.

First, I determine whether the adolescent potentially meets the inclusionary criteria for one of the subtypes of ADHD based on the number of items endorsed 2 or 3: (1) six or more odd-numbered items for ADHD, Inattentive subtype; (2) six or more even-numbered items for ADHD, Hyperactive/Impulsive subtype; or (3) six or more odd- and six or more even-numbered items for ADHD, Combined subtype.

Next, I compute summary scores: (1) the summary score of the 0–3 ratings for the inattention items and (2) the summary score of the 0–3 ratings for the impulsivity/hyperactivity items. Table 3.3 contains normative data for parents of all-age adolescents (DuPaul et al., in press) and for adolescents over age 17 (Murphy & Barkley, 1995). Scores at least 1.5 standard deviations above the mean are considered clinically elevated.

Analysis of discrepancies between adolescents and adults on the ADHD checklist can be enlightening. Often, adolescents report many fewer symptoms than parents, raising the possibility that they are either unaware or denying their actions. If I have other clinical information suggesting that the adolescent is minimizing the presence of the ADHD symptoms, I may also examine carefully the items endorsed as "sometimes."

ADHD School History Grid and Demographic Data

The ADHD School History Grid, illustrated in Table 3.4, represents a convenient way for parents to encode their recollections of which ADHD symptoms and related school problems have been occurring from preschool until the adolescent's current grade. It consists of a list of 24 items, including ADHD symptoms, ODD behaviors, and common school problems encountered by youngsters with behavioral and learning prob-

TABLE 3.2. ADHD Behavior Checklist

PARENT RATING TEEN'S PRESENT BEHAVIOR

Name of Person Being Rated _____

Date _____

Name of Rater _____

Circle the number that best describes your adolescent's behavior over the past 6 months.

	Never or rarely	Sometimes	Often	Very often
1. Fails to give close attention to details or makes careless mistakes in work.	0	1	2	3
2. Fidgets with hands or feet or squirms in seat.	0	1	2	3
3. Has difficulty sustaining attention in tasks or fun activities.	0	1	2	3
4. Leaves seat in classroom or in other situations in which seating is expected.	0	1	2	3
5. Doesn't listen when spoken to directly.	0	1	2	3
6. Feels restless or moves about excessively.	0	1	2	3
7. Doesn't follow through on instructions and fails to finish work.	0	1	2	3
8. Has difficulty engaging in leisure activities or doing fun things quietly.	0	1	2	3
9. Has difficulty organizing tasks and activities.	0	1	2	3
10. Feels "on the go" or "driven by a motor."	0	1	2	3
11. Avoids, dislikes, or is reluctant to engage in work that requires sustained mental effort.	0	1	2	3
12. Talks excessively.	0	1	2	3
13. Loses things necessary for tasks or activities.	0	1	2	3
14. Blurts out answers before questions have been completed.	0	1	2	3
15. Is easily distracted.	0	1	2	3
16. Has difficulty awaiting turn.	0	1	2	3
17. Is forgetful in daily activities.	0	1	2	3
18. Interrupts or intrudes on others.	0	1	2	3

Note. From Murphy & Barkley (1995). Copyright 1995 by The Guilford Press. Reprinted in *ADHD in Adolescents: Diagnosis and Treatment* by Arthur L. Robin. Permission to photocopy this table is granted to purchasers of *ADHD in Adolescents* for personal use only (see copyright page for details).

TABLE 3.3. Normative Data on the DSM-IV ADHD Behavior Checklist

Age	N	Inattention				Hyperactivity–impulsivity				Total score			
		Mean (SD)	90th %ile	93rd %ile	98th %ile	Mean (SD)	90th %ile	93rd %ile	98th %ile	Mean (SD)	90th %ile	93rd %ile	98th %ile
Parent normative data for males (DuPaul, Anastopoulos, Power, Reid, Ikeda, & McGoey, in press)—summation scores													
11–13 yr	149	6.70 (6.27)	18.0	18.5	24.0	4.79 (5.54)	14.0	16.0	21.0	11.50 (11.32)	31.0	34.0	47.0
14–18 yr	133	5.70 (5.36)	13.6	15.6	23.0	3.68 (4.32)	10.0	11.0	16.3	9.38 (8.96)	23.4	27.0	36.3
Parent normative data for females—summation scores													
11–13 yr	173	4.61 (6.27)	12.8	16.0	21.0	2.88 (5.54)	9.0	10.0	12.0	7.49 (11.32)	20.0	21.6	28.5
14–18 yr	225	4.07 (4.57)	12.2	14.0	16.5	3.29 (3.82)	10.0	11.0	16.0	7.36 (7.74)	22.0	24.0	32.5

Normative data for older adolescents and young adults (ages 17–29) on DSM-IV ADHD Behavior Checklist (Murphy & Barkley, 1996a)

	Mean	SD	+1.5 SD cutoff
Number of symptoms			
Inattention	1.3	1.8	4.0
Hyperactivity–impulsivity	2.1	2.0	5.1
Total ADHD score	3.3	3.5	8.6
Summation of symptom ratings			
Inattention	6.3	4.7	13.4
Hyperactivity–impulsivity	8.5	4.7	15.6
Total ADHD score	14.7	8.7	27.8

Note. SD, standard deviation.

TABLE 3.4. ADHD School Symptom History Grid

Name of Child _____ Today's Date _____

Form Completed by _____

Current School _____Grade _____

Please review each of the items listed below.

Place an "×" in the boxes which represent the grades in school when that item was a problem for the child named above. Leave the box blank if the item was not a problem in that grade.

SAMPLE

Making careless mistakes was a problem for Bill from second through fifth grades. Mrs. Jones placed ×'s in the appropriate boxes.

	P	K	1	2	3	4	5	6	7	8	9	10	11	12
Makes careless mistakes				×	×	×	×							
1. Makes careless mistakes														
2. Fidgets, is restless														
3. Doesn't pay attention														
4. Leaves seat in class														
5. Doesn't listen when spoken to directly														
6. Doesn't follow instructions														
7. Doesn't finish in-class assignments														
8. Doesn't finish homework														
9. Has difficulty with organization														
10. Talks too much														
11. Socializes too much in class														
12. Daydreams in school														
13. Blurts things out, interrupts														
14. Is impatient, can't wait turn														

(continued)

TABLE 3.4. *(continued)*

	P	K	1	2	3	4	5	6	7	8	9	10	11	12
15. Is easily distracted														
16. Doesn't bring materials to class														
17. Doesn't bring papers/notes home														
18. Has sloppy handwriting														
19. Has low test scores														
20. Asks for help when needed														
21. Is argumentative in class														
22. Gets in fights at school														
23. Cheats														
24. Steals														

Note. From *ADHD in Adolescents: Diagnosis and Treatment* by Arthur L. Robin. Copyright 1998 by The Guilford Press. Permission to photocopy this table is granted to purchasers of *ADHD in Adolescents* for personal use only (see copyright page for details).

lems. Each item has a grid with boxes for preschool through 12th grade. The parent puts x's in the boxes for all the grades during which that item applied. Although we have not yet collected normative data on this measure, we use it to increase our clinical efficiency in taking a detailed history of ADHD symptoms and school problems.

Most clinicians use a Demographic Data Form, which includes a variety of medical, developmental, and family history questions. Examples of such forms can be found in several texts (Barkley, 1997c; Gordon, 1995a).

Child Behavior Checklist

The Child Behavior Checklist (CBCL) is one of the most widely used and psychometrically sound parent rating scales in the assessment of ADHD (Achenbach & Edelbrock, 1983; Achenbach, 1991). The 138 items of the CBCL are broken down into 20 items which assess Social Competence and 118 items that comprise the Behavior Problems scales. The Social Competence scale generates scores for Activities, Social, and School; the Behavior

Problems scales generate eight factorially based scores: (1) Withdrawal, (2) Somatic Complaints, (3) Anxious/Depressed, (4) Social Problems, (5) Thought Problems, (6) Attention Problems, (7) Delinquent Behavior, and (8) Aggressive Behavior. The CBCL can be either hand-scored or computer-scored, yielding a profile of T-scores based on analyses of parent ratings of 2,300 clinically referred children and normed on 1,300 nonreferred children.

Selected CBCL Behavior Problem scores are excellent discriminators of ADHD with or without comorbidity (Anastopoulos, 1993; Biederman et al., 1993; Robin & Vandermay, 1996). The CBCL scores correlate highly with structured psychiatric diagnostic interviews and other comparable rating scales; discriminate accurately between ADHD, control, and other psychiatric groups; and are stable over long periods.

Clinically, a T-score elevation of 60 on the Attention Problems scale has been found to be optimal for diagnostic discrimination of ADHD; a T-score of 70, 2 standard deviations above the normative mean and the normally recommended cutoff is too stringent and fails to identify many patients diagnosed as ADHD based on structured interviews or clinician diagnosis (Biederman et al., 1993). ADHD teens without any other comorbid psychiatric disorders are also likely to have T-scores above 60 on Anxious/Depressed, Social Problems, and Aggressive Behavior (Biederman et al., 1993).

Not only can the CBCL distinguish between ADHD and non-ADHD children, but it can also help distinguish reliably between pure ADHD and ADHD plus comorbid children. Biederman et al. (1993) compared the CBCL profiles of 6- to 17-year-old boys with ADHD and no comorbid psychiatric conditions to those of four other groups: (1) ADHD plus Conduct Disorder, (2) ADHD plus Anxiety Disorders, (3) ADHD plus Major Depressive Disorder, and (4) ADHD plus more than two comorbidities. The children in all these groups were diagnosed based upon the DSM-III version of the Kiddie SADS-E (Orvaschel & Puig-Antich, 1987), a well-established structured psychiatric interview. Using T-score cutoffs of 60, they considered a CBCL scale to be a good predictor of diagnostic group membership if the total predictive value (percent cases diagnosed with Kiddie SADS correctly predicted by a scale) was greater than 70% and the odds ratio was greater than three, compared to the pure ADHD group (not to a control group). Table 3.5 summarizes their results. Based on these results, clinicians can use T-score elevations greater than 60 on Delinquent and Aggressive Behavior and Thought Problems as an indicator to screen for possible Conduct Disorder in an ADHD child, T-scores greater than 60 on Anxious/Depressed and Thought Disorders and Aggressive Behavior as an indicator to screen for a possible comorbid Anxiety Disorders in an ADHD child, and a T-score greater than 60 on Thought Disorders alone as an indicator to screen for a possible comorbid Major Depressive Disorder. Of course, Biederman's results were obtained only with males, and with a

TABLE 3.5. CBCL Scales with Total Predictive Value >70% and Odds Ratio Greater Than 3 in ADHD + Comorbidity Groups Compared to Pure ADHD Group (Biederman et al., 1993)

	ADHD + Conduct Disorder	ADHD + Anxiety Disorders	ADHD + Major Depression	ADHD + 2 or more comorbidities
Scale				
Withdrawn				Yes
Somatic Complaints				Yes
Anxious/Depressed		Yes		Yes
Social Problems				
Thought Problems	Yes	Yes	Yes	Yes
Attention Problems				
Delinquent Behavior	Yes			Yes
Aggressive Behavior	Yes	Yes		Yes

broad age range of children; these limitations should be taken into account when interpreting adolescent data. Finally, clinicians should never use the CBCL in place of a thorough differential diagnostic interview but, rather should use it to corroborate interview-based impressions or suggest additional hypotheses for verification.

In a further study of the comorbidity of Major Depressive Disorder and ADHD, Biederman, Faraone, Mick, Moore, and Lelon (1996) compared the CBCL scores of four groups of carefully screened and diagnosed youngsters: (1) ADHD alone, (2) Major Depressive Disorder alone, (3) ADHD + Major Depressive Disorder, and (4) normal controls. Using more stringent T-score cutoffs of $T - 70$ and the predictive value/odds ratio methodology from the earlier investigation, Biederman, Faraone, Mick, et al. (1996) found that children with Major Depressive Disorder with or without comorbid ADHD differed significantly from those with ADHD on the Withdrawn and Somatic Complaints scales. Children with ADHD were significantly elevated on the Attention Problems scale irrespective of comorbidity with major depression in comparison to those with Major Depressive Disorder only. Finally, the group with comorbid ADHD and Major Depressive Disorder differed from both the Major Depressive Disorder and ADHD alone groups in higher rates of Aggressive Behavior and from the ADHD alone group in higher rates of Delinquent Behavior.

The CBCL is also useful in helping to differentiate between youngsters with ADHD and comorbid Bipolar Disorder versus ADHD alone or Bipolar Disorder alone (Biederman, Faraone, Mick, Wozniak, et al., 1996). Although there is no pathognomonic CBCL profile specific for Bipolar Disorder, such children tend to have elevations on Delinquent Behavior, Aggressive Behavior, Somatic Complaints, Anxious/Depressed, and Thought Problems. ADHD children with Bipolar Disorder tended to have higher CBCL scores than did other ADHD children, particularly on Delinquent Behavior, Aggressive Behavior, and Social Problems. ADHD children with or without Bipolar Disorder had higher scores on Attention Problems than either children with Bipolar Disorder alone or controls.

Conners Parent Rating Scale—Revised

All the Conners rating scales recently underwent a major revision and restandardization, resulting in a total of 11 long and short versions for parents, teachers, and also adolescents (Conners, 1997, 1997a, 1997b). The measurement development and validation process was similar for the parent, teacher, and new adolescent self-report versions. I briefly describe the process here and refer to it in later discussions of the teacher and adolescent self-report versions. Each scale consisted of a large number of items generated from the original Conners rating scales, other versions such as the Iowa Conners, the DSM-IV ADHD criteria, and recent literature on ADHD. These items were administered to more than 8,000 parents, teachers, or adolescents in a carefully selected, representative sample. For each agent, the sample was divided in half, and a seven-factor structure was first derived through exploratory factor analysis with half of the sample, then tested for goodness of fit through confirmatory factor analysis with the other half. Items retained in the final scales loaded .30 on only one factor. A long and a short form were constructed for each agent. The short forms consisted of a subset of the scales, and for these scales, it included the items that loaded highest on the original factors.

In addition to the seven factor scales, an ADHD index was constructed through discriminant analysis by selecting the 12 items for each agent that best discriminated between groups of ADHD and matched control children. The ADHD Indix was cross-validated on separate samples and found to have very high sensitivities, specificities, and overall correct classification rates. The 10-item Hyperactivity Index from the original Conners questionnaires was renamed the Conners Global Index and factor-analyzed to derive two factor scores: Restless/Impulsive and Emotional Lability. Finally, rationally derived scales with the 18 DSM-IV ADHD symptoms were also constructed.

The resulting Conners Parent Rating Scale—Revised (CPRS-R; Conners, 1997a) comes in a long form of 80 items (CPRS-R:L) and a short form of 27 items (CPRS-R:S), with separate norms by sex and age in 3-year intervals. The CPRS-R:L includes the following 14 scales (scales followed by an asterisk are also included in the CPRS-R:S):

1. Oppositional*
2. Cognitive Problems*
3. Hyperactivity*
4. Anxious/Shy
5. Perfectionism

6. Social Problems
7. Pychosomatic
8. Conners Global Index (CGI) (formally Hyperactivity Index)
9. CGI Restless/Impulsive
10. CGI Emotional Lability
11. ADHD Index*
12. DSM-IV Total Score
13. DSM-IV Inattentive Subscale
14. DSM-IV Hyperactive–Impulsive Subscale

Easily scored by hand using a carbonless quick-scoring form, the CPRS-R:L yields a profile of *T*-scores such that *T*-scores of 60–65 are mildly atypical, 66–70 are moderately atypical, and over 70 are markedly atypical. Validation research done as part of the restandardization effort indicated that the long and short forms have good criterion-related and concurrent validity and good internal validity. Further research is needed to determine whether the CPRS-R can differentiate between adolescents with pure ADHD versus ADHD and various comorbidities, as can the CBCL.

BASC Parent Rating Scale

The Behavior Assessment System for Children–-Parent Rating Scale (BASC-PRS; Reynolds & Kamphaus, 1992) is a comprehensive measure of an adolescent's adaptive and problem behaviors in community and home settings, consisting of 131 items using a four-choice response format. The BASC-PRS has three forms with items targeted at three age levels: preschool (4–5), child (6–11), and adolescent (12–18), and takes the average parent 10–20 minutes to complete. The measure yields a number of broad-band composite and individual scale *T*-scores, along with an F (fake bad) index designed to detect parental negative response sets. The scales for the adolescent, parent, and teacher versions are listed in Table 3.6, along with the Mean *T*-scores for a group of ADHD children.

The parent responds on a carbonless quick-scoring form. *T*-scores are obtained such that high scores are negative for the clinical scales and low scores are significant for the adaptive scales. For the clinical scales, *T*-scores of 60–69 are considered "at risk," and 70 or above clinically significant; for the adaptive scales, *T*-scores of 31–40 are considered "at risk," and 30 or below are considered clinically significant.

The BASC-PRS was developed through a comprehensive norming process with a theoretically driven factor structure. It has good internal consistency, test–retest reliability, and correlates reasonably well with the CBCL, the CPRS, and several others. The test manual gives clinical profiles for children and adolescents with various diagnoses, but only data for children (mean age = 8.7) were available in the area of ADHD. The manual

TABLE 3.6. BASC Scales and Mean *T*-Scores for ADHD Children

Scale	Parent	Mean score	Teacher	Mean score
Externalizing Problems	Yes	66.9	Yes	60.0
Aggression	Yes	63.0	Yes	58.9
Hyperactivity	Yes	68.0	Yes	60.5
Conduct Problems	Yes	62.6	Yes	58.0
Internalizing Problems	Yes	54.9	Yes	57.4
Anxiety	Yes	50.0	Yes	56.7
Depression	Yes	61.0	Yes	58.6
Somatization	Yes	49.3	Yes	53.4
School Problems	No		Yes	62.1
Attention Problems	Yes	65.7	Yes	62.5
Learning Problems	No		Yes	60.8
Other Problems				
Atypicality	Yes	55.2	Yes	56.9
Withdrawal	Yes	49.9	Yes	58.5
Adaptive Skills	Yes	39.0	Yes	40.3
Leadership	Yes	43.4	Yes	42.2
Social Skills	Yes	40.9	Yes	43.4
Study Skills	No		Yes	39.3
Behavioral Symptoms Index	Yes	65.3	Yes	61.2
F (Fake Bad) Scale	Yes	N.A.	Yes	N.A.

Note. Data from Reynolds & Kamphaus (1992).

does not provide any statistical comparisons of these profiles. Table 3.8 provides the mean *T*-scores for 52 children diagnosed with ADHD based on DSM-III-R criteria or other research criteria. This sample received high scores on Hyperactivity and Attention Problems and lower but nonetheless elevated scores on Aggression, Conduct Problems, and Depression, as well as a low score on adaptive skills. I am not aware of any specific research using the BASC-PRS with ADHD adolescents.

Parental Psychopathology Measures

Because parental psychopathology, particularly maternal depression and marital strife, significantly complicates the clinical picture in families with ADHD adolescents, I include at least one marital and one general psychopathology screening measure. Practitioners have many good measures to choose from. I use the Beck Depression Inventory (Beck, 1976), the Symptom Checklist 90—Revised (SCL-90-R; Derogatis, 1983) and the Marital Satisfaction Inventory—Revised (Snyder, 1997). I administer the Global Distress and Conflict over Childrearing scales from the Marital Satisfaction Inventory rather than the entire questionnaire.

Adolescent Rating Scales

As pointed out in the earlier discussion of parent rating scales, the adolescent rates him- or herself on an appropriately worded version of the DSM-IV ADHD Behavior Checklist (Table 3.2). In addition, the adolescent completes the Brown ADD Scales and the Conners–Wells Adolescent Self-Report Scale.

Brown ADD Scales

The Brown Adolescent and Adult Attention Deficit Disorder scales (Brown, 1996) are excellent examples of user-friendly, self-report measures that tap highly salient, clinically important dimensions of ADHD symptoms. Administered either as a paper-and-pencil measure or a structured clinical interview, the Brown Adolescent ADD Scale consists of 40 items grouped into five clusters of conceptually related ADHD symptoms:

1. *Activating and organizing to work*—nine items tapping excessive difficulty getting organized and started on school or work-related tasks, along with undue problems in self-activating for daily routines such as getting out of bed.
2. *Sustaining attention and concentration*—nine items tapping chronic problems in sustaining attention to work-related tasks (e.g., daydreaming or distractibility when listening or reading).
3. *Sustaining energy and effort*—nine items assessing trouble keeping up consistent energy and effort for work-related tasks, daytime drowsiness, slow processing of information, inadequate task completion, and inconsistent performance.
4. *Managing affective interference*—seven items assessing mood and sensitivity to criticism.
5. *Utilizing working memory and accessing recall*—six items inquiring about forgetfulness in daily routines and problems in recall of learned information.

The scales can be used for initial screening of individuals suspected of having ADHD, for comprehensive diagnostic assessment, and for monitoring of treatment responses to medical and psychosocial interventions (see Chapter 8, this volume, for use in monitoring medication). The adolescent version is normed on 12- to 18-year-olds, whereas the adult version, with slight rewording of several items, is normed on individuals age 18 and over. The individual responds on a carbonless ready score form, which is easily hand-scored to obtain a raw summary score and cluster *T*-scores reflecting comparisons to a normative population of non-ADHD adolescents. When the Brown ADD Scale is administered in an interview format, Brown recommends that parents and adolescents be seen together, and that after the adolescent has responded to each item, the interviewer ask the parent to rate the adolescent. Parent responses are used clinically, as no normative data have yet been collected for quantitative analysis of these scores. Brown did compare total scores for parents and adolescents and found them to be correlated .84.

The five clusters are based on a model that emphasizes that the cognitive impairments of ADHD are multifaceted and provides a component analysis of these impairments. However, the measure does not, tap the behavioral disinhibition component of ADHD. Brown (1996) provided ample data supporting the concurrent, criterion-related, and construct validity of the measure, as well as its internal consistency and test–retest reliability; he found no significant age, sex, socioeconomic status, or ADHD subtype differences and thus developed a single set of norms for adolescents. He also provided a comprehensive diagnostic form and a method to analyze IQ scores for ADHD-related problems to accompany the questionnaire.

Clinically, a total raw score of 50 is the most reasonable cutting score for screening for possible ADHD; this score results in a 10% false-negative rate and a 22% false-positive rate for the adolescent measure and a 4% false-negative and a 6% false-positive rate for the adult measure. Brown carefully analyzed the sensitivity and specificity of the scales to obtain this recommended cutting score. For adolescents, total scores below 45 suggest that ADHD is possible but not likely; scores between 45 and 59 suggest that ADHD is probable but not certain; and scores above 60 indicate that ADHD is highly probable. Cluster T-scores of 65 or above (1.5 standard deviations over the normative mean of 50) are taken as clinically significant.

Conners–Wells Adolescent Self-Report Scale

The Conners–Wells Adolescent Self-Report Scale (CASS; Conners & Wells, 1997) was first developed in 1985 and in its first version has been part of my battery of questionnaires for a long time (Robin & Vandermay, 1996). As described earlier, it was recently updated and standardized as part of the Conners restandardization project (Conners, 1997b). The 84-item long form of the CASS includes the following scales (scales followed by an asterisk are also included in the 27-item short form):

1. Family Problems
2. Emotional Problems
3. Conduct Problems*
4. Cognitive Problems*
5. Anger Control
6. Hyperactivity*
7. ADHD Index*
8. DSM-IV Symptom Total

    9. DSM-IV Inattention

   10. DSM-IV Hyperactivity–Impulsivity

Internal consistencies ranged from .83 to .92, and test–retest reliabilities over 6 weeks ranged from .68 to .89. All six scales were significantly elevated in a group of 86 adolescents with ADHD and no comorbidities compared to a matched control group. Sensitivity was 81.4%, specificity was 83.7%, positive predictive power was 83.3%, and negative predictive power was 81.8%.

    Although there is some overlap between the CASS and the Brown ADD Scales, the Conners–Wells Adolescent Self-Report Scale taps a number of dimensions beyond inattention but does not provide coverage of the components of inattention on the Brown ADD Scales. Thus, we find it clinically useful to administer both adolescent self-report measures. Research is needed to correlate these two measures with each other.

Teacher Rating Scales

Assessing teachers' perceptions of ADHD symptoms and school performance in middle and high school youngsters is difficult because the adolescent typically has five to eight teachers, each of whom sees the adolescent for one class period per day in one subject area. Secondary education teachers do not have as comprehensive a picture of the average adolescent as do elementary school teachers, who see the younger student in a variety of activities. In addition, many of the crucial behaviors that contribute to academic success in high school occur outside the classroom (e.g., completing homework, reading textbooks, collecting reference information in the library, writing papers, organizing books and materials, and studying for examinations), so the average teacher does not have an opportunity to observe the adolescent's level of performance of these behaviors. The overt motor overactivity and disruptive behavior of many younger ADHD children diminishes and/or transforms into mental restlessness during adolescence, further limiting the potential sample of ADHD behaviors available to be observed during a single class period in middle or high school. The majority of teacher rating scales normed and validated for use with ADHD children contain items that rely heavily on direct observations of ADHD symptoms. Therefore, they do not yield clinically useful information for many adolescents and in many cases do not have adequate normative databases for students above age 12.

    Yet, teacher input is crucial for diagnosing and managing ADHD in adolescents, particularly for the determination of educational impairment and prescription of classroom accommodations. Ideally, the clinician conducts a telephone interview with the teachers, but this is really not practical. The clinician is advised to administer at least one ADHD symptom checklist to all of the adolescent's teachers, to request copies of all of the adolescent report cards and any other written documentation on file at the school, and to administer a questionnaire assessing classroom performance to each teacher. It is important to encourage teachers to write in anecdotal comments on the bottom of the rating scales; I often find that their anecdotal comments are more useful than their formal quantitative ratings in building a picture of a given adolescent's performance deficiencies in school.

I administer the Classroom Performance Survey and one of the following rating scales: (1) Attention Problems Scale—Teacher Report Form, (2) Conners Teacher Rating Scale—Revised, or (3) BASC Teacher Rating Scale. I do not routinely administer the entire Teacher Report Form (TRF) because I find it impractical to computer score and interpret five to eight of them on a routine basis. However, in certain cases, parental reports of adolescent psychopathology on the CBCL are suspect, and it is important to attempt to obtain such information from a full TRF.

Attention Problems Scale—Teacher Report Form

The Attention Problems Scale consists of the 20 items listed in Table 3.7. In an attempt to create subscales useful for making diagnoses of DSM-IV ADHD subtypes, Achenbach (1996) factor-analyzed this scale separately for boys and girls at ages 5–11 and 12–18, using his 1991 sample of 2,815 clinically referred children. He derived a 10-item inattention factor on the left side of Table 3.7 and a 6-item hyperactivity–impulsivity factor in the middle of the table. However, he found that the four additional items at the right of the table were strongly associated with both the inattention and hyperactivity–impulsivity factors. Practically, he recommended adding them to each of the factors when computing summary scores. The practitioner should use the 95th percentile cutoffs for deviance given in Table 3.8 to judge the clinical significance of elevations on these two subscales.

The Child Attention Profile (CAP; Barkley, 1991a), a 12-item teacher questionnaire also derived from the TRF (which I have used extensively), contains many of the same items in Table 3.7. However, the normative data available for adolescents are not separated by age on this measure, although they are separated by sex. In using these measures with the teachers of adolescents, I find that the inattention scores are typically elevated clinically but the hyperactivity/impulsivity scores usually are in the normal range. Readers should not interpret such results to mean that the adolescent does not display restlessness or impulsivity. The examples of restlessness and impulsivity evidenced by most adolescents are not easily observed by secondary education teachers who have the students for a single class period per day; such characteristics are better ascertained from parent and adolescent reports.

TABLE 3.7. Attention Problems Scale—TRF Subanalysis

Inattention items	Hyperactivity–Impulsivity items	Core items associated with both subsets
Fails to finish things he or she starts	Acts too young for his or her age	Can't concentrate, can't pay attention for long
Is confused or seems to be in a fog	Hums or makes other odd noises in class	Has difficulty following directions
Daydreams or gets lost in his or her thoughts	Can't sit still, is restless or hyperactive	Does messy work
Has difficulty learning	Fidgets	Is inattentive, easily distracted
Is apathetic or unmotivated	Is impulsive or acts without thinking	
Does poor schoolwork	Is nervous, high-strung, or tense	
Is poorly coordinated or clumsy		
Stares blankly		
Underachieves, does not work up to potential		
Fails to carry out assigned tasks		

Note. Adapted from Achenbach (1996). Copyright 1996 by The Guilford Press. Adapted by permission.

TABLE 3.8. 95th Percentile Cutoffs for Deviance for the TRF Attention Problems

	Boys		Girls	
Scale	5–11 yr	12–18 yr	5–11 yr	12–18 yr
Inattention	19	21	16	15
Hyperactivity–Impulsivity	15	14	10	9

Conners Teacher Rating Scale—Revised

Like the new parent questionnaire, the Conners Teacher Rating Scale—Revised (CTRS-R) comes in a long form (59 items) and a short form (28 items). The CTRS-R includes the same scales as the parent version, with the single omission of Psychosomatic Problems. Given the fact that the average adolescent has six or seven teachers, we find the short form of this measure more practical.

BASC Teacher Rating Scale

The Behavior Assessment System for Children—Teacher Rating Scale (BASC-TRS) is formatted in a manner identical to the parent version discussed earlier. As indicated in Table 3.8, the BASC-TRS includes all the scales on the parent version plus scales for Learning Problems, Study Skills, and a School Composite Scale. It has similar psychometric properties to the BASC-PRS. No data are available specifically on adolescents with ADHD. Inspection of the mean T-scores for a group of 68 children (mean age = 8.6) with ADHD shows milder elevations than were obtained on the parent measure. Scores were elevated somewhat for Attention Problems, Hyperactivity, Learning Problems, and the School Composite Score, and were lowered for Study Skills and Adaptive Skills. The length of this measure may render it impractical when the adolescent has six or seven teachers.

Classroom Performance Survey

The Adolescent Subcommittee of CH.A.D.D.'s Public and Professional Education Committee developed the Classroom Performance Survey as part of a presentation on ADHD in secondary education for the 1995 National CH.A.D.D. Conference (CH.A.D.D., 1996). Presented in Table 3.9, the Classroom Performance Survey consists of 20 items which identify a student's strengths and concerns in the classroom, tapping areas such as bringing materials to class, completing homework on time, recording assignments consistently, arriving to class on time, taking notes regularly, demonstrating respect for property, and so on. These are the types of behaviors that are salient in middle and high school but have not been sam-

TABLE 3.9. Classroom Performance Survey

Teacher_____ Subject_____

Period _____ Student_____ Date_____

Please complete the following ratings to help us identify the student's strengths and areas of concern in the classroom and collect data about the student's academic performance, participation, and behavior.

	Always		Sometimes		Never
1. Brings necessary materials to class	1	2	3	4	5
2. Completes class assignments	1	2	3	4	5
3. Completes homework on time	1	2	3	4	5
4. Records assignments consistently	1	2	3	4	5
5. Turns in completed work	1	2	3	4	5
6. Completes long-term assignments	1	2	3	4	5
7. Attends to instructions in class	1	2	3	4	5
8. Arrives to class on time	1	2	3	4	5
9. Cooperates/participates in class	1	2	3	4	5
10. Demonstrates skills in reading assigned tests and materials	1	2	3	4	5
11. Demonstrates adequate spelling and writing skills in work	1	2	3	4	5
12. Takes notes in class to study	1	2	3	4	5
13. Performs satisfactorily on tests	1	2	3	4	5
14. Completes assigned work with accurate computation/detail	1	2	3	4	5
15. Completes assignments legibly	1	2	3	4	5
16. Relates positively to teacher(s)	1	2	3	4	5
17. Demonstrates respect for property	1	2	3	4	5
18. Relates positively to peers	1	2	3	4	5
19. Communicates own needs or asks questions	1	2	3	4	5
20. Accepts assistance when needed or offered	1	2	3	4	5

Please add any additional skills, behaviors, or concerns that you feel have an impact on this student's classroom performance and achievement:

In the past month, what percentage of this student's assignments were turned in completed and on time?_____

What percentage of assignments are handed in completed and on time by the average student in your class?_____

Please list all test and quiz scores received by this student within the past month:

Is this student working up to potential: YES   NO pled on any published teacher rating scales. Each of the adolescent's teachers indicates the extent to which each item applies to the student on a five-point Likert scale. Although no normative data have been collected on this measure to date, I administer it routinely to all the adolescent's teachers. I consider ratings of three or higher to be in the problem range. I inspect the individual items to construct a profile of the particular deficits a student has across classes.

I have also added several items to the Classroom Performance Survey, asking each teacher to indicate (1) the percentage of the student's assignments turned in on time over the past month, (2) the percentage of similar assignments turned in on time by the average student in the class, (3) all quiz and test scores from the past month, and (4) whether the teacher believes the student is "working up to potential." This information is helpful in determining the degree of educational impairment experienced by the student, as discussed in Chapter 5 (this volume).

The Classroom Performance Survey is similar to Barkley's (1991a) Academic Performance Rating Scale, which was developed primarily for elementary school children. Psychometric research on this type of measure for secondary education is sorely needed.

Integrating Multiple Teacher Questionnaires

No guidelines have been published for clinicians regarding the manner in which to integrate findings from multiple teacher rating scales collected on an adolescent undergoing evaluation for possible ADHD. In fact, even when published norms exist for the adolescent age range (e.g., the TRF), no attempt has been made to determine whether ratings would vary by the content area of the regular education teacher. For example, are there base rate differences in ADHD symptoms between English, math, chemistry, foreign language, or history classes, or is this variable irrelevant?

In the case of elementary school children with a single teacher, we are looking for elevations on rating scales of ADHD symptoms to corroborate the cross-situational nature of these symptoms. In the case of secondary education, adolescents may not display equal degrees of difficulty with concentration, organization, follow-through, and behavioral disinhibition in all their classes. When the Attention Problems Scale—TRF and Classroom Performance Survey have been administered to several teachers, the clinician should tabulate the data or construct profiles that permit easy comparison across classes. Mean scores and standard deviations can be computed across teachers. Then, the clinician should inspect the profiles and look for consistency across classes. Does the student receive high scores across all of his or her classes? If there is inconsistency such that one class is an outlier compared to all the others, is there a logical explanation for this pattern? Consistency or an explanation for lack of consistency across classes on teacher ratings is essential in supporting a diagnosis of ADHD.

Table 3.10 gives Inattention and Hyperactivity–Impulsivity scores (on TRF) from seven teachers for William Jones, a 16-year-old 11th-grade student undergoing an ADHD evaluation. Five of William's seven teachers rated him above the cutoff for the 95th percentile of Inattention. On further investigation, the low score in gym was explained by the nature of this subject, which required active involvement and left less opportunity for daydreaming and off-task behavior. However, the low score in algebra was at first perplexing, as William's academic grade in this subject was a D, and it required sustained attention. When questioned, William pointed out that his algebra teacher was a very attractive blond lady, and that he always paid careful attention to her. Thus, there may be many idiosyncratic reasons for teachers to perceive high school students as paying or not paying attention. Six out of William's teachers did not report elevations in hyperactivity–impulsivity above the 95th percentile; in history, where the teacher reported a great deal of restlessness, the teacher dimmed the lights and gave lectures in a monotone, using overhead transparencies, which the students were expected to copy. Such a situation is a setup for restlessness. In summary, William's scores on the Attention Problems Scale—TRF support clinically significant problems with inattention and follow-through but not hyperactivity–impulsivity. This is the most common finding on this measure with ADHD high school students.

Questionnaires for Family Interactions

Following the behavioral family systems model discussed in Chapter 2, the clinician should assess the following dimensions of family functioning: (1) specific disputes between parents and adolescents, (2) problem-solving communication skills, (3) distorted cognitions and irrational beliefs about family life, and (4) problems in the family structure (coalitions, triangulation).

TABLE 3.10. TRF Attention Problem Ratings for William Jones

Subject	Inattention	Hyperactivity–Impulsivity
English	28	15
History	25	22
Chemistry	30	11
Algebra II	10	7
Economics	22	12
Pottery	35	12
Gym	13	7
Mean score	23	12
95th percentile	21	14

Issues Checklist

The Issues Checklist (IC) is a measure of the topics of specific disputes between parents and adolescents, a type of Home Situations Questionnaire for family interactions. It consists of 44 issues that may lead to disagreements between parents and adolescents. It assesses both conflictual issues and the perceived anger intensity of disputes over these issues and takes the place of the Home Situations Questionnaire (Barkley, 1990), which is most useful with younger children. Parents and adolescents complete identical versions of the IC by recalling discussions of issues such as curfew, chores, and drugs. For each topic, the respondent indicates whether the issue has been broached during the previous 4 weeks. For each topic endorsed as having occurred, the respondent rates the anger intensity of the discussions on a 5-point scale from calm to angry, and estimates how often the topic arose.

The IC yields three scores for each respondent: (1) the quantity of issues, obtained by summing the number of issues circled "yes"; (2) the mean anger-intensity level of the endorsed issues, obtained by averaging the anger-intensity ratings for all of the endorsed issues; and (3) the weighted average of the frequency and anger intensity of the endorsed issues, obtained by multiplying each frequency estimate by its associated intensity, summing these cross-products, and dividing by the total of all the frequency estimates. This gives an estimate of anger per discussion, whereas the intensity score reflects merely the average anger per issues, regardless of the frequency with which the issue was discussed. The reliability and the validity of the IC have been extensively researched (Robin & Foster, 1989). Clinically, the IC is useful for pinpointing sources of conflict and targets for family intervention. As reviewed in Chapter 2, Barkley, Anastopoulos, et al. (1992) found that families with adolescents diagnosed as having ADHD and ODD reported more frequent and intense conflicts with their parents than did matched controls, but that those with ADHD alone did not differ from the controls

Because the mean intensity and the weighted intensity score correlate very highly (.80), the practitioner can save time scoring the IC and obtain an adequate picture of the level of specific parent–adolescent disputes from the number of conflicts and the mean anger-intensity score.

Conflict Behavior Questionnaire

The Conflict Behavior Questionnaire (CBQ) is a 20-item questionnaire of perceived negative communication and poor problem solving between parents and adolescents (Barkley, 1991a; Robin & Foster, 1989). Parents and adolescents complete parallel versions of the CBQ, retrospectively recalling their interactions over the past 2 weeks. They are asked to read and decide whether each item is "mostly true" or "mostly false" for their relationship.

Scoring is accomplished by counting the number of items endorsed in a negative direction; it is convenient to construct a transparent overlay corresponding to the item keys, such that high scores represent negative perceptions. The practitioner should convert the raw scores to *T*-scores, using published tables (Barkley, 1991a). A *T*-score over 65 indicates of significant family conflict. The CBQ has been found to be a highly internally consistent (alpha = .90), valid indicator of conflict and negative interaction, which discriminates well between families with and without conflict and which correlates moderately with observations of parent–teen interactions (Robin & Foster, 1989). Barkley, Anastopoulos, et al. (1992) found that mothers of ADHD adolescents reported more conflict than did matched controls, but mothers of ADHD/ODD adolescents reported even greater conflict than the ADHD alone group. For adolescents, only those with ADHD plus ODD reported more conflict than the controls.

Parent–Adolescent Relationship Questionnaire

To assess belief systems and family structure, and to explore deficits in problem-solving communication skills in greater depth, the clinician can administer the Parent–Adolescent Relationship Questionnaire (PARQ; Robin et al., 1990). The PARQ is a multidimensional measure consisting of 250 and 285 true–false items, respectively, for parents and adolescents, divided into 16 scales tapping three broader dimensions of family functioning: (1) skill deficits/overt conflict (global distress, communication, problem solving, warmth/hostility, cohesion, school conflict, sibling conflict, conventionalization), (2) faulty belief systems/distorted cognitions (parents: ruination, obedience, perfectionism, self blame, malicious intent; teenagers: ruination, unfairness, autonomy, perfectionism, approval), and (3) family structure problems (coalitions, triangulation, somatic concerns, hierarchy reversal) (Robin et al., 1990). The clinician can administer only those scales that are needed or the entire instrument. Parents and adolescents complete the PARQ independently; there are slight differences in wording between the parent and adolescent PARQ, and the adolescent belief scales differ slightly from the parent belief scales.*

Although individual scales of the PARQ may be scored by hand, microcomputer scoring is the only practical method when the entire instrument has been administered; a microcomputer program is available. *T*-scores based on a normative sample of adolescents are obtained, yielding profiles of family functioning for mothers, fathers, and adolescents. *T*-scores above 60 are considered significantly elevated.

The PARQ has been found to have good internal consistency (alpha for most scales above .80), to discriminate well between families with ex-

---

*The PARQ is available from the author.

ternalizing behavior disorders and no psychiatric problems (Robin et al., 1990) and mother–adolescent dyads with ADHD and nondistressed controls (Robin, Kraus, Koepke, & Robin, 1987), to correlate well with interview-based and observational ratings of similar constructs (e.g., have good construct validity) (Koepke, 1986; Koepke, Robin, Nayar, & Hillman, 1987; Webb, 1987), and to be sensitive to treatment changes produced by behavioral family systems therapy (Robin, Siegel, & Moye, 1995). Factor analysis of the 16 scales yielded three factors that corresponded well to the theoretically derived constructs underlying the measure.

Conclusion

Whenever possible, I score all the rating scales and construct a preliminary picture of the adolescent and his or her family before starting the interview. Then, the rating scales can be used to guide the interviewing process efficiently. As I describe the interviewing process in Chapter 4, I refer back to particular rating scales.

CHAPTER FOUR

—————— O ——————

Interviewing and Determining Comorbidities/ Differential Diagnoses

The clinical interview is the primary tool for evaluating whether an adolescent has ADHD and/or other conditions. Specifically, I interview to determine: (1) the presence of sufficient DSM-IV ADHD criteria to say that the adolescent meets the inclusionary criteria for ADHD, (2) the comorbidity and/or differential diagnosis of other psychiatric conditions, and (3) the extent and nature of family interaction problems. I usually interview the parent and the adolescent separately with regard to the first two purposes. However, with older adolescents, who are beyond the early adolescent rebellion/individuation stage, it is more efficient to conduct conjoint family interviews of ADHD symptoms and comorbidities as long as a brief separate interview with the adolescent is also conducted to probe for sensitive material (e.g., substances, sexuality, and suicide). In such cases, the clinician explains that the ADHD evaluation is a collaborative exploration, and enlists the parents and adolescent as an investigative team. Clinicians should always conduct a conjoint interview to assess family interaction.

In the discussion that follows, I highlight my methods and procedures, emphasizing what is unique to the adolescent stage of development. Readers interested in a more detailed discussion of interviewing for ADHD diagnosis in general should consult Barkley (1997c, 1998) or Gordon (1995b). Barkley (1997c) provides a comprehensive, step-by-step protocol for such an interview.

PARENT INTERVIEW

The parent interview has four phases:

1. Listen to the parents' presenting concerns. Parents need a few minutes to ventilate their anxieties and concerns about their adolescents so that they feel understood.
2. Review of the inclusionary criteria for ADHD (i.e., DSM-IV criteria). Use the Past and Present History of ADHD Symptoms (Table 4.1).
3. Collect developmental, medical, and school history information.
4. Explore possible comorbidities and differential diagnoses. Use the key questions in Table 4.2 or follow guidelines in Barkley (1997c).

I try to steer a middle course between the extremes of being too encyclopedic and being too cursory. Usually, this parent interview can be completed in approximately 60 minutes.

Barkley (1997c) has correctly pointed out the importance of being sensitive to ethnic and cultural factors in conducting these interviews. He suggested that when interviewing parents of minority children and adolescents, the clinician should often ask the following question: "Do you consider this to be a problem for your child compared to other children of the same ethnic or minority group?" I concur with Dr. Barkley on this point.

ASSESSING INCLUSIONARY CRITERIA FOR ADHD

Table 4.1 presents the Past and Present History of ADHD Symptoms (PPHS-ADHD), which I have developed as my semistructured interview of the ADHD symptoms. I tried a variety of approaches for assessing the 18 DSM-IV ADHD symptoms before settling on the current format. Many authors prefer an approach that permits the assessor to check off the presence or absence of each symptom (e.g., Barkley, 1997c). I prefer to rate the frequency and pervasiveness of each symptom on a Likert scale, after collecting explicit examples that serve as the basis for these ratings. This approach recognizes the many faces of ADHD in adolescence, permitting the assessor to record the broad range of manifestations of these symptoms in adolescents. Before beginning the interview, the clinician transfers the mother's, father's, and adolescent's ratings for each of the 18 DSM-IV ADHD symptoms from the appropriately completed ADHD Behavior Checklists (Chapter 3, Table 3.2) to the appropriate spaces at the bottom of each item on PPHS-ADHD, for convenience. The clinician begins the interview as follows:

> "We are now going to review the symptoms of ADHD, to determine the extent to which they apply to your son/daughter now and over the

TABLE 4.1. Past and Present History of ADHD Symptoms

Name of Adolescent_____   Birthdate/Age_____

Interviewer_____   Date_____

Ask for clear examples of each symptom, and rate the presence of each symptom currently and during childhood according to the following scale:

3 = Clearly present in more than two different settings many times per week.
2 = Clearly present in two situations several times per week.
1 = Occasionally present, primarily in one setting, intermittent, infrequent.
0 = Rarely or never present

1. Has difficulty sustaining attention in work-related tasks (unable to keep paying attention for long periods)

Parent:

    A. Present:

    B. Past:

Teen:

Ratings: __Mother __Father __Teen __Clinician— Currently __Clinician—In Past

2. Fails to follow through on instructions and finish schoolwork or chores on time

Parent:

    A. Present:

    B. Past:

Teen:

Ratings: __Mother __Father __Teen __Clinician—Currently __Clinician—In Past

(continued)

TABLE 4.1 *(continued)*

3. Is easily distracted by extraneous stimuli (other things going on)

Parent:

    A. Present:

    B. Past:

Teen:

Ratings: __Mother __Father __Teen __Clinician—Currently __Clinician—In Past

4. Fails to give enough attention to details, or makes many careless mistakes in schoolwork, work, or other activities

Parent:

    A. Present:

    B. Past:

Teen:

Ratings: __Mother __Father __Teen __Clinician—Currently __Clinician—In Past

5. Has difficulty organizing tasks or activities (loses track of assignments and has trouble organizing homework)

Parent:

    A. Present:

    B. Past:

Teen:

Ratings: __Mother __Father __Teen __Clinician—Currently __Clinician—In Past

(continued)

TABLE 4.1 *(continued)*

6. Misplaces or loses things necessary to tasks or activities (keys, pencils, notes, books, school assignments)

Parent:

    A. Present:

    B. Past:

Teen:

Ratings: __Mother __Father __Teen __Clinician—Currently __Clinician—In Past

7. Is forgetful in daily activities

Parent:

    A. Present:

    B. Past:

Teen:

Ratings: __Mother __Father __Teen __Clinician—Currently __Clinician—In Past

8. Avoids, dislikes, or is reluctant to engage in tasks that require sustained mental effort

Parent:

    A. Present:

    B. Past:

Teen:

Ratings: __Mother __Father __Teen __Clinician—Currently __Clinician—In Past

(continued)

TABLE 4.1 *(continued)*

___

9. Does not seem to listen when spoken to directly

Parent:

    A. Present:

    B. Past:

___

Teen:

___

Ratings: __Mother __Father __Teen __Clinician—Currently __Clinician—In Past

10. Blurts out answers before questions have been completed

Parent:

    A. Present:

    B. Past:

___

Teen:

___

Ratings: __Mother __Father __Teen __Clinician—Currently __Clinician—In Past

11. Interrupts or intrudes on others (butts into conversations and games)

Parent:

    A. Present:

    B. Past:

___

Teen:

___

Ratings: __Mother __Father __Teen __Clinician—Currently __Clinician—In Past

(continued)

TABLE 4.1 *(continued)*

12. Has difficulty awaiting turn (lines, traffic, taking turns to speak, waiting for services in stores)

Parent:

    A. Present:

    B. Past:

Teen:

Ratings: Mother   Father   Teen   Clinician—Currently Clinician—In Past

13. Fidgets with hands or feet or squirms in seat (plays with objects in hands)

Parent:

    A. Present:

    B. Past:

Teen:

Ratings: __Mother __Father __Teen __Clinician—Currently __Clinician—In Past

14. Is easily bored, feels very restless

Parent:

    A. Present:

    B. Past:

Teen:

Ratings: __Mother __Father __Teen __Clinician—Currently __Clinician—In Past

(continued)

TABLE 4.1 *(continued)*

15. Talks excessively
Parent:

    A. Present:

    B. Past:

Teen:

Ratings: __Mother __Father __Teen __Clinician—Currently __Clinician—In Past

16. Is on the go or acts as if driven by a motor
Parent:

    A. Present:

    B. Past:

Teen:

Ratings: __Mother __Father __Teen __Clinician—Currently __Clinician—In Past

17. Leaves seat in classroom or other situations where remaining seated is
expected; has difficulty sitting for long time
Parent:

    A. Present:

    B. Past:

Teen:

Ratings: __Mother __Father __Teen __Clinician—Currently __Clinician—In Past

(continued)

TABLE 4.1 *(continued)*

18. Has difficulty engaging in leisure activities quietly

Parent:

    A. Present:

    B. Past:

Teen:

Ratings: __Mother __Father __Teen __Clinician—Currently __Clinician—In Past

INTERVIEW SUMMARY

Number of Attention Symptoms Rated 2 or 3, Presently _____
   (Items 1–9)

Number of Attention Symptoms Rated 2 or 3, In the Past _____
   (Items 1–9)

Number of Hyperactivity/Impulsivity Symptoms Rated 2 or 3 _____
   in the Present (Items 10–18)

Number of Hyperactivity/Impulsivity Symptoms Rated 2 or 3 _____
   in the Past (Items 10–18)

Impairment Rating:

Have ADHD symptoms created impairment in any of the following settings? If yes, give several examples:

___ School:

___ Family (chores, getting along, siblings):

___ Hobbies, sports:

___ Peer relationships:

___ Self-care:

(continued)

TABLE 4.1 *(continued)*

Considering all areas, assign a single rating of impairment according to the following scale:

3 = Very impaired 2 = Impaired 1 = Mildly impaired 0 = No impairment

Rating_____

Inclusionary criteria met for:

ADHD, Inattentive Type _____
ADHD, Hyperactive–Impulsive Type_____
ADHD, Combined Type _____

Note. From *ADHD in Adolescents: Diagnosis and Treatment* by Arthur L. Robin. Copyright 1998 by The Guilford Press. Permission to photocopy this table is granted to purchasers of *ADHD in Adolescents* for personal use only (see copyright page for details).

course of his/her life. You already rated these symptoms on a 4-point scale, where 0 was 'not at all' and 3 was 'very much.' I will read you each symptom, tell you your rating, and ask you to give me clear examples of the symptom at home, at school, and in the community, at the present time, and then in the past. After you have given me any examples you recall, I will ask you to tell me how this symptom gets in the way of your adolescent's life, that is, creates impairment. Any questions?"

The clinician then reads the first item and asks for examples at the present time and in the past, recording the responses in the appropriate spaces on the form. He or she asks follow-up questions to clarify the examples and establish the intensity, frequency, and severity of the behaviors.

The clinician rates each symptoms 0, 1, 2, or 3 based on all of the available information. This information includes the parent's response to the interview, the previously completed ratings scales, and previous reports from the school or other professionals, and any direct observations of the adolescent. The clinician completes his or her ratings according to the criteria for cross-situational consistency and frequency outlined here. A separate rating is completed for the presence of the symptom at the current time in the adolescent's life, and for the presence of the symptom since childhood (defined to include ages 6–10). Separate ratings for the present and the past are necessary because the nature of ADHD changes with maturity and development. Moreover, even if the criteria were met both in the past and at the present time, it is unlikely that they were met with exactly the same absolute symptom constellation. Ratings are assigned as follows:

3 = Clearly present in more than two different settings many times per week.
2 = Clearly present in two situations several times per week.

1 = Occasionally present, primarily in one setting, intermittent, infrequent.
0 = Rarely or never present.

The clinician goes through each of the 18 symptoms in this manner, assigning ratings for the present and for childhood.

Since the DSM-IV does not adequately sample impulsivity in adolescence, I usually supplement my inquiry on items 10–12 with several general questions. I explain to parents the heuristically helpful distinction between behavioral impulsivity (poor judgment and acting rashly), cognitive impulsivity (sloppily rushing through academic tasks with careless mistakes), and emotional impulsivity (temper control problems and emotional over-reactions). Then, I inquire about the extent to which each of these types of impulsivity occurs in the adolescent.

Also, I find that people may provide information about several symptoms when responding to my inquiry about one. When this happens, I record the information under the appropriate symptoms, and abbreviate my inquiry of those additional symptoms when I reach them later in the interview.

Afterward, the clinician explicitly assesses whether the ADHD symptoms have created impairment in school, in the family, in hobbies, in peer relationships, or in self-care activities. He or she records examples of impairment. Taking all these examples into account, the clinician completes the four-point rating of impairment.

When this interview is completed, the clinician has surveyed extensively the DSM-IV ADHD symptoms, both at the present time and over the course of the adolescent's development. The clinician adds up the number of Inattention and Hyperactivity–Impulsivity criteria rated 2 or 3 and puts these numbers in the appropriate spaces in the summary section. I find it helpful to give the parents feedback about the current status of my diagnostic exploration, as a transition to the next phase. I might make the following types of statements:

1. *Inclusionary criteria met*: "At this point, we have surveyed the diagnostic criteria for ADHD, and your son/daughter clearly meets enough of them now and in the past, to seriously consider that s/he has ADHD. We now need to look at what else could explain that state of affairs, or be going on in addition to ADHD, before we can reach a definitive conclusion."
2. *Inclusionary criteria not met*: "At this point, we have surveyed the diagnostic criteria for ADHD, and your son/daughter does not appear to meet enough of them for me to consider ADHD to be the problem. We now need to look for what else may be going on that sometimes appears as if it is ADHD."

TAKING A DEVELOPMENTAL, MEDICAL, AND SCHOOL HISTORY

Next, the clinician takes a medical, developmental, and school history. Demographic data forms completed by the parents can guide this history. Questions are asked about the mother's pregnancy (including use of drugs, alcohol, and tobacco, and the mother's emotional status); the adolescent's birth, any birth complications or medical conditions in infancy; major developmental milestones such as walking, speech, and toilet training, and so forth. Any chronic and acute medical problems are reviewed. It is important to ask explicitly about temperament, activity level prior to age 2, early onset of temper tantrums and oppositional behavior, and how the parents reacted to these phenomena. School history is assessed chronologically, starting with nursery school and utilizing report cards and any other materials which the parents brought. The clinician should have the ADHD School Symptom History Grid (Table 3.4) handy during the review of school history. Readers interested in more detailed models of how to conduct the medical, developmental, and school histories might consult several detailed published protocols (e.g., Barkley, 1997c; Gordon, 1995a).

ASSESSING COMORBIDITY/ MAKING A DIFFERENTIAL DIAGNOSIS

The clinician's task is to determine which conditions might be comorbid to ADHD or which could be alternative explanations for the symptoms that look like ADHD. This is an important determination because many of these conditions may masquerade as ADHD look-alikes. Sloppy diagnostic practices resulting in incorrect diagnoses may in part account for the perception that the incidence of ADHD is increasing. Incorrect diagnoses may also lead to ineffective and even harmful treatments.

I systematically assess the extent to three classes of variables may explain the presence of ADHD-like symptoms: (1) environmental variables such as family adversity, divorce, and poverty; (2) educational problems such as learning disabilities; and (3) formal psychiatric comorbidities such as ODD, CD, Mood Disorders (Major Depressive Disorder, Dysthymia, Bipolar Disorder), Anxiety Disorders (Generalized Anxiety Disorder, Panic Disorder, Specific Phobias, Obsessive–Compulsive Disorder, Posttraumatic Stress Disorder), and Substance Use Disorders. Less common conditions may also occur, including Tic Disorders, Eating Disorders, Sleep Disorders, Speech/Language Disorders, Schizophrenia or other psychotic disorders, organic brain disorders, and/or chronic illnesses or medications that can induce ADHD-like behaviors.

In some cases, the clinician may decide that the teenager displays some of the symptoms of a disorder comorbid to ADHD and the symptoms are clinically meaningful, but the teenager does not meet the full DSM-IV criteria for the disorder. In such cases, the categorical diagnostic model does not adequately reflect the spectrum of behavioral problems. As mentioned in Chapter 1, the clinician can use the new *Diagnostic and Statistical Manual for Primary Care, Child and Adolescent Version* (American Academy of Pediatrics, 1996) to characterize subclinical problems.

Determining the Role of Environmental Variables, Family Adversity

How can a clinician determine when environmental variables such as family adversity cause an adolescent to look as if he or she has ADHD? I usually ask the parent to list the five most stressful events throughout the adolescent's entire life. Then, I ask the parents to tell me when in the adolescent's life these major stressful events occurred, and for how long the events and the resulting stresses continued. Then, I look for temporal covariation between the ADHD symptoms and the occurrence of the major stressors. For example, did the adolescent fail to complete schoolwork and receive lower grades primarily during the year after her parents separated and divorced? Does she get restless and moody mainly when her asthma is acting up? Does the adolescent act more defiant when his father comes home drunk, or after his parents have a bad argument? For how long after the teenager's best friend moved to England did she continue to do worse in school? At age 6, when the child was removed from the natural parents for abuse and neglect, did his high frequency of hyperactive behavior change? Over the next 6 months? In a foster care home? If ADHD symptoms are primarily a response to environmental situations, the clinician should be able to establish a clear pattern of temporal covariation between the symptoms and the environmental stressors, both at the present time and over the course of the youngster's life.

By contrast, in the case of a positive ADHD diagnosis, the clinician typically reaches one of two conclusions from the analysis of temporal covariations: (1) most commonly, the developmental course of the ADHD symptoms is a gradual but constant pattern of escalation from a starting point pinpointed in early childhood, despite any environmental stressors; or (2) the environmental stressors were associated with a temporary worsening of the ADHD symptoms, but the ADHD symptoms nonetheless ran a course of basically steady escalation over the course of development, worsening or intensifying long after the environmental stresses were ameliorated. Sometimes, in cases of chaotic families with multiple environmental stresses (e.g., abuse, neglect, homelessness, poverty, violence, and parental mental illness and substance abuse), it is virtually impossible for the clinician to analyze this temporal covariation because the environmental stresses have been severe and constant for the adolescent's entire life. In such cases, I usually defer the diagnosis of ADHD and work toward helping the adolescent deal with the environmental stresses. Only when the adolescent's life situation is more stable can I even attempt to make a differential diagnosis such as ADHD. Let us examine two contrasting cases regarding the role of environmental stresses on ADHD symptoms.

Case Example 1

Mandy Siegel presented as a vivacious, highly talkative 15-year-old high school sophomore with difficulties completing her schoolwork, particularly homework, papers and long-term assignments, poor school grades, periodic moodiness, moderately defiant behavior toward her parents, and mental (but not physical) restlessness. I quickly learned that Mandy's parents were divorced when she was 11, following 3 years of a bitter separation and legal fight, including a custody battle over Mandy and her younger sister. Mrs. Siegel now has custody, and Mandy visits her father twice a month on weekends. Mandy's difficulties with schoolwork began around the time of the divorce, when she entered middle school, and have continued and worsened until the present time. Mrs. Siegel took Mandy to two psychologists regarding these school difficulties, at ages 12 and 14. In both cases, the psychologists indicated that Mandy did not have ADHD but was reacting to the stresses of her parents' divorce by not completing her schoolwork, and that this was an expression of a masked depression. Mandy liked the therapists and willingly participated in 6 months of individual therapy in each case, but she showed no consistent improvement in her academic functioning. Mrs. Siegel is convinced that Mandy has ADHD, based on everything she has observed and read, and she is also convinced that her ex-husband has ADHD. A careful analysis of the temporal covariation between Mandy's ADHD symptoms and the stresses of the divorce reveals that: (1) Mandy's ability to complete assignments and her grades had slowly dropped since middle school and the divorce, but the drop was much more precipitous in the past year, since she entered high school; (2) Mandy used to be upset by her parents' problems and think they were her fault, but she has now moved on with her life and no longer gets so upset by these old issues; (3) Mandy has a great deal of mental restlessness and difficulty with distraction, which seriously interferes with the concentration necessary for completing assignments, and she always had this restlessness, although it did not interfere with her functioning during the elementary school years. Mandy's sister was equally upset by the divorce but has adjusted to it, reinforcing the impression that the negative impact of the divorce is unlikely to be the major factor underlying Mandy's current school difficulties. Rating scales support the presence of ADHD. The clinician concludes that the ADHD symptoms preceded the marital problems and the divorce. Although the divorce was a major stressor, the fact that Mandy is no longer upset by it and now has more severe difficulties with concentration, distraction, and mental restlessness supports the diagnosis of ADHD. The clinician diagnosed ADHD in Mandy. In families with a major stressor such as a divorce, many therapists assume that any ADHD-like symptoms must represent a continued reaction to the stress for many years after the original stressful event occurred. However, this hypothesis must be carefully scrutinized in each case.

Case Example 2

Ted Jamison presents as a 14-year-old Korean youngster adopted by Mr. and Mrs. Jamison when he was 6. Ted has a difficult time accepting his mother's authority; he argues incessantly with her and defies her requests. In school, he acts defiant, primarily toward female teachers, although he occasionally defies males too. Ted says his mother and some teachers single him out and treat him unfairly compared to the other students. His difficulties accepting authority began within several months of his adoption but were tolerable until he entered adolescence, when they escalated considerably. Ted is receiving C's and D's in most of his subjects. He is very inconsistent about completing his homework and completing chores around the house. He often gets moody, throws major tantrums, after which he storms out of the house and walks around the neighborhood. He apologizes for his outbursts and seems to experience remorse but cannot prevent them from happening again and again. He is a loner who has not made any close friends in school or the neighborhood. Ted won't talk at all about his life in Korea, and he clams up when anyone tries to ask him about it. No information was available about Ted's natural parents or his life in Korea other than the fact that he somehow got to an orphanage at age 4, where he lived until he was adopted. Mr. and Mrs. Jamison had to wait 4 years for a child available for adoption, and have done their best to provide a warm, nurturing home. They are relatively easy-going, laid-back people who do not naturally discipline strongly. They are very upset by Ted's problems and feel they have been bad parents. They read about ADHD and thought that perhaps this was Ted's problem.

Although Ted exhibits some of the symptoms of ADHD, there is a clear-cut temporal covariation between his adoption and the onset of oppositional behavior. In addition, there appears to be a temperament mismatch between Mr. and Mrs. Jamison, who are laid-back individuals, and Ted, who is much more intense and highly reactive. Such a mismatch could easily lead to the shaping of coercive behavior over time, as the parents alternated between giving in and trying to discipline when Ted became defiant and had emotional outbursts. Also, in Korea, boys are given a great deal of power in the family over their mothers, and accepting female authority is often a major issue for many Korean boys adopted at an older age by families in the United States. The family told a vivid story about what happened when they first picked up Ted at the airport, when he was 6. When they escorted him to the back seat of their car and Mrs. Jamison sat in the front, he immediately threw a major tantrum. Later, they learned that he expected to sit in the front seat and that Mrs. Jamison would sit in the back.

The clinician concluded that the adoption and acculturation are major environmental issues for Ted and his parents. He diagnosed Ted as having ODD. He does not feel he can justify an ADHD diagnosis but wishes to note that Ted does have some attention problems, so he diagnosed him under the DSM-PC criteria as having an Inattention Problem. The clinician began a course of family and individual therapy. In such cases, after working with the youngsters for several months in therapy and really getting to know them and their families well, I often revisit the issue of possible ADHD. Sometimes, after the emotional and acculturation issues have been addressed, poor task completion and concentration problems persist. Then, I diagnose ADHD.

Assessing Educational, Psychiatric Comorbidities/ Differential Diagnoses

To determine whether the teenager has a learning disability requires the administration of an intellectual ability and an achievement test; this determination is discussed in Chapter 5. All the other comorbidities/differential diagnoses can be investigated through a combination of interviews and analysis of the already-administered rating scales and questionnaires, which were discussed in Chapter 3. Ideally, structured psychiatric interviews with good psychometric characteristics, such as the Schedule for Affective Disorders and Schizophrenia for School-Age Children (K-SADS-E; Orvaschel & Puig-Antich, 1987), the Diagnostic Interview Schedule for Children—2 (DISC-2; Schwab-Stone, Fischer, Piacentini, Shaffer, Davies, & Biggs, 1993), the Diagnostic Interview for Children and Adolescents (DICA; Herjanic & Reich, 1982), or the Structured Clinical Interview for DSM-III-R (SCID; Spitzer, Williams, Gibbon, & First, 1990), are used. Such interviews are the "gold standard" for selecting subjects in clinical research. In reality, although highly effective, such interviews are too cumbersome and time-consuming for routine administration to every case in these days of a managed care mental health environment. The SCID and the DICA, however, are available in computerized versions. The computerized version of the SCID, known as the SCID Screen Patient Questionnaire (First, Gibbon, Williams, & Spitzer, 1996), is designed for an adolescent (seventh-grade reading level or higher) or an adult to complete sitting at a personal computer, in about 15 minutes. It screens (but does not give definitive diagnoses) for Mood Disorders, Anxiety Disorders, Substance Use Disorders, Eating Disorders, Schizophrenia and other psychotic disorders, and Somatiform Disorders. The computerized version of the DICA (Reich, Welner, Herjanic, & MHS Staff, 1997) can be completed by a parent or an adolescent in 30 minutes and yields diagnoses for the following disorders:

TABLE 4.2. **Key Questions for Assessing Comorbidity/ Differential Diagnosis**

Name of Adolescent_____ Date_____

Name of Respondent_____

Please respond to each of the following questions by circling YES or NO.

OPPOSITIONAL DEFIANT DISORDER

1. Which of the following negativistic, hostile, and defiant behaviors is your adolescent currently exhibiting, and has he or she been exhibiting them for at least 6 months? (Circle YES if the behavior occurs now and has occurred for at least 6 months.)

   a. Often loses temper   YES   NO

   b. Often argues with adults   YES   NO

   c. Often actively defies or refuses to comply with adults' requests or rules
                                            YES   NO

   d. Often deliberately annoys people   YES   NO

   e. Often blames others for his or her mistakes or misbehavior
                                            YES   NO

   f. Is often touchy or easily annoyed by others
                                            YES   NO

   g. Is often angry and resentful   YES   NO

   h. Is often spiteful or vindictive   YES   NO

CONDUCT DISORDER

2. Which of the following behaviors is your adolescent currently exhibiting, and has your adolescent been exhibiting for the past 6–12 months? (Circle YES if behavior is currently exhibited and has occurred over the past 6–12 months.)

Aggression to people and animals

   a. Often bullies, threatens, or intimidates others
                                            YES   NO

   b. Often initiates physical fights   YES   NO

   c. Has used a weapon that can cause serious physical harm to others (e.g., a bat, brick, broken bottle, knife, gun)   YES   NO

   d. Has been physically cruel to people   YES   NO

   e. Has been physically cruel to animals YES   NO

   f. Has stolen while confronting a victim (e.g., mugging, purse snatching, extortion, armed robbery)   YES   NO

   g. Has forced someone into sexual activity   YES   NO

(continued)

TABLE 4.2 *(continued)*

Destruction of property

   h. Has deliberately engaged in fire-setting with the intention of causing serious
      damage   YES   NO
   i. Has deliberately destroyed others' property (other than by fire-setting)
                                                YES   NO

Deceitfulness or theft

   j. Has broken into someone else's house, building, or car
                                                YES   NO
   k. Often lies to obtain goods or favors or to avoid obligations (i.e., "cons"
      others)   YES   NO

MOOD DISORDERS

   3. In the past month, has your adolescent felt or acted depressed, most of the
      day, every day, for any period of time?   YES   NO

   4. If YES, did the depressed mood last at least 2 weeks?
                                                YES   NO

   5. Did the depressed mood interfere with daily functioning in school, at home,
      with peers, or in recreation?   YES   NO

   6. Have there been any other periods of depressed mood earlier in your
      adolescent's life, lasting most of the day, every day, for at least 2 weeks?
                                                YES   NO

   7. Has your adolescent been depressed, most of the time, for the past year?
                                                YES   NO

   8. Has your adolescent become depressed, for several days, in response to any
      acutely upsetting event (e.g., breakup with boyfriend/girlfriend, failing a test,
      argument with you)?
                                                YES   NO

   9. Has there been any period, within the past month, when your adolescent felt
      or acted abnormally irritable (e.g., screaming, shouting, yelling, etc., with
      extreme intensity)?   YES   NO

  10. Did this period of irritability last for more than a few hours, even for days or
      weeks?   YES   NO

  11. Has there ever been any other period, earlier in your adolescent's life, when he
      or she was abnormally irritable for long periods of time?
                                                YES   NO

  12. Has there been any period, within the past month, when your adolescent
      felt or acted very elated, manic, or in a high mood (not connected with
      drugs)?   YES   NO

(continued)

TABLE 4.2 *(continued)*

13. Did this period of elation or mania last more than a few hours, even for days or weeks?   YES   NO

14. Has there ever been any other period, earlier in your adolescent's life, when he or she was abnormally elated, manic, or in a high mood (not connected with drugs) for long periods?   YES   NO

ANXIETY DISORDERS

15. Has your adolescent ever had a panic attack, in which he or she suddenly felt very frightened, anxious, or extremely uncomfortable?
                                                     YES   NO

16. Has your adolescent ever been afraid of going out of the house alone, being in a crowd, standing in line, traveling on buses, trains, or riding in cars?
                                                     YES   NO

17. Has your adolescent ever been afraid of doing things in front of other people, like speaking, eating, or writing, or of interacting with other people?
                                                     YES   NO

18. Has your adolescent ever been afraid of going to school (e.g., truly afraid, not trying to avoid school)?   YES   NO

19. Has your adolescent ever been very afraid of things like flying, heights, seeing blood, thunder, lightening, closed places, animals, or insects?
                                                     YES   NO

20. Has your adolescent ever been bothered by thoughts that didn't make any sense and kept coming back even when he or she tried not to have them?
                                                     YES   NO

21. Has your adolescent ever had things that he or she had to do over and over again and couldn't resist (e.g., compulsive acts such as washing hands, checking something, touching things in a certain order, walking a certain way)?   YES   NO

22. Has your adolescent ever been in a very dangerous/traumatic situation, or witnessed firsthand a very dangerous/traumatic situation? (violence, physical/sexual abuse, accident, near-death situation, etc.)
                                                     YES   NO

23. If YES to 22, has your adolescent ever had these things come back over and over again in nightmares, flashbacks, or obsessive thoughts?
                                                     YES   NO

24. In the past 6 months, has your adolescent been generally worried, anxious, and nervous for at least half of the time (not in response to just one event)?
                                                     YES   NO

TIC/ MOVEMENT DISORDERS

25. Has your adolescent ever had any tics (involuntary, rapid, recurrent movements such as eye blinking, twitches, or head turning, etc.)?
                                                     YES   NO

(continued)

TABLE 4.2 *(continued)*

---

26. Does your adolescent ever say words or make other sounds, besides burping or hiccups, that are not intended, that keep repeating, and that he or she can't stop?   YES   NO

27. Has your adolescent ever had any unusual habits, movements, etc.?
                                                      YES   NO

EATING/SLEEP DISORDERS

28. Has your adolescent ever had a period of being underweight? For girls, during this time, did she stop menstruating or have irregular periods?
                                                      YES   NO

29. Has your adolescent ever been afraid of getting fat or believed that he or she is fat when in reality he or she is not?   YES   NO

30. Has your adolescent ever engaged in out-of-control eating (e.g., eating a lot in a short time and feeling out of control about it)?
                                                      YES   NO

31. Has your adolescent ever gotten rid of unwanted food and calories through vomiting, using laxatives, excessive exercise, or fasting?
                                                      YES   NO

32. Does your adolescent have any difficulty with sleep (getting to sleep, staying asleep, waking up)?   YES   NO

PSYCHOTIC SYMPTOMS

33. Has your adolescent ever reported seeing, hearing, smelling, or feeling things that were not based in reality?   YES   NO

34. Has your adolescent ever reported having any of the following possibly delusional beliefs:

    a. People were taking special notice of him or her
                                                      YES   NO

    b. Receiving special messages from TV, radio, newspaper, etc.
                                                      YES   NO

    c. Feeling important and having special powers that others don't have
                                                      YES   NO

    d. Something strange happening to his or her body despite doctor finding nothing   YES   NO

    e. Feeling he or she committed a crime and should be punished
                                                      YES   NO

    f. Something external to the teenager is controlling his or her thoughts and actions against his or her will (beyond normal complaints that parents are too controlling)   YES   NO

    g. Thoughts that are not his or her own are being put into his or her head
                                                      YES   NO

(continued)

TABLE 4.2 *(continued)*

   h. Thoughts are being broadcast so others can hear them
                                        YES   NO

DRUGS/ ALCOHOL

35. Does your adolescent have any problems with alcohol or drugs?
                                        YES   NO

Note. From *ADHD in Adolescents: Diagnosis and Treatment* by Arthur L. Robin. Copyright 1998 by The Guilford Press. Permission to photocopy this table is granted to purchasers of *ADHD in Adolescents* for personal use only (see copyright page for details).

ADHD, ODD, CD, Substance Use Disorders, Mood Disorders, Anxiety Disorders, Posttraumatic Stress Disorder, Eating Disorders, Somatization Disorders, Enuresis, Encopresis, Psychotic Symptoms, and Gender Identity Disorders.

I screen for all the major Axis I disorders, by interview or a combination of computerized and in-person interviews. First, I review the full criterion sets for ODD and CD, the most likely comorbidities. Then, I review the broad, first-order questions for Mood, Anxiety, Substance Use, Eating, Tic, and Psychotic disorders. If I uncover positive indicators from the broad review, I explore particular disorders in more depth, using the entire DSM-IV criterion sets. Barkley (1997c) provides a detailed structured interview that facilitates in-depth interviewing around the major childhood and adolescent disorders. Table 4.2 summarizes the questions I routinely ask. I often ask parents to complete these questions as a self-report questionnaire and then go over it during my interview.

Following are suggestions for assessing particular disorders.

Oppositional Defiant Disorder

Up to 65% of children and adolescents with ADHD develop ODD (Barkley, 1990) (in Barkley, Fischer, et al.'s [1990] follow-up study of ADHD children into adolescence, the exact figure was 54%). ODD consists of a pattern of negativistic, hostile, defiant behavior, which is more frequent than that typically observed in teenagers of a similar age and developmental level, and which persists for at least 6 months. The eight items in the first question in Table 4.2 represent the specific DSM-IV criteria for ODD; at least four need to be present to make a positive diagnosis. These four symptoms need to (1) have been present for at least 4 months; (2) be more frequent than is observed in other adolescents of the same age; and (3) be causing clinically significant impairment in social, academic, or occupational functioning. In essence, ODD consists of two elements: (1) defiant, argumentative behavior in opposition to demands typically made by adult authority figures and (2) negative, hostile, angry mood.

The clinician should review each of the eight criteria with the parents and determine whether they currently apply and whether they have applied for at least 6 months. None of these criteria involve either overt aggression and fighting or such covert antisocial behavior as stealing and lying, which are part of CD. Because most adolescents lose their temper, argue with their parents, and can be touchy or easily annoyed anywhere from several times a month to once or twice a week, here the term "often" means five to seven times a week or virtually daily, to meet the criterion of being more than is typical for that age. Also, the stage of adolescent development should be used as a reference point. The base rate of defiant behavior is higher in early adolescence (ages 12–14) than in middle (15–17) or later (18–20) adolescence. Clinicians should ask themselves the following key question: "Is the adolescent's primary mode of response defiant behavior and an angry, hostile mood, and has it been this way for at least six months?" Regarding the criterion of significant clinical impairment, which DSM-IV does not define further, I typically evaluate the nuisance value and bothersomeness of the defiant behavior to the adults in the adolescent's environment. When a teacher must stop teaching to deal with defiant behavior whenever it occurs, or when a parent must significantly alter his or her routines to deal with defiant behavior whenever it occurs, the impairment criterion is met. Furthermore, if the adolescent is losing friends, making enemies, or losing part-time jobs because of defiant behavior, clinical impairment is significant.

In addition to the categorical criteria, the adolescent must meet the quantitative, dimensional criteria of obtaining an elevation on an aggression, conduct, or conflict scale of a major parent or teacher-report rating scale. T-scores above 65 on the Aggression or Delinquency Scale of the CBCL or Teacher Report Form, or the Conflict Behavior Questionnaire or the Global Distress Scale of the PARQ are examples of such criteria. When the adolescent exhibits fewer than three of the ODD criteria several times a week with moderate negative impact on his or her environment, I now apply the *DSM-PC, Child and Adolescent Version* criteria and diagnose the adolescent as having an Aggressive/Oppositional Problem or, in the case of frequent hostile mood outbursts, a Negative Emotional Behavior Problem.

How does a clinician determine whether ODD or ADHD is the differential diagnosis for an adolescent? Families that present primarily for parent–adolescent conflict whose teenagers do not have school problems often have adolescents who meet criteria for ODD but not ADHD. The absence of a pattern of increased difficulty with task completion, organization, and follow-through, over time, in a youngster with significant argumentative, rebellious behavior is the tip-off for ODD without ADHD. Such youngsters typically do not have problems getting schoolwork done because of forgetfulness, misplaced materials, and disorganization. If they fail to do schoolwork, it was a purposeful decision.

Conduct Disorder

Forty to 60% of adolescents with ADHD meet the clinical criteria for CD (Barkley, 1990). CD consists of a persistent pattern of behavior in which the basic rights of others or major age-appropriate societal norms or rules are violated. Such behaviors include aggressive conduct that causes or threatens physical harm to other people or animals, destruction of property, covert antisocial acts such as deceitfulness or theft, and serious rule violations. CD differs from and is more severe than ODD: CD includes elements of physical aggression and direct or clandestine antisocial acts in addition to defiance and rebelliousness. Typically, those meeting criteria for CD also meet criteria for ODD; in such cases CD takes precedence as a diagnosis. Table 4.2 lists the 11 DSM-IV criteria for CD; at least 3 need to have been present for the past 12 months, with at least one present for the past 6 months. The clinician should carefully review these items with the parent and look for evidence of clinical impairment. However, clinical impairment in educational and family functioning is almost self-evident if a sufficient number of CD criteria are met. The clinician should also look for two of the hallmarks of CD: (1) lack of remorse for antisocial behavior and (2) extreme self-centeredness. CD is also associated with the early onset of sexual behavior, smoking, drinking, marijuana, and other drug use in the adolescent, as well as a history of CD, Antisocial Personality Disorder, Substance Use Disorders, and Major Depressive Disorder in other family members. Thus, if a positive history of several of the CD criteria emerges, further evaluation for these high-risk behaviors in the adolescent and the family is warranted.

CD has two subtypes: childhood onset and adolescent onset. The childhood-onset CD teen, defined by the onset of at least one criterion prior to age 10, is frequently male, with more physical aggression, poor peer relationships, prior ODD, full-blown CD prior to puberty, and a poorer prognosis, with a high probability of continuing into Antisocial Personality Disorder in adulthood. Those with adolescent onset subtype, defined by the absence of any criteria prior to age 10, are less likely to have physical aggression and disturbed peer relationships, have a lower male-to-female ratio, and have a better prognosis. Research suggests that adolescents with ADHD and CD more commonly have childhood-onset CD (onset between ages 6 and 8), with an even earlier onset of antisocial behavior and a greater number of arrests than adolescents with CD alone (Forehand, Wierson, Frame, Kempton, & Armistead, 1991; Moffitt & Silva, 1988), with higher persistence into adulthood, and with a poorer prognosis (Barkley, 1990). By adolescence, many of the childhood-onset ADHD/CD youngsters have left a tremendous trail of destruction in their families, schools, and communities. Moreover, the clinician should not assume that most adolescents with ADHD/CD come from severely disrupted families characterized by parental strife, substance abuse, and pathology. A significant minority who had difficult temperaments and severe hyperactivity and aggression from a very early age come from affluent, upper-middle-class families with reasonably skilled, empathetic parents who have in fact raised other children without such problems. Often, such youngsters have been adopted.

CD is not a diagnosis to apply lightly as it has serious implications for prognosis and treatment. Clinicians wishing to categorize adolescents with CD tendencies who do not meet full criteria might turn to the DSM-PC behavior clusters. Adolescents who are displaying one or two of the CD criteria intermittently, with less adverse impact on their environments, may qualify for a DSM-PC diagnosis of Aggressive/Oppositional Problem or Secretive Antisocial Behavior Problem. For example, Secretive Antisocial Behavior Problem, under the Secretive Antisocial Behavior Cluster, may include relatively infrequent, less intense actions such as shoplifting candy and gum, keying cars, and writing graffiti on walls. In these cases, there is some destruction of property but not enough to warrant a CD diagnosis.

The differential diagnosis between ADHD and CD is fairly straightforward. ADHD adolescents do not normally engage in the kinds of antisocial behaviors that are criteria for CD. ADHD typically involves an early onset of behavioral disinhibition, whereas CD reflects an early negative temperament, family and social adversity, and premeditated rather than impulsive aggressive and antisocial behavior.

Mood Disorders

Overview. It is rare to find adolescents with ADHD who do not have periods of depression, especially if they have only recently been diagnosed and/or are not receiving effective treatments to help them cope with their disability and its impact on their lives. However, it is important for the clinician to distinguish between "depressed" as an adjective and "Depression" as a noun. It is also important to distinguish between moodiness as a symptom of ADHD and moodiness as part of a mood disorder. For adolescent females, the role of hormones and Premenstrual Syndrome must also be considered when assessing for comorbid Mood Disorders. Epidemiological research suggests that the overlap between ADHD and Mood Disorders ranges from 25% to 75% in referred samples and 15% to 19% in nonreferred children (Biederman et al., 1992). The most common Mood Disorders comorbid to or differential from ADHD are (1) Major Depressive Disorder, (2) Bipolar Disorder, (3) Dysthymic Disorder, and (4) Cyclothymic Disorder. Mood Disorders secondary to substances and medical conditions, and Adjustment Reactions with Depressed Mood may also occur. Finally, some adolescents may have Mood Disorders that fluctuate with the seasons (e.g., they are depressed primarily in the winter). DSM-IV handles this fluctuation by adding a modifier, "with Seasonal Pattern," to Major Depressive Disorder, Bipolar I Disorder, and Bipolar II Disorder.

In DSM-IV, Major Depressive and Bipolar Disorders are built from four types of Mood Episodes plus additional criteria: (1) Major Depressive Episode; (2) Manic Episode; (3) Hypomanic Episode; and (4) Mixed Episode. A Major Depressive Episode includes five or more of the following symptoms for at least 2 weeks (but must include depressed mood or loss of interest in pleasurable activities):

- Depressed or irritable mood most of the day
- Diminished interest or pleasure in activities
- Weight loss or appetite loss
- Insomnia
- Psychomotor agitation or retardation
- Fatigue or lethargy
- Feelings of worthlessness or guilt
- Diminished concentration
- Recurrent thoughts of death or suicide

A Manic Episode consists of a period of abnormally, persistently elevated expansive mood or abnormally, persistently irritable mood, lasting at least 1 week, including three or more of the following symptoms for expansive moods or four or more for irritable moods (those that overlap with ADHD are *italicized*):

- Inflated self-esteem, grandiosity
- Flight of ideas
- *Decreased need for sleep*
- Thoughts racing
- *More talkative than usual*
- *Distractibility*
- Psychomotor agitation or increase in goal-directed activity
- *Excessive involvement in pleasurable activities with high potential for painful consequences*

A Hypomanic Episode is similar to a manic episode but less intense, lasting 4 instead of 7 days, without psychotic or delusional thought content, and causing less severe impairment. A Mixed Episode is one that satisfies the criteria for both a Manic and a Major Depressive Episode. Mood disorders are built from mood episodes, as indicated in the following table:

Disorders	Types of episodes			
	Major Depressive	Manic	Hypomanic	Mixed
Major Depressive Disorder	Yes			
Bipolar I	Yes	Yes		Yes
Bipolar II	Yes		Yes	

A Major Depressive Disorder consists of at one or more Major Depressive Episodes, without any Manic, Hypomanic, or Mixed Episodes. Bipolar I Disorder consists of a clinical course characterized by the occurrence of one or more Manic Episodes or Mixed Episodes, and in some subtypes, one or more Major Depressive Episodes. There is a subtype of Bipolar I (Single Manic Episode) in which no Major Depressive Episodes are necessary. Bipolar II Disorder is characterized by one or more Major Depressive Episodes accompanied by at least one Hypomanic Episode. DSM-IV provides even more detailed subtyping of Mood Disorders.

In Dysthymic Disorder, another common Mood Disorder, the adolescent is chronically depressed or irritable most of the day for at least 1 year (2 years in adults). During the course of the depression and/or irritability, the adolescent also exhibits at least two of the following: poor appetite or overeating, insomnia or hypersomnia, low energy or fatigue, low self-esteem, poor concentration or difficulty making decisions, and feelings of hopelessness. There must not be any asymptomatic period of 2 or more months during the year of the symptoms, any Major Depressive Episode during the first year, and any previous Manic, Hypomanic, or Mixed Episodes, and the criteria for Cyclothymic Disorder must not have been met. In Dysthymic Disorder, depression and/or irritability becomes a way of life, a chronic, unremitting condition that just goes on interminably.

By contrast, in Cyclothymic Disorders, the adolescent experiences a chronic, fluctuating course of numerous periods of hypomanic symptoms and numerous periods of depressive symptoms, but none meet the criteria for either a Major Depressive or a Manic Episode. In adolescents, this fluctuating course needs to go on for at least 1 year to be considered Cyclothymic Disorder.

Major Depressive Disorder, Dysthymic Disorder, and ADHD. A number a methodologically sophisticated studies using converging criteria have now demonstrated what clinicians have known for some time: A substantial minority of youngsters have comorbidities for depression and ADHD (Angold & Costello, 1993; Biederman, 1996; Milberger, Biederman, Faraone, Murphy, & Tsuang, 1995). Biederman, Faraone, Mick, Moore, and Lelon (1996) also found that the overlapping symptoms between ADHD and depression could not account for these comorbidities.

In screening for depression, the clinician should review the patterns of elevations on the CBCL, keeping in mind the data discussed in Chapter 3, and should ask the parents the key questions in Table 4.2. Affirmative answers to questions 3–6 suggest a Major Depressive Episode and should be followed up by a detailed inquiry covering the specific symptoms enumerated earlier. An affirmative answers to question 7 suggests Dysthymic Disorder and should be followed up by a detailed inquiry of the relevant specific criteria. An affirmative answer to question 8 should be explored further to determine whether the adolescent has an Adjustment Reaction with Depressed Mood.

If the adolescent meets some but not all the criteria for a Major Depressive Disorder or a Dysthymic Disorder, and the clinician believes that the sadness or depression exceeds the normal range of development, the clinician might invoke the Sadness and Related Symptoms Cluster of the DSM-PC and consider the diagnosis of a Sadness Problem. A Sadness Problem is defined as sadness or irritability that includes some symptoms of Major Depressive Disorder in milder form; the symptoms must be more than transient and have a mild negative impact on the child's functioning.

Often, the question arises as to how to determine whether depressive symptoms represent a Mood Disorder or are part of ADHD. On the surface, sleep problems, poor concentration, and psychomotor agitation are parts of ADHD and Major Depressive Disorder. The poor concentration of the ADHD adolescent is situational, appearing only when the tasks are boring and monotonous, not when the tasks are highly stimulating and intrinsically interesting. By contrast, the depressed adolescent's poor concentration occurs in all situations and represents a morbid preoccupation with his or her own thoughts and inner feelings. Depressed individuals lose interest in pleasurable activities as well as effortful activities. ADHD individuals do not lose interest in highly reinforcing activities. Likewise, the psychomotor agitation of the depressed individual is episodic, whereas the hyperactivity of the ADHD individual is chronic. Fewer than 30% of ADHD children have sleep problems; many depressed adolescents have sleep difficulties. Keeping these guidelines in mind should help the clinician when depression is a differential diagnosis from ADHD.

Bipolar Disorder. If the answers to screening questions 9–14 in Table 4.2 are Yes, the clinician needs to inquire further about the possibility of a Bipolar Disorder (BPD), exploring in detail the criteria for Manic and Hypomanic Episodes. BPD is not an easy diagnosis to make in adolescents, either as a comorbidity or as a differential diagnosis (Carlson, 1990; Bowring & Kovacs, 1992). Often, a diagnosis of BPD is better made after working with an adolescent for a number of weeks or months. Until recently, clinicians did not think it possible for preadolescents or even early adolescents to have BPD, and they certainly did not consider it possible for any individual to have ADHD and BPD, but recent research has changed our thinking.

A number of studies have investigated the comorbidity of ADHD and BPD. In the only study done exclusively with teenagers, West, McElroy, Strakowski, Keck, and McConville (1995) reported that 57% of adolescents with BPD also had ADHD. Biederman, Faraone, Mick, Wozniak, et al. (1996) conducted the most comprehensive investigation of the comorbidity of BPD and ADHD. Using a thorough diagnostic procedure based on the K-SADS-E and a clinical review and consensus by senior experienced clinicians, they studied 140 ADHD children, ages 6–17, and 120 non-ADHD control children at baseline and at a 4-year follow-up. At baseline, they identified 15 (11%) of the ADHD children as comorbid for BDP (significantly higher than 0% controls), and at follow-up, they identified an additional 15 (12%) of the ADHD children as comorbid for BPD (again significantly higher than the controls: 1.8%). Thus, there was a 21% lifetime comorbidity for BPD in their ADHD group. The ADHD/BPD group had strikingly higher rates of severe depression, multiple anxiety disorders, conduct disorders, oppositional defiant disorders, mean numbers of comorbidities, and psychiatric hospitalizations than did the ADHD alone group; the ADHD/BPD group also was more elevated than the ADHD alone group on the CBCL scales of Anxiety/Depression, Delinquency, and Aggression but equal on Attention.

The clinical picture of these ADHD/BPD children was primarily irritable rather than euphoric, with an onset of BPD at a mean age of 5 for the group identified at baseline and 11 for the group identified at follow-up. They exhibited multiple episodes, severe agitation and violent behavior, rapid cycling, and a mixed picture of simultaneous Manic and Major Depressive Episodes. Examining the factors at baseline that predicted the onset of BPD in ADHD children by follow-up, Biederman, Faraone, Mick, Wozniak, et al. (1996) found that ADHD children who developed BPD 4 years later had higher initial rates of other comorbidities, more symptoms of ADHD, worse scores on all the CBCL scales, and a greater family history of bipolar and nonbipolar mood disorders compared with the non-BPD/ADHD children. They also found that adjusting the diagnoses for overlapping symptoms did not change the results substantially. Biederman, Faraone, Mick, Wozniak, et al. (1996) concluded by raising the intriguing nosological questions of whether these ADHD/BPD children are truly cases of BPD or cases of ADHD with severe affective dysregulation. Whatever the answer, ADHD/BPD children do exist and have a syndrome of severely disabling psychopathology that frequently leads to hospitalization and marked impairment.

In addition to the formal criteria for BPD, the key point to remember when considering BPD as a comorbidity to ADHD is *severity*. ADHD/BPD adolescents have violent temper outbursts of astounding intensity, during which they may commit serious aggressive acts. These outbursts accompany a continuous pattern of episodes of irritability, for days or weeks on end. Irritability is much more common than expansive grandiosity, but when grandiosity occurs, it may look different in children and adolescents than in adults. For example, one 11-year-old with BPD had manic episodes during which she firmly believed that all of the children in her class were her good friends, and she had major affective outbursts when they did not respond to her as she wished. When she was not in a manic episode, she displayed low self-esteem and complained that no one liked her and she had no friends. Young, Biggs, Ziegler, and Meyer (1978) constructed and validated a scale for clinicians to rate mania which may be helpful in making the BPD diagnosis.

Practitioners should keep several points in mind when considering

Bipolar Disorder as a differential diagnosis for ADHD. ADHD typically has an early onset prior to age 7, whereas the majority of BPD cases have a later onset; (2) ADHD is a chronic condition with the symptoms continuously present, and by adolescence the individual usually has a history of escalating difficulty at school and at home, whereas BDP has an episodic course, often with relatively clear points of onset and offset, and certainly with long periods when the adolescent is symptom free; (3) BPD is primarily a disorder of mood, and the irritability of BPD is much more severe than the irritability associated with moodiness in ADHD, whereas ADHD includes a much broader set of symptoms than moodiness alone; and (4) there is no psychotic thinking in ADHD, whereas psychotic thought processes are often associated with BPD.

Anxiety Disorders

Like depression, anxiety may be applied to adolescents with ADHD both as an adjective and a noun, and the clinician needs to determine whether the degree of anxiety qualifies for a comorbid psychiatric diagnosis. Epidemiological research suggests that the overlap between ADHD and Anxiety Disorders ranges from 27% to 30% in referred samples and 8% to 26% in nonreferred samples (Biederman et al., 1992). Generalized Anxiety Disorder, Panic Disorder, Obsessive–Compulsive Disorder (OCD), Social Phobia, and Posttraumatic Stress Disorder are the five most common types of anxiety disorders found as comorbid conditions. Generalized Anxiety Disorder and Posttraumatic Stress Disorder (PTSD) are the two most likely to be seriously considered differential diagnoses.

The practitioner should ask the key questions focused on anxiety (15–24, in Table 4.2) during the parent interview. If the answer to question 15 is affirmative, the clinician should review the full criterion set for Panic Disorder with the parent. If the answer to question 16 is affirmative, the clinician should review the criteria for Agoraphobia. If the answer to question 17 is affirmative, the clinician should review the criteria for Social Phobia. If the answer to question 18 is affirmative, the clinician should review the criteria for School Phobia. If the answer to question 19 is affirmative, the clinician should review the criteria for specific phobias such as blood, animals, or insects. If the answers to questions 20–21 are affirmative, the clinician should review the criteria for OCD. If the answers to question 22–23 are affirmative, the clinician should review the criteria for PTSD. If the answer to question 24 is affirmative, the clinician should review the criteria for Generalized Anxiety Disorder.

The differential diagnosis between ADHD and Anxiety Disorders is usually not problematic. Most children with ADHD do not classically manifest a great deal of anxiety about their performance; in contrast, onlookers who witness their behaviorally disinhibited performance often are amazed that they are not more anxious about the impact of their actions on the environment and themselves. Most children with Anxiety Disorders do not show the pervasive pattern of impaired delayed responding, poor impulse control, and hyperactivity seen in ADHD. The restlessness of ADHD is qualitatively different than the restlessness associated with Anxiety Disorders. In addition, Panic Disorder, Agoraphobia, Social Phobia, and Simple Phobias are relatively straightforward because these forms of Anxiety Disorders have clear-cut presentations whose symptoms do not typically overlap with ADHD.

Differential diagnoses between ADHD and OCD, PTSD, and Generalized Anxiety Disorder can be more problematic. In the case of OCD, confusion can arise because ADHD individuals may compensate for their impairments by developing repetitive routines which seem obsessive–compulsive to the onlooker. One of my adult patients, for example, spends hours sorting and re-sorting the materials she needs for her teaching job. Onlookers consider her compulsive, but in reality her chronic disorganization makes her repetitive sorting necessary. In ADHD, such actions do not have an imperative quality (e.g., the person cannot stop them without great distress). In OCD, such an imperative quality is clearly present. In fact, successfully compensating ADHD adults often develop a healthy degree of obsessive–compulsive traits in their personality.

In the case of PTSD, flashbacks to traumatic events may be associated with distractibility, poor concentration, and difficulty completing the tasks of daily life. However, these difficulties are much more circumscribed and situational than the broad-based distractibility and follow-through problems of the ADHD individual. The individual with Generalized Anxiety Disorder may appear restless and on edge a great deal of the time, preoccupied with worries that interfere with concentration and task completion. Careful inquiry of ADHD adolescents reveals, however, that their poor concentration is not due to worries; they usually cannot tell the interviewer why they cannot concentrate. If they do have worries, the worries are a consequence of poor concentration rather than an antecedent to it.

Other Comorbidities and Differential Diagnoses

Table 4.2 provides the leading questions to screen for Tic Disorders, Eating Disorders, Sleep Disorders, Psychotic Disorders, and Substance Use Disorders. The first three are likely to show up as comorbidities; psychotic disorders are generally considered differential diagnoses, not comorbidities, with respect to ADHD, but some research suggests that there may be a form of psychosis that develops as a result of the cumulative effect of ADHD on cognitive and social development (Bellack, Kay, & Opler, 1987). Tic Disorders usually have their onset prior to adolescence, and in younger children the question is sometimes whether hyperactivity is an early symptom of a tic disorder or part of ADHD.

Very little has been written about the comorbidity of eating disorders and ADHD. Schweichert, Strober, and Moskowitz (1997) described a case of a 25-year-old female who had had bulimia nervosa and ADHD since childhood. Her ADHD was diagnosed at age 7, and her bulimia nervosa was diagnosed at age 13. As an adult, she was successfully treated for ADHD and bulimia nervosa with methylphenidate and psychotherapy. Hallowell and Ratey (1994a, 1994b) provide a clinical discussion of co-morbid ADHD and eating disorders. In my experience working with many adolescents with Eating Disorders, it is rare to see a comorbidity of re-stricting Anorexia Nervosa and ADHD. Perhaps this comorbidity is rare because girls who develop restricting Anorexia Nervosa typically have a great deal of excellent self-control and focused attention. They could not starve themselves unless they had the self-control to deny themselves food. By contrast, girls who develop Bulimia Nervosa or Binge Eating Disorder have poor self-control and a great deal of impulsivity, both the hallmarks of ADHD. When a girl with ADHD goes on a diet, she has poor impulse control and could easily develop a pattern of bingeing and/or purging. Anorexia Nervosa, Bulimic subtype, also might develop. Thus, especially in adolescent females, the clinician should ask the basic screening questions in Table 4.2 for Eating Disorders. Similarly, whenever a clinician is work-ing with adolescents who have Bulimia Nervosa or Anorexia Nervosa, Bu-limic subtype, it is wise to screen for ADHD.

The most unusual comorbidity to ADHD is ADD Psychosis (Bellak, 1985, 1994; Bellak et al., 1987). Bellak argues that ADHD across the life span is a developmental risk factor for a type of organic psychosis. He points out that the attentional cognitive symptoms interfere with the order-ly acquisition of data and hence the maturation and integration of normal intellectual operations. The low stimulus barrier associated with ADHD may lead to sensory overload and cognitive disorganization, and problems in relationships are made worse by impulsivity. In short, the neurobiology of ADHD and its secondary emotional problems may play a significant role in the formation of personality and may lead to a psychotic disorder which is a primary result of the effects of ADD. There is no indication that ADD Psychosis will be present during adolescence, and this concept is not at all well established in the field, so that the practitioner does not need to screen for it. I mention it here mainly as a way of alerting readers to the range of comorbidity which has been studied.

ADOLESCENT INTERVIEW

The interview with the adolescent is usually shorter and less formal than the interview with the parents. The clinician leads off the interview with a rapport-building phase designed to set the adolescent at ease and establish the clinician as seriously interested in the adolescent as a person, not just as another controlling adult. I usually open with the following type of remark: "I'd like to get to know you and what you are interested in. Tell me how you like to spend your free time and what you like to do for fun." As the adolescent discusses his or her hobbies and recreational interests, I listen intently and share any commonalities which might arise with my own recreational interests and hobbies. Often, opportunities for a smooth transition into the diagnostic phase of the interview arise, as when an ADHD symptom appears to be interfering with a recreational interest:

RANDALL: I really enjoy playing tennis, but I get so frustrated when I lose that I throw a fit on the court. My friends get really bummed out.

DR. ROBIN: Is getting frustrated something that happens other times too?

RANDALL: Yes!! Teachers, nerds, parents, lots of people piss me off.

DR. ROBIN: That brings us to the reason why we are here today. We need to take a look at what is happening that is causing your frustration, school and home difficulties, and what we can do to help you deal with them. I've been looking at these checklists you filled out and I really appreciate all the work you did. I'd like to ask you about some things you wrote down.

The clinician then reviews the DSM-IV inclusionary criteria for ADHD, using the PPHS–ADHD interview. The clinician is looking for general confirmation of the presence or absence of each symptom, not as detailed an analysis as is elicited from the parents. One good example per symptom is sufficient, and when symptoms overlap, I often record the information for both overlapping symptoms, reducing redundant questioning. For example, in responding to the item about blurting things out, the adolescent may also give examples of interrupting other people, so the clinician does not need to ask about interrupting separately.

Some 12- to 14-year-olds deny the presence of most symptoms because of their need to be omnipotent or because they may not be aware of the occurrence of the ADHD symptoms. In such cases, the clinician can ask about the symptoms indirectly through specific situations rather than general questions. Consider the following example:

DR. ROBIN: Do you get easily distracted by things going on around you?

JENNIFER: No, my mind is sharp and I pay attention all the time.

DR. ROBIN: So what happens if you are trying to read your Algebra book and there is a lot of noise around you?

JENNIFER: I don't read my Algebra book. It's a bore.

DR. ROBIN: What do you mean by "It's a bore"?

JENNIFER: I end up daydreaming and reading the same sentence over and over again. Algebra is just too boring. I don't see why I have to take it.

Jennifer could not openly admit that she got easily distracted. However, when given a more specific example, she was able to describe her distractibility, externalizing blame on the subject matter rather than taking personal responsibility for it. The clinician learns about the adolescent's readiness to accept ADHD from these types of interactions during the interview.

After reviewing the inclusionary criteria for ADHD, the clinician conducts a selective differential diagnostic interview. I review only the comorbidities and/or differential diagnoses that appear likely based on the parent interview and the rating scales. If I am considering Mood Disorders, I also do an assessment for suicidal ideation. Whenever possible, I have the adolescent complete the SCID Screen Patient Questionnaire or DICA on a laptop computer, a task most adolescents enjoy. I use the same questions in Table 4.2 and the earlier section of this chapter to verify hypotheses about comorbidities and differential diagnoses.

The adolescent interview is also the setting in which to assess peer relationships, sexuality, and substance use. I ask frank and open questions about exploration and use of alcohol, marijuana, and other drugs, as well as degree of involvement in sexual activities. I also ask adolescents to describe their relationships with their closest friends.

The interview usually lead naturally into the next phase of assessment, the formal psychological testing. Chapter 5 discusses psychological testing.

FAMILY INTERACTION ASSESSMENT

After I complete the adolescent interview and the psychological testing, I interview the parents and the adolescent together to assess family interactions. The family assessment is typically a broad, 15- to 20-minute interview designed to map out the major landmarks and land mines of the parent–teen relationship, not to get all the details. Following the biobehavioral family systems model outlined in Chapter 2, I organize my interview around five topics: (1) specific issues of dispute, (2) problem-solving skills, (3) communication patterns, (4) extreme beliefs and cognitive distortions, and (5) family structure problems. My goal is to be able to begin to paint a mental picture of the family interaction along these five dimensions, and I move flexibly between them in the ensuing questions. I carefully review all the family questionnaires beforehand (Issues Checklist, Conflict Behavior Questionnaire, PARQ) and formulate any hypotheses I can about the family based on the questionnaires. I then test these hypotheses during the interview. I start by asking each family member to respond briefly to the general question, "How well do the three (two) of you get along?" As they give their answers to this question, I review each person's Issues Checklist, looking particularly at the issues with intensity levels of 4 or 5. As a way of pinpointing problem solving and communication habits, I pick one of these issues, and ask each family member to give me a blow-by-blow description of a recent discussion concerning the issue. I am interested in how the issue came up, who said what, how the argument proceeded, and how it ended up. Do family members exhibit any problem-solving skills (e.g., clearly defining the topic under consideration, thinking of several ideas for solving it, discussing the ideas and trying to negotiate a compromise, or planning how to implement an agreement)? Does the family constantly change topics in response to each new criticism they make of each other, completing forgetting the original topic and bringing up all the accumulated dirty laundry from the past few years? Is the discussion basically a shouting match with each person attempting to coerce the others to get his or her own way? Does the discussion start in a civil manner but rapidly deteriorate in a burst of negative communication characterized by put-downs, accusations, interruptions, defensive comments, and sarcastic criticism? Which negative communication habits predominate, and who takes the lead to sidetracking the discussion? Does one person usually get his or her way and the other gives in?

If common extreme belief themes do not spontaneously arise from the blow-by-blow description of the disagreement, I specifically ask the parents and then the adolescent to what extent they adhere to beliefs such as ruination, perfectionism, obedience, self-blame, malicious intent, or approval. For example, a typical question might be:

> "Many parents worry that if their adolescent doesn't learn to clean up his room now, he will never amount to anything when he grows up and will be a worthless, aimless, unemployed adult. Do you have any such worries?"

To an adolescent, I might say:

> "Most kids your age think they ought to have as much freedom as they want and think their parents are too controlling? Do you agree? In what ways?"

In this brief family interview, I usually learn only a little bit about family structure. I look for any obvious examples of coalitional or triangulated behavior in the session and inquire about who takes sides with whom at home. I also look for examples of overinvolvement by one parent and disengagement by another. Sometimes, subtle factors such as how the family seats itself (person in the middle may be triangulated; person further back from others may be disengaged) suggest hypotheses about family structure to be confirmed over time. However, it usually takes more time before I begin to truly understand the family structure.

At the close of the family assessment interview, I summarize what I learned, couched in terms that try to show how ADHD affects family interactions and point the family toward setting goals for change. The following example illustrates the summary statement:

> "ADHD is really doing your family in when issues come up between you. Bill, you get really intense and lose it when your parents bring stuff up. You say things that you regret later on. Your parents come right back, bringing up everything you ever did wrong. It ends up in a shouting match and nothing gets accomplished. Everyone overreacts. It seems like the world is going to come to an end. We have to work on communication, problem solving, and managing anger. Any questions?"

Interview and questionnaire-based assessment of family interaction can be supplemented with direct observation methods taken in naturalistic or analog settings; Chapter 5 summarizes such observational methods. Readers interested in more detailed guidelines and additional examples of how to conduct family assessment interviews might consult *Negotiating Parent–Adolescent Conflict: A Behavioral–Family Systems Approach* (Robin & Foster, 1989, Chap. 4).

CONCLUDING COMMENT

This chapter provides detailed, specific guidelines for using parent, adolescent, and family interviews to assess ADHD symptoms, comorbidity for other psychiatric conditions, differential diagnoses of other conditions, and family interactions. I demonstrated how the practitioner might integrate some of the rating scale and questionnaire data into the interview process and pointed out potential shortcuts through the use of computerized interview protocols.

In addition to interviews and questionnaire, the comprehensive ADHD evaluation typically includes cognitive ability and achievement testing, a continuous performance measure, and at times direct observational data. I now turn to these sources of information.

CHAPTER FIVE

—————— O ——————

Cognitive Testing, Educational Impairment, and Laboratory/ Observational Measures

Gathering objective data from cognitive tests and schoolwork samples is an indispensable and critically important aspect of a comprehensive assessment of ADHD. Such data are necessary to determine the presence of educational impairment arising from ADHD, and such a determination is necessary to seek remedial educational services for the adolescent. Continuous performance tests and direct observational techniques are also helpful in the evaluation process. This chapter provides the practitioner with a detailed discussion of these areas.

COGNITIVE TESTING AND LEARNING PROBLEMS

To characterize the relationship between ADHD and learning disabilities and advise practitioners about the use of cognitive ability and achievement tests, we first must discuss some definitional issues surrounding learning problems. There remains a great deal of confusion and heterogeneity in how the term "learning disability" has been defined. In most educational settings, the term "learning disabled" usually refers to the child who fails to learn despite a normal capacity to learn, with a quantitative discrepancy between intellectual ability and academic achievement serving as the defining yardstick of a learning disability.

Learning disabilities have been defined as disorders in one or more of the basic psychological processes involved in understanding or using spoken or written language; these disorders may impair the ability to listen, think, speak, write, spell, or do mathematics and include conditions such as perceptual handicaps, brain injury, minimal brain dysfunction, dyslexia, and developmental aphasia (National Advisory Committee on Handicapped Children, 1968). Learning disabilities exclude learning problems that are primarily the result of sensory or motor problems, mental retardation, emotional disturbance, cultural or environmental factors. This definition has been refined over time to refer to individuals who fail to learn and/or accomplish academic and selected interpersonal tasks that others can accomplish despite average ability, when this lack of accomplishment is due to biological factors rather than poor teaching, environmental deprivation, or limited experience (Kavanaugh, 1988).

A great deal of factor-analytic research on the subtypes of learning disabilities has concluded that there are two broad types of skills necessary for learning (Goldstein, 1997; Rourke, 1989):

1. *Auditory–verbal processes.* Weaknesses in these areas lead to reading disorders and other language-based disorders. The majority of learning-disabled youngsters have problems with reading and language, and these difficulties have a lasting impact on their functioning in adolescence and adulthood (Goldstein, 1997).
2. *Visual, perceptual, and motor (nonverbal) processes.* Weaknesses in these areas may lead to reading problems but are more likely to lead to mathematics, handwriting, and selected social skills problems. Often, individuals with these types of learning disabilities can compensate more easily for them as adolescents and adults than can the majority, who have trouble with reading and language.

Practically, researchers and clinicians studying ADHD and learning disabilities have typically relied on the definition of learning disabilities as a significant discrepancy between scores on an IQ and an achievement test. The size of the discrepancy may vary from study to study or school system to school system, but a 1.5 or 2.0 standard deviation discrepancy is fairly common. Readers interested in further discussion of these definitional issues and their implications for assessment and treatment should consult Goldstein (1997) and Reynolds (1985, 1990).

Learning Disabilities and ADHD

What exactly is the incidence of comorbidity for learning disabilities (LD) in children and adolescents with ADHD? Studies have reported rates of LD ranging widely from 10% to 90% in ADHD populations (Biederman et al., 1992). The accurate answer to the LD comorbidity questions depends upon exactly which definition of LD one chooses to use. Two studies have compared the comorbidity of LD to ADHD using different definitions of LD. Barkley (1990) compared the applications of three different definitions of LD to Wechsler Intelligence Scale for Children—Revised (WISC-R) and Wide Range Achievement Test—Revised (WRAT-R) data he collected on 42 ADHD children and 36 normal controls: (1) a 15-point discrepancy between IQ and achievement, (2) achievement falling 1.5 standard deviations below the normal mean (7th percentile), and (2) a combination of the first two definitions. Barkley points out that the IQ/achievement discrepancy approach may overestimate the prevalence of LD in children performing normally in school who have gifted IQ (e.g., IQ = 130 while Reading SS = 100); the achievement cutoff approach may include borderline to mildly retarded children in the LD category. His third, combined approach avoids this pitfalls and is most rigorous.

Table 5.1 presents the results of Barkley's study. The percentage of children in each group defined as learning disabled varied considerably with each approach. With the discrepancy approach, a large number of the ADHD and normal children were defined as learning disabled in reading, spelling, or mathematics. This is clearly not a rigorous approach to defining LD. Considerably lower percentages of ADHD children (19–28%) and

TABLE 5.1. Comparisons of ADHD/LD Comorbidities with Different Definitions of LD

Formula	Barkley (1990) ADHD %	Control %
Reading		
IQ–Achievement discrepancy	40.5	20.6
Achievement cutoff score	21.4	0.0
Combined formula	19.0	0.0
Spelling		
IQ–Achievement discrepancy	59.5	38.2
Achievement cutoff score	26.2	2.9
Combined formula	23.8	0.0
Math		
IQ–Achievement discrepancy (15 pts.)	59.5	35.3
Achievement cutoff score	28.6	2.9
Combined formula	26.2	2.9

Formula	Biederman, Faraone, & Lapey (1992) ADHD %	Psychiatric controls %	Normal controls %
Reading			
IQ–Achievement discrepancy (10 pts.)	38	43	8
IQ–Achievement discrepancy (20 pts.)	22	10	2
Combined formula (achievement 85 or less; 15-pt. discrepancy)	15	3	0

very few normal children were defined as LD using the achievement cutoff or the combined approaches.

Biederman and his colleagues (Biederman et al., 1992; Semrud-Clikeman et al., 1992) compared the rates of reading learning disabilities in 60 clinically referred ADHD children, 30 psychiatric controls, and 36 normal controls using three different definitions of LD: (1) a 10-point standard score difference with Full Scale IQ higher than reading achievement, (2) a 20-point standard score difference with Full Scale IQ higher than reading achievement; and (3) a 15 point scaled score difference between full scale IQ and reading achievement, and a achievement score less than 85. The first two approaches are similar to Barkley's discrepancy definition; the third is similar to his combined formula. Inspection of Table 5.1 shows that similar to Barkley's results, the discrepancy formulae identify high rates of learning disability whereas the combined formula identifies lower rates. Significantly more ADHD children were identified as having a reading learning disability with method 1 than with methods 2 or 3, which did not differ from each other. I did not locate any similar studies done specifically with adolescents, so at this time we must make generalizations based on the studies done with children.

Readers should also note that these two studies focused on LD in reading, mathematics, or spelling but did not address other areas such as written expression. Clinically, many adolescents with ADHD manifest difficulties in putting their ideas in writing when they have to complete papers and essays in high school and college. Low scores on Spelling subtests do not necessarily provide a mechanism to screen for such written expression difficulties. In the future, researchers need to administer direct measures of written expression such as the Test of Written Language (TOWL-3) to older adolescents with ADHD to formally determine the extent of LD in written expression in this population.

The practitioner can draw two conclusions from these studies: (1) using more conservative definitions, approximately 20–25% of ADHD children have comorbid learning disabilities; and (2) in clinical practice, practitioners should use an approach that combines an IQ/achievement discrepancy with an absolutely low achievement score. Ideally, practitioners should use a regression method that computes expected achievement for ability to measure IQ/achievement discrepancy, taking test measurement error into account. However, in practice, this may not always be possible. Practitioners should become familiar with the criteria for learning disabilities used in their local school districts, so that they can gear their reports to these criteria.

Cognitive Assessment Battery

I routinely administer either the Wechsler Intelligence Scale for Children (third edition) (WISC-III; Wechsler, 1991) or the Wechsler Adult Intelligence Scale—III (WAIS-III; Wechsler, 1997b). The Wechsler scales provide a good overall measure of verbal and performance ability.

When I need specific measures of memory, I administer the Wide Range Assessment of Memory and Learning (Adams & Sheslow, 1990), which includes nine subtests tapping verbal and visual memory, as well as verbal, visual, and verbal–visual learning over four trials. The instrument has normative data for childhood through 16 years of age. For older adolescents I administer the Wechsler Memory Scales—III (Wechsler, 1997c), which offers a summary score, measures of visual and verbal memory, learning, and attention. (The attention score has not been found to correlate with the diagnosis of ADHD, however.)

When adolescents are referred for evaluation and/or treatment, whether or not an ADHD diagnosis has already been made, it is wise to obtain an updated IQ measure. Unless someone else has administered the WAIS-III or the WISC-III within the past 6 months, I administer it.

By contrast, I do not routinely administer memory tests unless there is some indication from other testing, clinical evaluation, or history of the need to do so.

Achievement Tests

There are a wide range of achievement tests from which to choose (Reynolds, 1990). The educational standard for a comprehensive evaluation is the Woodcock–Johnson Psycho-Educational Battery—Revised (however, I do not use the ability sections of this battery). (Woodcock & Johnson, 1989). The Woodcock–Johnson gives a detailed analysis of visual or verbal strengths and weaknesses; highlights specific deficits in reading, mathematics, or written expression; and has norms from childhood through adulthood. However, it takes a long time to administer and may not be practical in many private practice or managed care settings, which provide little or no insurance reimbursement for educational testing. Much shorter tests (e.g., the WRAT-III) may estimate achievement but give too cursory a view and do not have wide enough coverage (e.g., reading comprehension and written expression).

A reasonable compromise which I have been using consistently for the past few years is the Wechsler Individual Achievement Test (WIAT; Wechsler, 1992). The WIAT is a comprehensive achievement battery with norms up through age 19. It includes eight subtests: (1) Basic Reading (phonics), (2) Mathematics Reasoning, (3) Spelling, (4) Reading Comprehension, (5) Numerical Calculations, (6) Listening Comprehension, (7) Oral Expression, and (8) Written Expression. The WIAT is linked through co-norming to the WISC-III and the WAIS-III, which permits easy determination of discrepancies between ability and achievement. In fact, the WIAT manual contains tables permitting two methods of determining ability/achievement discrepancies between Full Scale IQ and each subtest of the WIAT: (1) the simple difference between the standard scores on the IQ and achievement tests, and (2) a regression method, which computes achievement in each area predicted by Full Scale IQ and compares that to actual achievement. After computing the discrepancy, the practitioner checks for whether it is significant and then considers the result together with other factors in determining the presence of a learning disability.

Administration of the entire WIAT takes 40–50 minutes. Administration of a shorter screener version consisting of Basic Reading, Mathematics Reasoning, and Spelling takes 10–15 minutes. I typically administer five subtests in approximately 30 minutes: Basic Reading, Mathematics Reasoning, Spelling, Reading Comprehension, and Numerical Calculation. I add one or more of the remaining subtests (most commonly Written Expression) when history warrants it.

Freedom-from-Distractibility Factor

The third factor of the WISC-III IQ test, consisting of Arithmetic and Digit Span, is known as the Freedom-from-Distractibility (FFD) Factor. With the previous version of the Wechsler IQ test, the WISC-R, this factor consisted of Arithmetic, Digit Span, and Coding. The FFD was often been touted as a measure of attention and distractability in children and adolescents and has been adopted by some as a clinical diagnostic measure of ADHD. There is no compelling evidence, however, that the FFD factor reliably and validly distinguishes ADHD individuals from those with LD alone and/or normal controls (Barkley, 1990). In addition, reviews of the research on the FFD factor suggest that it measures myriad executive functions, including short-term memory, facility with numbers, arithmetic calculations, and visual–spatial skills (Wielkiewicz, 1990). It should not be routinely used to make a diagnosis of ADHD, even though it may be lower than the Verbal Comprehension and the Perceptual Organization factors in some individuals diagnosed as having ADHD.

Brown (1996) further analyzed discrepancies between these IQ subtests thought to have particular relevance to ADHD and the Verbal or Performance factors in adolescents with ADHD. He computed Bannatyne Index Scores as follows for the WISC-III or the WAIS-R, designed to yield a mean of 100 and a standard deviation of 15:

<u>WISC-III</u>

Verbal Index = (Vocabulary + Comprehension + Similarities) × 1.8 + 47

Spatial Index = (Picture Completion + Block Design + Object Assembly) × 1.8 + 46

Concentration Index = (Digit Span + Arithmetic + Coding) × 2.2 + 34.

WAIS-R

Verbal Index = (Vocabulary + Comprehension + Similarities) × 1.9 + 43

Spatial Index = (Picture Completion + Block Design + Object Assembly) × 2 + 40

Concentration Index = (Digit Span + Arithmetic + Digit Symbol) × 2.1 + 37.

He compared the differences between the Verbal and Concentration, and the Spatial and Concentration Indices in a sample of 191 adolescents diagnosed with ADHD. These differences were highly significant. Examination of the percentage of ADHD adolescents with large differences indicated that 66% of the ADHD adolescents had either Verbal or Spatial Index scores at least one standard deviation higher than their Bannatyne Concentration Index, which was more than three times the rate of such differences in the general population.

Preliminary data comparing ADHD (N = 30) individuals to the standardization sample was collected as part of the standardization of the WAIS-III (Wechsler, 1997a). The mean overall intellectual functioning of the ADHD group was within the average range, but there were intraindividual differences in WAIS-III index scores. ADHD individuals scored an average of 8.3 points lower on the Working Memory Index than on the Verbal Comprehension Index, and an average of 7.5 points lower on the Processing Speed Index than on the Perceptual Organization Index. These findings were consistent with Brown's results.

Both Brown (1996) and the author of the WAIS-III (Wechsler, 1997a) are very careful to point out that such differences may often result from cognitive problems other than ADHD, and therefore should not be used to diagnose ADHD. Nonetheless, it may be instructive to note how frequently these differences go along with ADHD. Brown interprets these results as supporting a wide umbrella model of ADHD including a variety of cognitive deficits. Practitioners might compute the Bannatyne indices and assess the significance of the difference as one additional aspect of the adolescent's cognitive profile, as long as they do not use such differences to make a differential diagnosis.

Concluding Comment

In my comprehensive differential diagnostic work-up for ADHD in adolescents, I routinely conduct a "screening" for LD by giving a Wechsler IQ test and an achievement test such as the WIAT. I believe that no ADHD workup for an adolescent is really complete without such a screen, although, as mentioned in the Introduction to Section II, there may be compelling practical reasons in a managed care environment to try to get the school to conduct the testing. If I uncover a significant discrepancy between expected and actual achievement suggestive of a learning disability, I typically attempt to get the adolescent's school system to conduct a thorough psychoeducational workup for the specific deficiency, using finer-grain educational tests. Most of the families I see do not wish to pay privately for such evaluations, and I have not encountered any third-party payers that cover testing for LD per se. Furthermore, it is, after all, the public school's responsibility to conduct full psychoeducational workups when there is reasonable suspicion of a learning disability.

ELIGIBILITY FOR EDUCATIONAL SERVICES

Once the clinician diagnoses an adolescent as having ADHD and a learning disability, how does he or she determine the youngster's eligibility for educational services and report the results to the school in a manner that maximizes the chances that the adolescent will receive the needed services? This is a complicated question that goes beyond the scope of this book to answer in detail. However, the practitioner needs to have a general awareness of two areas to maximize the chances that his or her patients will receive the educational services they need: (1) the legal rights of the student and the legal obligations of the school system and (2) the determination of educational impairment in adolescents with ADHD.

Legal Rights of the Student and Obligations of the School District

Three federal laws cover adolescents with ADHD: (1) the Individuals with Disabilities Education Act, Part B (IDEA); (2) Section 504 of the Rehabilitation Act of 1973; and (3) the Americans with Disabilities Act of 1990 (ADA). The U.S. Department of Education has the legal authority to interpret and enforce IDEA, and the Office of Civil Rights of the Department of Education has the right and authority to interpret and enforce the provisions of Section 504 and the ADA that pertain to education.

The Department of Education issued a Policy Clarification Memorandum on September 16, 1991 (Davila, Williams, & MacDonald, 1991), which has become the single most important governmental document outlining the conditions under which adolescents with ADHD are eligible for special education and/or related services under IDEA and Section 504. IDEA, Part B requires public schools in the United States to provide a free and appropriate education for all children with disabilities. To be eligible under IDEA Part B, the evaluation must show that the child has one or more specified physical or mental impairments, and these impairments must be such that they require special education (Davila et al., 1991). Being diagnosed with ADHD does not automatically qualify an adolescent for special services; ADHD must impair the adolescent from benefiting from education.

The Memorandum indicates that children with ADHD may be eligible for special education services under three categories defined by IDEA: (1) other health impaired, (2) specific learning disability, and (3) serious emotional disturbance. Adolescents with ADHD may be eligible for special education services under "other health impaired" because ADHD is viewed as a chronic or acute health problem that results in limited alertness, which adversely affects educational performance. Adolescents with ADHD may receive services solely on the basis of ADHD, not having to qualify under any other categories, under the "other health impaired" category. Adolescents with ADHD may also qualify for special education services if they meet criteria because of either a coexisting specific learning disability or a serious emotional impairment. Serious emotional impairments are defined to mean that the adolescent has an unexplained inability to learn, unsatisfactory personal relationships with teachers and peers, inappropriate behavior and feelings, general depression, and physical symptoms or fears resulting from personal or school problems, and that these problems markedly impair educational performance over a long period.

Schools are required, under IDEA, Part B, to find adolescents with ADHD and use the multidisciplinary team/individualized education program (IEP) process to evaluate the educational needs and plan an IEP tailored to each adolescent. The IEP must describe the nature of the child's disability, how it adversely impacts educational performance, and how a variety of multidisciplinary services and aids will be used to meet the child's unique needs and achieve a free and appropriate education. The IEP must specify how these needs will be met in the least restrictive environment, starting with regular education. Parents are given legal rights to impartial hearings and court challenges where they can disagree with the school system's evaluations and recommendations.

Section 504 of the Rehabilitation Act is a civil rights law that prohibits discrimination, in federally funded programs, against otherwise qualified persons with disabilities solely on the basis of the person's disability. Unlike IDEA, which has specific disability categories, Section 504 broadly defines a disability as a "physical or mental impairment which limits one or more major life activities," including learning. Unlike IDEA, no funding follows along with Section 504. Like IDEA, Section 504 requires public schools to provide a free and appropriate education, using regular and special education and related aids and services, tailored to the student's unique needs, based on a multidisciplinary evaluation. Regular education is to be used to the maximum extent possible. Failure to meet Section 504 requirements can result in a cutoff of federal funds to a school district. The clarification memorandum indicated that full protection of Section 504 applied to students with ADHD suspected of having a disability in school; it outlines the school district's responsibilities to conduct a multidisciplinary evaluation and write an educational plan. The memorandum gives explicit examples of accommodations in regular education under a Section 504 plan:

1. Providing a structured learning environment.
2. Repeating and simplifying instructions about in-class and homework assignments.
3. Supplementing verbal instructions with visual instructions.
4. Using behavioral management techniques.
5. Adjusting class schedules.
6. Modifying test delivery.
7. Using tape recorders, computer-aided instruction, and other audiovisual equipment.
8. Selecting modified textbooks or workbooks.
9. Tailoring homework assignments.

These federal regulations specify the minimum legal rights of children with ADHD, and have typically been incorporated into state laws. Some state laws go beyond the minimal federal requirements and have even recognized ADHD as a disability. It behooves the practitioner to become familiar with the laws in his or her state by asking the state department of education to send him or her a copy of its regulations regarding disabilities.

What obligations do private schools have to meet the needs of adolescents with disabilities? The ADA extends the protections of Section 504 to all public and private schools, but religious schools are exempt from these requirements. ADA prohibits discrimination at work, at school, and in public accommodations and is not limited to those organizations and programs that receive federal funding. ADA uses the same definitions, eligibility criteria, and types of accommodation specified by Section 504. To be eligible for protection under ADA, an individual with ADHD must disclose his/her disability to the appropriate authority.

At the postsecondary level, older adolescents with ADHD are protected by Section 504 and ADA, not IDEA. Colleges and professional schools do not have to lower their admission standards, but they do have to make reasonable accommodations in their courses and procedures. Unfortunately, in some cases sloppy diagnostic practices or inadequate documentation results in inappropriate requests for accommodation. Even worse, unscrupulous individuals have seen an opportunity for profit by advertising that they will raise clients' scores on national professional examinations through a combination of tutoring and requests for special accommodation, when the clients may not truly have ADHD or a learning disability. Such situations make it more difficult for clients who truly deserve accommodation to obtain them.

In one case involving the National Board of Medical Examiners, when the board denied the request for accommodation, the students sued (Gordon, Barkley, & Murphy, 1997). The Judge upheld the board's decision, and indicated in his ruling that to be eligible for accommodation under the ADA, there must be solid evidence of abnormality relative to the general population. Gordon et al. (1997) appropriately caution practitioners to be thorough in documenting requests for accommodation at the postsecondary level under ADA. They recommend that the practitioner do the following:

1. Establish evidence that ADHD-type symptoms arose in childhood.
2. Establish evidence that the symptoms currently meet DSM-IV criteria in their nature and severity.
3. Establish evidence that current remediation does not lead to sufficient improvement in function.
4. Provide a rationale for the kinds of accommodation requested.
5. Indicate why he or she is qualified to render this diagnosis (especially if he or she is not a physician or does not hold a terminal degree in clinical psychology).

The bottom line is that not every student who has trouble taking standardized examinations truly has a disability or qualifies for accommodation.

Readers interested in a more detailed discussion of the school's legal obligations might consult Cohen (1996) or Latham and Latham (1992, 1993, 1997). Zeigler Dendy (1995) wrote an excellent chapter for parents, guiding them through the legal/educational maze. Gordon and Keiser (1998) provide the practitioner with detailed guidelines for accommodations in higher education.

Determining Adverse Effects of ADHD on School Functioning

Not all adolescents with ADHD are eligible for accommodation and/or more intensive interventions under either Section 504 or IDEA. Only when the family or school can demonstrate that ADHD has an adverse effect on the child's education is an ADHD individual eligible for such assistance. Unfortunately, neither federal nor state laws provide a clear-cut definition of "adverse effect on education," nor do the laws outline procedures for local school districts to follow in determining such an adverse impact. Thus, local school districts have been left to establish their own criteria, and not surprisingly, there is a great deal of variability, with unfortunate results in some cases when children with obvious difficulties are denied services. During the congressional inquiry that eventuated in the 1991 clarification memorandum, a group of ADHD researchers and professionals (called PGARD) formulated and submitted to the U.S. Congress what has become one of the most widely known and intuitively reasonable definitions of the "adverse effects of ADHD on education." I routinely use this definition, published in the *CH.A.D.D. Educator's Manual* (Fowler, 1995, p. 27) and have found that most of the schools to which I present it find it reasonable: "ADD adversely affects educational performance to the extent that a significant discrepancy exists between a child's intellectual ability and that child's productivity with respect to listening, following directions, planning, organizing, or completing academic assignments which require reading, writing, spelling, or mathematical calculations." Constructed to be parallel to the definition of a specific learning disability, this definition emphasizes the discrepancy between what a child is capable of producing and what a child is indeed producing as the key aspect of the adverse impact of ADHD on educational performance. This definition operationalizes one of the most common complaints of teachers about ADHD students: They are failing to work up to potential. It focuses on planning, organization, timely completion of assignments, and following directions, all areas in which ADHD adolescents fall down the most in middle and high school. This definitions fits intuitively with the problems most teachers and parents encounter with ADHD students: not completing tasks in class or completing homework. Cumulative academic achievement, grades, and knowledge are not the primary outcome variables; how much the student gets done is.

To apply the PGARD definition, we need to assess IQ and productivity, compute a discrepancy measure, and make a decision about what size discrepancy is educationally significant and worthy of intervention. We also need to decide what percentage of assignments children of different IQs should be expected to compute. Should a child of average IQ, for example, be expected to complete 90% of the assigned work? Should children of superior IQ be expected to complete 100% of the work, and so on?

IQ is readily assessed through the use of the standardized measures discussed earlier. Productivity must be assessed through work samples of the adolescent's homework and classwork, along with the teachers' records of the timeliness of completion of the work. However, we have no universal standards or published tables for assessing productivity. Should productivity standards be absolute and set by each teacher (e.g., every adolescent is expected to complete 80%, 90%, or 100% of the assigned homework)? Or should productivity standards be based on the normative standard for the class (e.g., the mean productivity for the class)? Should only the mean for those students who do not have any disabilities (i.e., a "nondistressed" control group) be taken? The assessment of productivity also has to take into account the particular subject matter, teacher, and school systems; standards for productivity might be different in English, chemistry, and algebra, and in a private prep school versus a public school, for example. Many of these questions remain to be answered by future research. Educators need to develop normative data for productivity similar to the normative data for IQ and cumulative achievement used to compute the discrepancies on which learning disabilities are based.

In the meantime, the clinician needs to make determinations about productivity deficits in patients, based on currently incomplete standards. To take teacher, subject matter, and classroom environmental factors into account, it is clear that we somehow need to compare the ADHD adolescent's productivity to that of the peers of similar intellectual ability in a particular classroom. Until school systems develop standardized local norms for productivity, the clinician is advised to follow these procedures, which may be less than ideal but nonetheless have proven useful:

1. Calculate the percentage of work completed on time and the percentage completed correctly in each of the adolescent's classes over a 2-week period.
2. Determine what percentage of work is expected to be completed by adolescents of a similar IQ to the patient by doing one or both of the following: (a) obtain the mean percentage productivity for the whole class or for a subset of the class of similar IQ to the patient; or (b) ask the teacher what percentage productivity he or she expects. Ideally, the teacher provides the clinician with the mean and the standard deviation of productivity for the class, so that the clinician can compute cutoffs for 1.5 standard deviations below the mean, but realistically, few teachers are willing to provide such detailed information.
3. Compute a discrepancy by subtracting the ADHD adolescent's percentage work done from the class mean or the teacher's expected standard. Compute this discrepancy for each class.
4. Decide whether the discrepancy is educationally meaningful. If standard deviations are available, the formula common in the literature of 1.5 standard deviations below the mean as the cutoff for clinical significance may be applied. If standard deviations are not available, the teachers might be asked what size discrepancy is educationally significant for that setting.
5. Repeat steps 2–4 for the percentage accuracy of the assignments completed.
6. Summarize in which of the adolescent's classes ADHD causes significantly adverse effects on education for the quantity and the accuracy of work completed. The last few items on the Classroom Performance Survey in Table 3.9 are designed to prompt teachers to provide the information needed to assess productivity.

Let us consider the case of Nadia Smith, a 16-year-old high school junior recently diagnosed with ADHD, Inattentive Type. Nadia has been having a great deal of trouble keeping up with homework, papers, and lab reports in chemistry, English, history, and algebra. Her teachers were asked to supply data on her productivity during the past 2 weeks compared to her peers. Table 5.2 summarizes the data which Nadia's teachers provided.

TABLE 5.2. Productivity Data for Nadia Smith, Last 2 Weeks

	Nadia % homework done	Class mean % done	Class SD %	Discrepancy %	Teacher expects %
Chemistry	40	75	10	35	100
English	45	80	15	35	90
History	60	90	25	30	95
Algebra	65	75	15	27	100
Mean	53	80		33	96

In chemistry, Nadia completed 40% of her homework, 35% below the class mean of 75%, a highly significant difference of 3 standard deviations. This discrepancy is highly significant by conventional statistical standards. The teacher's expectation of 100% is probably unrealistic for the current classroom conditions, given the class mean of 75%. In English, Nadia completed 45% of her assignments, 35% less than the class mean of 80, or over 2 standard deviations below the class mean. Again, this is a highly significant discrepancy. The teacher's expectations of 90% are not unreasonable given the class mean of 80%. In history, Nadia completed 60% of her assignments, 30% less than the class mean of 90%, but only a little over 1 standard deviation off the class mean. One might argue that the size of the discrepancy is not educationally significant given the high variability in the class. Finally, in algebra, Nadia completed 65% of her assignments, only 10% less than the class mean of 75%, less than 1 standard deviation and not educationally significant. In summary, using the class means and standard deviations as a basis for comparison, ADHD has an adverse impact on Nadia's productivity in chemistry and English but not in history and algebra. Using absolute teacher standards, Nadia is far behind in all classes, but in several cases, teacher standards are not reasonable for the class as a whole, and the teachers need to reexamine their instructional procedures or adjust their standards.

The PGARD definition also mentions productivity with respect to listening, following directions, planning, and organizing in addition to completing of assignments. We do not have any standardized measures of these forms of productivity in the classroom but could potentially use behavioral observations, teacher rating scales, or laboratory analog measures such as continuous performance tests as alternatives.

This discussion may have raised more questions than it answered, because educators and researchers really have not paid sufficient attention to operationally defining the adverse effects of ADD on the performance of secondary education students. In closing, I recommend using some version of work samples with comparisons to peers and/or absolute standards, taking IQ into account, to determine when ADHD is creating an educational impairment in need of intervention.

LABORATORY MEASURES

Laboratory Measures (LMs) have increasingly been used to assess inattention and impulsivity as part of the diagnostic process with ADHD individuals (Barkley, 1991b; Goldstein & Goldstein, 1990; Gordon, 1987, 1993a). Such measures have included continuous performance tests (CPTs), cancellation tasks, matching familiar figure tasks, subtests of IQ tests, card sort tasks, color association tests, and direct observations of ADHD symptoms in analogue laboratory situations. LMs have great potential as one component of a multimethod assessment because of their objectivity; that is, they are not subject to the possible biases of teachers or parents completing rating scales or clinicians conducting interviews. In addition, a great deal of rigorously standardized normative data can potentially be collected for such measures. To be useful to the clinician, however, LMs not only need to meet the traditional standards of reliability and validity, but, as Barkley (1991b) has pointed out, they need to have ecological validity and practicality. Ecological validity refers to the extent to which we can generalize from the results of an LM to the same behaviors of ADHD adolescents in the natural environment. Practicality refers to the degree to which an assessment procedure fits comfortable into the daily practice of a busy clinician in a managed care environment (Gordon, 1987).

Few LMs for adolescents have been researched. Those that have been evaluated (e.g., the Matching Familiar Figures Test [MFFT] and Wisconsin Card Sort) have not yet been able to differentiate between ADHD and non-ADHD adolescents (Fischer et al., 1990). A number of continuous performance tests have been employed with children and adolescents (Conners, 1995; Gordon & Mittelman, 1988; Greenberg & Waldman, 1993).

Gordon Diagnostic System

The Gordon Diagnostic System (GDS) is a popular CPT that has been subjected to careful empirical scrutiny in studies with ADHD adolescents. The GDS is one of the few LMs that meets the dual criteria of psychometric validity and practicality in clinical work with adolescents. The GDS is a portable, solid-state, child-proofed microprocessor-based CPT which can be programmed to administer multiple tasks. Three tasks are commonly administered to adolescents. The Vigilance task requires the child to inhibit responding under conditions that make demands for sustained attention. A series of digits flashes one at a time on an electronic display, and the adolescent is told to press the button every time a "1" is followed by a "9." The GDS records the number of correct responses, the number of omission errors (number of times the adolescent failed to respond to the "1/9" combination), and the number of commission errors (number of extraneous button presses). The Delay task requires the adolescent to inhibit responding in order to earn points, according to a Differential Reinforcement of Low Responding (DRL) schedule. The adolescent is instructed to press a button, wait a while, and then press the button again. If he or she waits for at least 6 seconds, a light flashes and the point counter increments; if the adolescent responds is less than 6 seconds, the timer resets and no points are earned. The Delay task yields three primary scores: the number of responses, the number of correct responses, and the efficiency ratio (percentage of correct responses). The Distractibility task is similar to the Vigilance task and yields the same scores but has additional digits flashing on the screen to the right and left of the target digits. The adolescent must ignore these distractors and look for a "1/9" combination in the middle position. For all three tasks, the GDS also records quantitative features of the adolescent's performance for individual time blocks as well as the total session, permitting analysis of the performance within the session. These three tasks take approximately half an hour to administer, and because of the portability of the GDS, they can be easily administered in virtually any setting.

Extensive normative data have been collected for the GDS (Gordon & Mettleman, 1987, 1988), and research indicates that it distinguishes ADHD from non-ADHD children, is sensitive to changes produced by stimulant medications, and correlates to a modest extent with other measures of sustained attention and impulsivity (Barkley, 1991b). Several of these studies have been conducted specifically with adolescents. In their follow-up study of hyperactive children into adolescence, Fischer et al. (1990) compared the ADHD and the control groups on the GDS Vigilance and Distractibility tasks. The standard 9-minute Vigilance task was lengthened to 12 minutes, but the Distractibility task was administered in its original 9-minute version. The ADHD group made significantly more omission and commission errors on Vigilance than did the control group, but there were no significant differences between groups on Distractibility. However, the older adolescents made fewer commission and omission errors than did the younger adolescents on Distractibility. Gordon (personal communication, 1996) noted a high degree of variability with several outliers 4–9 standard deviations above the mean in Fischer et al.'s (1990) ADHD group on the Distractibility task. He reanalyzed their data after transforming the scores to percentiles to minimize the impact of the outliers on the results. He then found that the ADHD group made significantly more commission scores than did the control group on the GDS Distractibility task. Brown and Sexson (1988) found that the GDS vigilance score was sensitive to medication effects in a sample of 11 black male adolescents, mean age 13 years, 7 months, with intermediate and high doses producing greater effects than lower doses. In another analysis using the combined follow-up sample of ADHD and control adolescents, Barkley (1991b) found some evidence for the ecological validity of the GDS Vigilance task in adolescents but weaker evidence than in 6- to 12-year-olds. In adolescents, the commission errors correlated with off-task behavior recorded during an analog academic task. Although the GDS Vigilance scores did not correlate with teacher ratings or MFFT scores in adolescents (as they did in 6- to 12-year-olds), commission errors did also correlate .25 and .36 with parent hyperactivity ratings on the Conners Parent Questionnaire and the Child Behavior Checklist. Kashden, Fremouw, Callahan, and Franzen (1993) found that suicidal adolescents made more commission errors on the GDS Vigilance task than either a matched psychiatric group of nonsuicidal adolescents or a community control group.

Concerns have been raised that the GDS may underidentify children with ADHD (DuPaul, Anastopoulos, Shelton, Guevremont, & Metevia, 1992). Gordon (1993) has pointed out that the GDS was purposely developed in a conservative manner, designed to produce a low rate of false positives, but false negatives could range from 27% to 85% depending on the age of the children, the criteria on which they were selected, and the GDS scores used. For example, Gordon (1993a) found in one study that false negatives dropped from 45% to 25% when he used an abnormal score on any of the three GDS tasks rather than an abnormal score on Vigilance alone as the criterion. Adolescents tend to have a higher likelihood in general of receiving normal scores on the GDS and therefore a higher probability of a false negative.

Fischer, Newby, and Gordon (1995) systematically examined the manner in which diagnosed ADHD youngsters who received a false negative on the GDS differ from those who received a true positive. They examined agreements between a rigorous clinical/research diagnosis of ADHD and the GDS Vigilance task in 100 4- to 17-year-olds referred for a double-blind, placebo drug trial. They found that agreement dropped from 80% between ages 4 and 11 to 20% between ages 12 and 17. Compared to those for whom the GDS agreed with the clinical diagnosis, those with disagreements had higher parent ratings of conduct and psychosomatic problems, lower teacher ratings of inattention, and lower rates of observed off-task behavior in an analog academic situation. In addition, members of the disagreement group were twice as likely as members of the agreement group to be medication nonresponders and half as likely to receive a recommendation to remain on the higher Ritalin (methylphenidate) dose when continued medication maintenance was recommended at the end of the double-blind placebo trial. Fischer et al. (1995) interpreted these results as suggesting that ADHD children with normal GDS scores may be less impaired in the attentional area than are ADHD children with abnormal GDS scores but may be more likely to have other comorbid problems. The authors argued that for the practitioner, the clinical significance of the constellation of scores across the GDS and other measures may be more important than the mere fact of an agreement between the GDS and other measures.

Conners Continuous Performance Test Version 3.0

Conners (1995) noted that traditional CPTs have certain inherent problems which could limit their sensitivity. The events to which children are supposed to respond are typically relatively infrequent when the task requires the child to respond only to a target stimulus. Children may vary as to whether they have problems with high or low event rates, and a low-event rate task might miss such problems. In addition, the interstimulus interval is typically fixed in traditional CPTs. This may make the task too easy for adolescents and adults, reducing sensitivity. It is difficult to gauge reaction time meaningfully when the interstimulus interval is fixed because subjects may easily figure it out.

Conners (1995) designed his CPT to minimize these problems by requiring subjects to continuously respond for 14 minutes as single letters are flashed on the screen but to inhibit a response when a target stimulus (×) appears. Interstimulus rate varies, with 1-, 2-, and 4-second trials. In addition to the standard task, researchers have the option of creating multiple variations on the relevant parameters. The Conners CPT runs on a standard microcomputer rather than being a self-contained piece of equipment. The youngster responds by using the mouse or the keyboard. This has the disadvantage of introducing equipment variability compared to the GDS or the Test of Variable Attention, discussed next, where the equipment is standardized (Conners, 1996; Corman, 1995; Greenberg, 1996). The Conners CPT yields a variety of scores, which are automatically computed as soon as the software completes administration of the task. These scores include omission errors, commission errors, and a variety of reaction time and variability scores. This CPT was standardized on a large sample of 670 ADHD individuals and 520 individuals from the general population, ages 4 to 70, but primarily ages 4 to 17. All the scores were elevated in ADHD subjects compared to controls, in analyses of covariance which controlled for age and sex. Clinical norms and general population norms were derived. Upon cross-validation, for ages 6 to 17, false-positive rates were 13.5% and false-negative rates were 26.1%.

I am unaware of any published research using the Conners CPT Version 3.0 exclusively with adolescents, although Anastopoulos and Costabile (1995) reported promising pilot data in a sample of 6- to 11-year-olds. Conners (1997a, 1997b) did study the correlation between his CPT and his revised parent and teacher rating scales as part of the validation of the rating scales. Two nonclinical groups of children and adolescents (mean ages = 9 yars, 4 months, 8 years, 4 months) were administered the CPT. The parents of the first group filled out the revised Conners Parent Rating Scale, while the teachers of the second group filled out the teacher version.

The CPT overall index correlated in a low to moderate fashion with most of the parent and teacher ratings, particularly with Cognitive Problems and the DSM-IV Inattentiveness Scale.

Conners' strategy of having the subject respond continuously and inhibit responses to the target stimulus, instead of responding only to the target stimulus, is certainly consistent with contemporary reformulations of ADHD such as Barkley's (1997a) response inhibition theory. In my clinical experience using the Conners CPT with adolescents and adults, they find this approach more challenging than having to respond only when the target stimulus appears. In theory, the Conners CPT may prove more sensitive to ADHD in brighter, older adolescents than the GDS, but any definitive conclusions will have to await an appropriately designed comparison study of the GDS and the Conners CPT.

Test of Variables of Attention

The Test of Variables of Attention (TOVA) is a 23-minute CPT administered on a microcomputer, but with a special microswitch that the subject uses to respond, which standardizes the equipment more than using a keyboard or mouse (Greenberg & Waldman, 1993). The TOVA is a non-language-based CPT in which the subject watches for designated targets and ignores nontargets. The subject is to respond when a small square appears inside of a larger square. Like the Conners CPT, the TOVA has normative data available from childhood through adulthood, collected with over 2,000 individuals ages 4 to 80+. It provides scores for omission errors, commission errors, response time, variability, and anticipatory errors. The length of the task is thought to make it a more sensitive measure with older adolescents and adults, who may partially compensate and attend effectively during shorter continuous performance tests. An auditory version is also available.

The TOVA has been found to be sensitive to developmental changes in attention and impulse control in a cross-sectional study of the children and adolescents in the normative sample and able to correctly identify 90% of ADHD and 87% of normal controls in discriminant analysis, with 13% false positives and 10% false negatives (Greenberg & Waldman, 1993). Waldman and Greenberg (1992) found that the TOVA was able to discriminate between different types of disruptive behavior disorders. They compared the TOVA responses of 75 ADHD youngsters diagnosed under DSM-III-R, 33 youngsters diagnosed as Undifferentiated ADD (UADD) under DSM-III-R, 17 youngsters with CD, and 775 nondisordered controls. The ADHD group was more inattentive than the UADD group; the ADHD and CD groups were more impulsive than the UADD and nondisordered groups; and the UADD group was more inattentive than the control group. The TOVA has also been found to be sensitive to medication effects and suggested as a method of monitoring the effects of medication (Corman & Greenberg, 1996). A check with the publisher confirmed my finding that to date, there are no published studies using the TOVA specifically with adolescents or indicating the discriminant power of the measure specifically with ADHD adolescents. Adolescents were clearly included in the broader normative research, although it is not clear whether they were included in the studies showing differences between ADHD and non-ADHD individuals or the sensitivity of medication effects.

Concluding Comment

Given this discussion, should the clinician incorporate LMs into routine clinical practice? At present, the CPT is the only laboratory measure that has proven effective in routine clinical assessment of ADHD. Frankly, the differential diagnosis of ADHD can be made in a reliable and valid way without the administration of a CPT. However, the CPT adds another dimension of corroboration and important information about performance under standardized conditions. How should the practitioner interpret the results of a CPT with regard to making the diagnosis of ADHD? Abnormal scores on a CPT are almost always consistent with a positive diagnosis of ADHD. However, normal scores are associated with up to a 25% rate of false negatives. Fischer et al. (1995) suggest that ADHD children with normal CPT scores have milder attentional problems but higher rates of comorbid conditions. Given the dearth of specific CPT research with adolescents, I err on the conservative side and generally consider a normal CPT score to be a somewhat equivocal result. In such cases, I make my diagnosis based on other measures.

Which CPT is more sensitive, valid, and clinically useful in work with adolescents? There is no data-based answer to this question at the present time as there have been no comparison studies of the GDS, the Conners CPT, and the TOVA with adolescents. The GDS is the only CPT that has been researched specifically with adolescents, and it is the only major CPT that comes with its own hardware, eliminating the need for and the confounds of using a microcomputer. However, the brighter, video-game-wise adolescents inevitably do well on it, despite turning out to have ADHD, in some cases severe ADHD. For these reasons, I have been experimenting with the Conners CPT with these individuals, but it is too soon to say whether the Conners CPT will prove any more sensitive for this population.

Practitioners will also have to take cost into account in selecting a CPT. The GDS is a one-time expenditure of approximately $1,595; the Conners CPT is a one-time expenditure of $495; and the TOVA costs $495 to purchase, with five free tests/interpretations, plus $15 per additional interpretation. The Conners CPT and TOVA prices do not include the cost of the microcomputer. Although most practitioners have a microcomputer available, they may not have one available in the dedicated manner needed for routine use in a busy clinical practice.

Finally, I caution practitioners not to rely primarily on the CPT to titrate medication doses, despite what the CPT manuals might suggest. Yes, CPTs are sensitive to medication effects. However, we have few data on the ecological validity of these CPT medication effects. We have no real idea of how a CPT medication effect correlates with a medication effect on classroom performance or interpersonal relations. Until such information is readily available, titrating medication to maximize CPT performance could easily result in prescribing too much or too little medication for optimal effects in the classroom or at home.

DIRECT OBSERVATION

Informal observation of the adolescent in the interview and testing situation can provide useful information about the youngster's physical appearance, demeanor, interaction style, and general behavioral repertoire. However, clinicians should not base diagnostic decisions primarily on such information because behavior in the clinic settings may be atypical of behavior with natural caregivers in the classroom or home setting (Barkley, 1990).

By contrast, systematic, formal behavioral observations in naturalistic or standardized analogue settings may prove useful in the diagnostic and assessment process. Ideally, the clinician would observe the adolescent interacting with his or her parents and siblings in the home and the community, and with his or her teachers, peers, and academic materials in the school. In fact, such observations have been conducted with younger hyperactive and/or oppositional children and found to be sensitive measures of ADHD behavior in the classroom (Abikoff, Gittelman-Klein, & Klein, 1977) and opposition in the home (Patterson, 1982). Behavioral observations of adolescents with ADHD have also been successfully conducted in an intensive summer treatment program environment that has the resources to carefully train coders to record the frequency of a wide variety of negative and positive social and academic behaviors, and the degree of control to standardize the setting such that meaningful normative data can be collected to permit treatment decisions. In this specialized setting, such observations have proven reliable, valid, and highly sensitive to medication effects (Pelham, Vodde-Hamilton, Murphy, Greenstein, & Vallano, 1991; Smith et al., 1997). To my knowledge, no systematic observational studies of naturalistic interactions between ADHD adolescents and their parents in the home have been published.

Realistically, the average clinician has neither the time nor the resources to conduct systematic direct observation in the classroom or the home setting. Even if the clinician had the time and resources, school-based observations would have be conducted in five to seven classes per student and would be highly reactive at the adolescent age group, and local norms would have to be collected by teacher and school as a basis for comparison. Parent–adolescent interactions are so highly mobile and distributed widely in time that the observers would virtually have to move in with the family to be present at the salient times (e.g., 1 A.M. on Saturday morning when Sally comes home 2 hours after curfew, 8 P.M. on Sunday night when the trash is to taken to the curb).

Fortunately, analogue clinic observations provide a practical alternative which may lose some ecological validity but nonetheless can provide clinically useful information for diagnostic and treatment planning purposes. Two types of analogue observations have been sufficiently studied and found to be reliable and valid to recommend them to the clinician: (1) Restricted Academic Situation as a measure of ADHD behaviors; and (2) verbal discussion task as a measure of parent–adolescent interaction.

Restricted Academic Situation

The use of the Restricted Academic Situation for the assessment of ADHD in adolescents was developed and researched by Barkley and his colleagues (Barkley, 1990; Barkley, Anastopoulos, Guevremont, & Fletcher, 1991; DuPaul, Guevremont, & Barkley, 1991; Fischer et al., 1990). The adolescent is seated alone at a desk in a clinic room equipped with a one-way mirror and observed while attempting to complete a large set of boring mathematics problems. The math problems typically involve basic operations, with enough problems across difficulty levels provided to ensure that the adolescent does not finish the task within the 15-minute observation period. A stereo cassette tape player nearby plays rock music at a moderate volume to serve as a potential distractor. The adolescent is asked to complete as many of the mathematics problems as possible within 15 minutes. The adolescent is either observed live or videotaped through the one-way mirror while completing these tasks.

The live observations or videotapes are coded for the initial occurrence of five behaviors within 30-second intervals. A tape recording that contains cues for the beginning of each 30-second interval is either played or superimposed on the videotape to cue the observers. The observer records the first occurrence only of each behavior per interval. The five behaviors include (1) off-task—teen interrupts his or her attention to the tasks and engages in some other behavior; (2) fidgeting—any repetitive, purposeless motion of the legs, arms, hands, buttocks, or trunk (swaying back and forth, swinging arms at one's side, shuffling feet, shifting about in the chair, pencil tapping); (3) vocalizing—any vocal noise or verbalization (speech, whispering, singing, odd noises); (4) playing with objects—touching any object in the room besides his or her own clothes, the table, chair, math problems, and pencil; and (5) out of seat—any time the teen's buttocks breaks contact with the flat surface of the seat. The coding sheets, procedures, and elaborated definitions of the five behaviors have been published in two sources (Barkley, 1990, 1991a).

Two studies have examined the reliability and criterion-related validity of the Restricted Academic Situation with ADHD adolescents. As one aspect of the follow-up study described in Chapter 2 (this volume), Fischer et al. (1990) compared the behavior of 100 hyperactive and 60 control adolescents in the Restricted Academic Situation. Using a separate sample, Barkley, Anastopoulos, et al. (1991) also compared the behavior of 84 clinic-referred adolescents with ADHD to 77 demographically comparable community controls in the Restricted Academic Situation. Both studies found that the adolescents with ADHD exhibited more off-task behavior, fidgeting, and out-of seat behavior than did the controls. Fischer et al. (1990) also noted differences on vocalizing and playing with objects. Barkley, Anastopoulos, et al. (1990) found that the ADHD group completed fewer math problems than did the controls, but there were no differences on the accuracy of their work. A comparison of younger (mean age = 12 years, 9 months) versus older (mean age = 16 years, 9 months) adolescents indicated that younger adolescents were more likely to be off-task, out of seat, and playing with objects than the older adolescents, regardless of whether or not they had ADHD. Agreement reliabilities ranged from .83 for fidgeting to .99 for out-of-seat behavior. Barkley, Anastopoulos, et al. (1991) conducted a discriminant function analysis to compare the contributions to group discrimination of the Restricted Academic Measures, WRAT-R achievement scores, the Selective Reminding Test of memory, the MFFT-20, and the GDS. Most of the Restricted Academic Situation measures were among the most powerful discriminators of ADHD versus control subjects. However, the investigators did not compare the power of the Restricted Academic Situation to the clinical interview and rating scales to determine its clinical utility in making the initial diagnosis of ADHD. Such comparisons are necessary to inform the clinician about whether the effort and time involved in setting up, administering, and coding the Restricted Academic Situation yield a reasonable return in diagnostic accuracy.

It may also be instructive to record adolescent behavior with these five categories during the administration of a CPT such as the GDS. Barkley, DuPaul, and McMurray (1990) found such observations to be as powerful as the CPT itself in discriminating ADHD from non-ADHD children, although the investigators have not specifically looked at this effect with adolescents.

In clinical applications of the Restricted Academic Situation, we must keep in mind the natural decrease in overt hyperactive behaviors that occurs in adolescence. The significant age effect in the research reinforces this impression. Many ADHD symptoms become more subjective by middle or late adolescence. On the other hand, the Restricted Academic Situation is a good approximation of the homework setting, where the adolescent is in a room with distractions faced with boring, onerous academic tasks. However, clinicians must keep in mind that it may be necessary to add extra distraction (e.g., a television) to music to make the setting sensitive; many adolescents with ADHD routinely play music while doing homework. Product measures such as the number of mathematics problems completed may turn out to be most sensitive in the older adolescent age group. Further research is needed to clarify the utility of this measure across the entire age range of adolescence and to study variations such as having the adolescent bring in his or her own homework rather than using standardized math problems. Asking the older adolescent to rate his or her own subjective restlessness and concentration using a brief instrument such as the Conners–Wells Adolescent Self-Report Scale ADHD Index or the Sustained Attention subscales of the Brown ADD Scales at the end of the 15-minute observation may also prove illuminating.

Parent–Adolescent Verbal Discussion Tasks

I have extensively employed verbal discussion tasks as analogue measures of positive and negative communication and problem solving between parents and adolescents (Robin & Foster, 1989), and these measures have been validated for use with ADHD adolescents in the two studies discussed in Chapter 2 of this volume (Barkley, Anastopoulos, et al., 1992; Barkley, Fischer, et al., 1991). The parents and adolescent are asked to discuss and try to reach an agreement concerning several topics, for 10 minutes per topic. I usually employ one neutral topic (e.g., plan a family vacation) and one conflictual topic. I select the conflictual topic by examining the issues with the highest anger/intensity scores on the Issues Checklist (discussed in Chapter 3). Barkley, Fischer, et al. (1991) also add a positive discussion (e.g., describe the most positive characteristic of the other discussant). In a clinical situation with limited time, a single conflictual topic would suffice.

The discussions are audiotaped or videotaped for later coding. In research applications, I have coded these tapes with detailed, molecular coding systems such as the Parent Adolescent Interaction Code System (PAICS), which Barkley used in his two studies. The PAICS categorizes every utterance into positive or negative communication categories. However, it requires extensive training of coders and is not practical in clinical situations. Instead, a global inferential coding system such as the Interaction Behavior Code (IBC) might be used (Prinz & Kent, 1978; Robin & Foster, 1989). After listening to or watching an entire 10-minute discussion, the coder rates the presence of 32 behaviors such as yelling, negative exaggeration, making accusations, and compromise, each of which is accompanied by a brief definition. Table 5.3. presents the IBC. Twenty-two behaviors are rated "Present (1 point)" or "Absent (0 point)" if they occurred once or more during the discussion; 11 others are rated "Absent

TABLE 5.3. Interaction Behavior Code (IBC)

Family Name _____

Rater _____

Date _____

Please listen to or watch the entire discussion and then rate each of these items. Rate items 1–22 and 32–38 as absent (No) or present (Yes). Rate items 23–31 as Absent (1), A Little (2), or A Lot (3).

NEGATIVES	Mom	Teen	Dad
1. Repeating one's opinion with insistence	Y/N	Y/N	Y/N
2. Denying responsibility	Y/N	Y/N	Y/N
3. Disregarding the other person's points	Y/N	Y/N	Y/N
4. Interrupting with criticism	Y/N	Y/N	Y/N
5. Making quick, negative judgment of other's suggestion	Y/N	Y/N	Y/N
6. Humoring, discounting	Y/N	Y/N	Y/N
7. Asking accusing questions	Y/N	Y/N	Y/N
8. Ridiculing, making fun of	Y/N	Y/N	Y/N
9. Threatening	Y/N	Y/N	Y/N
10. Name calling (negative)	Y/N	Y/N	Y/N
11. Yelling	Y/N	Y/N	Y/N
12. Making demands	Y/N	Y/N	Y/N
13. Negatively exaggerating	Y/N	Y/N	Y/N
14. Giving short, unhelpful responses	Y/N	Y/N	Y/N
15. Using big words	Y/N	Y/N	Y/N
16. Arguing over small points	Y/N	Y/N	Y/N
17. Talking very little (throughout)	Y/N	Y/N	Y/N
18. Talking a great deal (throughout)	Y/N	Y/N	Y/N
19. Mind reading	Y/N	Y/N	Y/N
20. Dwelling on the past	Y/N	Y/N	Y/N
21. Abruptly changing of subject	Y/N	Y/N	Y/N
22. Failing to make eye contact	Y/N	Y/N	Y/N

	1 = Absent	2 = A Little	3 = A Lot
23. Anger	1 2 3	1 2 3	1 2 3
24. Personal attack	1 2 3	1 2 3	1 2 3
25. Criticism	1 2 3	1 2 3	1 2 3
26. Sarcasm	1 2 3	1 2 3	1 2 3
27. Demanding (coercive)	1 2 3	1 2 3	1 2 3
28. Acquiescence (over agree)	1 2 3	1 2 3	1 2 3
29. Silence; ignoring others	1 2 3	1 2 3	1 2 3
30. Lecturing; preaching	1 2 3	1 2 3	1 2 3
31. Fidgeting; slouching	1 2 3	1 2 3	1 2 3

TABLE 5.3 *(continued)*

POSITIVES	Mom	Teen	Dad
32. Stating the other's opinion	Y/N	Y/N	Y/N
33. Making suggestions	Y/N	Y/N	Y/N
34. Asking what the other would like, wants	Y/N	Y/N	Y/N
35. Praising, complimenting	Y/N	Y/N	Y/N
36. Joking (good natured)	Y/N	Y/N	Y/N
37. Listening	Y/N	Y/N	Y/N
38. Compromising	Y/N	Y/N	Y/N

SUMMARY SCORES

For each agent, convert the scores to points and sum the negative and positive item points separately. For items 1–22 and 32–38, "No" = 0 points and "Yes" = 1 point. For items 23–31, "Absent" or 1 = 0 points, "A Little" or 2 = .5 points, and "A Lot" or 3 = 1 point. Record the following summary scores.

Mother:　　Negative Behavior _____
　　　　　　Positive Behavior _____

Teenager:　Negative Behavior _____
　　　　　　Positive Behavior _____

Father:　　 Negative Behavior _____
　　　　　　Positive Behavior _____

Note. Adapted from Robin & Foster (1989). Copyright 1989 by The Guilford Press. Reprinted in *ADHD in Adolescents: Diagnosis and Treatment* by Arthur L. Robin. Permission to photocopy this table is granted to purchasers of *ADHD in Adolescents* for personal use only (see copyright page for details).

(0)," "A Little (0.5)," or "A Lot (1)." Points are totaled separately for positive and negative categories, as indicated in Table 5.3.

A single clinician can easily complete such ratings. In research, several coders rate each tape, and the mean of their ratings is used as the dependent variable. Reliabilities of the mean score have averaged .83 to .97, and the IBC has been found to be discriminate between families with and without conflict and to be sensitive to family treatment (Robin & Foster, 1989). To date, no studies using the IBC have been done solely with ADHD adolescents, but most of the adolescents in the existing research meet the DSM-III or DSM-III-R criteria for ODD.

Concluding Comment

Direct observation has become the hallmark of behavioral approaches to assessment and therapy (Mash & Terdal, 1997). Such approaches are more costly and difficult to apply to adolescents with ADHD than to younger children and may not always tap the most relevant content, as ADHD symptoms become more subjective by adolescence. Nonetheless, I have illustrated two areas in which clinician might choose to use behavioral observations.

GENERAL CONCLUSION

This chapter discusses how to conduct an LD evaluation, how to determine whether ADHD is creating educational impairment, how to use laboratory measures such as CPTs, and how to integrate direct observation into the comprehensive evaluation for ADHD. IQ and achievement tests are an essential part of the ADHD evaluation and should be administered either by the clinician or by the adolescent's school. By contrast, CPTs and direct observational techniques richly enhance the overall clinical picture of the adolescent and his or her family, but are not absolutely essential in the "stripped down, no frills" managed care ADHD evaluation. It is now time to turn our attention to the integration of all of the diverse sources of information, as the clinician reaches a diagnostic conclusion.

CHAPTER SIX

—————————— O ——————————

Integration of Data

After sifting through all the rating scales, interviews, continuous performance tests (CPTs), and direct observations, the practitioner must eventually come to a decision about the diagnosis of ADHD or a differential diagnosis, any comorbid conditions, and any educational impairments. I organize all the information in a worksheet such as Table 6.1 and then mull it over, looking for patterns and consistencies and attempting to explain any inconsistencies. Clinicians should ask themselves the following questions:

1. To what extent do the interview data, parent, teacher, and adolescent rating scales all converge upon a diagnosis of ADHD? If there are internal inconsistencies between these various sources of data, have we sufficiently explained them to nonetheless conclude that ADHD is present?
2. To what extent have we ruled out competing explanations of whatever ADHD symptoms we uncovered, or ruled them in as comorbid conditions?
3. To what extent can we rule out family and/or environmental factors as alternative explanations of ADHD symptoms?
4. How do we explain a CPT in the normal range?
5. What can we learn from the youngster's cognitive ability and achievement profile that will color our decision about the basic diagnosis?
6. Does the information show evidence of educational impairment?

The clinician must reach one of three conclusions regarding the ADHD diagnosis: (1) confirmed, (2) disconfirmed, or (3) deferred. He or she should defer the diagnosis when the information is incomplete, or there

173

TABLE 6.1. ADHD Diagnostic Worksheet

Name _____   Date of Evaluation _____
Date of Birth _____   Parents _____
Age _____   Examiner _____

WISC-III/WAIS-III

Full Scale IQ   _____
Verbal IQ   _____
Performance IQ   _____

Verbal Scaled Scores		Performance Scaled Scores	
Information	___	Picture Completion	___
Digit Span	___	Picture Arrangement	___
Vocabulary	___	Block Design	___
Arithmetic	___	Matrix Reasoning—WAIS-III	___
Comprehension	___	Object Assembly	___
Similarities	___	Digit Symbol/Coding	___
		Symbol Search	___

WIAT

Subtest	Predicted Standardized Score	Actual Standardized Score	Difference	Significance
Basic Reading	___	___	___	___
Math Reasoning	___	___	___	___
Spelling	___	___	___	___
Reading Comprehension	___	___	___	___
Numerical Operations	___	___	___	___

Gordon Diagnostic System (GDS)

Delay Task	Efficiency Ratio	____
Vigilance Task	Correct Responses	____
	Commission Errors	____
Distractibility Task	Correct Responses	____
	Commission Errors	____

DSM-IV ADHD Behavior Checklist

	Teen	Mom	Dad
Number of Inattention Items—2 or 3:	___	___	___
Summation Score—Inattention:	___	___	___
Number of Hyperactivity–Impulsivity Items—2 or 3:	___	___	___
Summation Score—Hyperactivity–Impulsivity:	___	___	___

Brown Attention Deficit Disorder Scale—Adolescent Version

Total Raw Score:	___	
Subscale *T*-Scores:	Activating to Tasks	___
	Sustaining Attention	___
	Sustaining Effort	___
	Managing Affect	___
	Working Memory	___

Beck Depression Inventory ___

TABLE 6.1 *(continued)*

Conners Parent Rating Scale—Revised Long Form (*T*-Scores)

	Mother	Father
Oppositional	——	——
Cognitive Problems	——	——
Anxiety/Shyness	——	——
Perfectionism	——	——
Social Problems	——	——
Psychosomatic	——	——
Conners Global Index (CGI)	——	——
CGI Restless/Impulsive	——	——
CGI Emotional Lability	——	——
ADHD Index	——	——
DSM-IV Total Score	——	——
DSM-IV Inattentive Score	——	——
DSM-IV Hyperactive–Impulsive Score	——	——

Child Behavior Checklist (*T*-scores)

Withdrawn	——
Somatic Complaints	——
Anxious/Depressed	——
Social Problems	——
Thought Problems	——
Attention Problems	——
Delinquent Behavior	——
Aggressive Behavior	——

Child Attention Profile	Inattention	Overactivity	Comments
(Subjects)	(7 is cutoff)	(5 is cutoff)	
———	——	——	
———	——	——	
———	——	——	
———	——	——	
	——	——	
Mean Score	——	——	

Percentage Assignments Completed on Time

	Student evaluated	Average student	Difference
———	——	——	——
———	——	——	——
———	——	——	——
———	——	——	——
———	——	——	——
Mean Score	——	——	——

ADHD History Grid (items were checked as problems)

—————————————
—————————————
—————————————

Note. From *ADHD in Adolescents: Diagnosis and Treatment* by Arthur L. Robin. Copyright 1998 by The Guilford Press. Permission to photocopy this table is granted to purchasers of *ADHD in Adolescents* for personal use only (see copyright page for details).

is so much environmental chaos that we cannot rule ADHD in or out. For example, youngsters removed by protective services or caught in the middle of a bitter divorce may really have ADHD, but it may be impossible to rule it in or out until their environment stabilizes. I usually require at least 6 months of a relatively stable environment in such cases before I make a definitive diagnosis. Of course, each case is a little different, and I sometimes make exceptions to this rule.

The best way to help the practitioner answer these questions is to present case examples. I present two case studies to help the practitioner see how to integrate all the data sources, reach a conclusion, and make recommendations. I personally evaluated each of these adolescents; the cases have been slightly modified to ensure anonymity. I present the cases studies here in the form of the evaluation report, which was completed after each evaluation, followed by a brief commentary.

These reports are representative of the level of detail I put into such a report. Although a much more detailed report might be more helpful to some audiences, and in fact such detailed reports have been presented as models in other professional books (Goldstein, 1997), most referral sources, therapists, and school systems are going to look primarily at the data page, conclusions, and recommendations rather than all the details. More important, in this era of managed care, practitioners do not get paid adequately for the time it takes to write such reports, to justify writing them routinely. Practitioners must achieve a reasonable compromise between being comprehensive and being realistic about what they can afford to do on a routine basis. I always give parents the option of having a more encyclopedic report if they wish to pay for the time it takes to write it; none have ever taken advantage of this option. In the cases that follow, the data tables are sometimes more comprehensive than those in the original reports to help the reader understand the cases. Typically, I send out a data page consisting of the IQ, achievement, and CPT scores, but not the scores on the ratings scales and questionnaires. It should also be noted that these cases include older versions of several measures such as the WAIS-R. Today. I use the updated versions, which have been incorporated into Table 6.1.

CASE 1: ADHD, INATTENTIVE SUBTYPE

ADHD Consultation Report

Name: Sylvie Nichols
Date of Evaluation: 5/12/96
Date of Birth: 1/31/80; Age: 16 years, 3 months
Parents: David and Joan Nichols
Examiner: Arthur L. Robin, PhD, Licensed Psychologist

Referral Question

Sylvie Nichols was referred by her therapist, Mrs. Jennifer Snead, for an evaluation to determine whether she has Attention-Deficit/Hyperactivity Disorder (ADHD), in addition to depression, oppositional behavior, and family conflict.

Background Information

Sylvie presented as a 16-year-old attending 11th grade at Franklin High School in Bloomfield Hills, who is currently experiencing serious academic difficulties. She reports that she has a difficult time getting focused on school and homework, is unable to consistently complete academic tasks, is unable to get or remain organized in school and at home, is forgetful in many situations, and is easily distracted. Although present since at least fifth grade, these difficulties really began to create educational impairments upon Sylvie's entry into ninth grade, when the demands for performance increased tremendously. There is no current or past history of impulsive behavior, hyperactivity, or significant conduct problems, and Sylvie has a close, loving relationship with her parents. Conflicts and disagreements between Sylvie and her parents are primarily limited to school-related matters.

Born following her mother's normal pregnancy, Sylvie's early medical and developmental histories were within the normal developmental range. She walked somewhat early at 9½ months, spoke single words by 11 months, spoke sentences by 20 months, and was toilet trained by 24 months. Bedwetting, however, continued to be a problem until age 11, and Sylvie was reported always to have been a very deep sleeper. She has no history of chronic illnesses or unusual acute illnesses and has not required any surgery, but she did break and dislocate her left wrist at age 5 (she is right-handed). In the second year of life, she had frequent ear infections.

Mrs. Nichols indicated that from birth Sylvie always had a very easy-going temperament and was happy, quiet, easy to please, and smiled a lot. She has no history of emotional outbursts, significant defiant behavior, or any other unusual behavioral patterns as a young child.

School history revealed that Sylvie did well in elementary school, completing her homework and following teacher instructions, until fifth grade. During her fifth-grade year, her teacher began to report that Sylvie was frequently daydreaming, not keeping up with the class, and not paying attention. There were, however, no concerns about her behavior or social adjustment. Her fifth-grade teacher was highly structured and expected a great deal of independent effort and work from her students to prepare them for middle school. Throughout middle school, Sylvie had an increasingly difficult time keeping up with her assignments, listening in class, and getting and staying organized. Her mother recalled many trips back to the school to get books and papers which Sylvie forgot to bring home, and a lot of credit lost due to misplaced or late assignments. She had the most difficulty with math and science, and the least difficulty with English and language arts. The difficulties with organization, follow-through, and assignments worsened considerably in 9th and 10th grade, to the point where Sylvie's marginal grades (C's, D's) were beginning to interfere with her participation in school sports.

During the middle school years Sylvie blossomed into a world-class athlete. Always highly coordinated in terms of gross motor and visual–motor acuity, she joined the swimming team in sixth grade and by the end of eighth grade was considered a champion swimmer. Throughout high school, she has swum on the junior varsity and then the varsity team, and competed in regional and statewide meets. During the summer she works as a life guard and swims on a team at a local pool. Her goal is to make the Olympics, and judging from the fact that she is being recruited by several college swimming coaches in 11th grade, it is possible that she might achieve this goal some day.

Several traumatic events occurred during the first few weeks of her 11th-grade year. She broke up with her first serious boyfriend, with whom she had been going for 10 months. The swimming team got a new coach, who showed favoritism toward several other girls on the team and replaced Sylvie in a number of meets, which upset her a great deal. Her closest girlfriend moved to Georgia, and her pet cat, which she had since she was 6, was run over and killed by a car. Taken together, these events lead Sylvie to become quite depressed and frustrated, feeling as if her whole world was caving in. This depressive period lasted for several weeks. She did not want to go to school or do anything. She ran away from home and stayed with a friend for 3 days. Her parents then took her to her current therapist, who after several sessions also recommended this evaluation. Sylvie has established good rapport with her therapist, and is feeling much less depressed now. However, her academic difficulties at school are worsening.

Measures Administered (See Table 6.2)

Wechsler Adult Intelligence Scale—Revised (WAIS-R)
Wechsler Individual Achievement Test (WIAT)
Gordon Diagnostic System (GDS)
DSM-IV ADHD Behavior Checklist (Parents and Teen)
Brown Attention Deficit Disorder Scales
Beck Depression Inventory
ADHD History Grid
Conners Parent Rating Scale
Child Behavior Checklist

TABLE 6.2. Psychological Test Scores for Sylvie Nichols

Name <u>Sylvie Nichols</u>   Date of Evaluation <u>5/12/96</u>
Date of Birth <u>1/31/80</u>   Parents <u>David and Joan Nichols</u>
Age <u>16-3</u>   Examiner <u>Arthur L. Robin, PhD</u>

WAIS-R

Full Scale IQ	102	Average
Verbal IQ	99	Average
Performance IQ	104	Average

Verbal Scaled Scores		Performance Scaled Scores	
Information	8	Picture Completion	7
Digit Span	10	Picture Arrangement	10
Vocabulary	9	Block Design	10
Arithmetic	6	Object Assembly	13
Comprehension	8	Digit Symbol	10
Similarities	9		

WIAT

Subtest	Predicted Standardized Score	Actual Standardized Score	Difference	Significance
Basic Reading	101	102	−1	N.S.
Math Reasoning	102	121	−19	N.S.
Spelling	101	104	−3	N.S.
Reading Comprehension	101	97	4	N.S.
Numerical Operations	101	109	−8	N.S.

Gordon Diagnostic System (GDS)

Delay Task	Efficiency Ratio	.89 (>.83 is normal)
Vigilance Task	Correct Responses	43 Normal
	Commission Errors	2 Normal
Distractibility Task	Correct Responses	32 Borderline
	Commission Errors	3 Normal

DSM-IV ADHD Behavior Checklist

	Teen	Mom	Dad
Number of Inattention Items—2 or 3:	9*	9*	9*
Number of Hyperactivity–Impulsivity Items—2 or 3:	1	1	1
Number of ODD Items—2 or 3:	0	0	0

Brown Attention Deficit Disorder Scale—Adolescent Version

Total Raw Score:	98*	
Subscale *T*-Scores:	Activating to Tasks	80*
	Sustaining Attention	74*
	Sustaining Effort	87*
	Managing Affect	63
	Working Memory	88*

(*continued*)

TABLE 6.2 *(continued)*

Beck Depression Inventory 16

Conners Parent Rating Scale (*T*-scores)

	Mother	Father
Conduct Problems	39	39
Learning Problems	100+*	93*
Psychosomatic	41	41
Impulsive–Hyperactive	38	38
Anxiety	40	40
Hyperactivity Index	61	55

Child Behavior Checklist (*T*-scores)

Activities	46
Social	55
School	35*
Withdrawn	70*
Somatic Complaints	56
Anxious/Depressed	50
Social Problems	50
Thought Problems	63*
Attention Problems	69*
Delinquent Behavior	51
Aggressive Behavior	50

Child Attention Profile	Inattention	Overactivity	Comments
(Subjects)	(7 is cutoff)	(5 is cutoff)	
French	7*	1	Incomplete Assignments
Algebra	12*	4	Incomplete Assignments, Daydreams
English	2	0	None
Chemistry	9*	3	Doesn't pay attention
History	4	2	Excellent student
Mean Score	6.8	2.0	

Percentage Assignments Completed on Time

	Sylvie	Average student	Difference
French	65	85	−20
Algebra	25	80	−55
English	80	85	−5
Chemistry	55	85	−40
History	90	85	10
Mean Score	63	84	21

ADHD History Grid (3 items were checked as problems from 5th through 11th grades)

Paying attention
Completing classwork
Sloppy schoolwork

* Significant elevation.

ADHD Symptoms

On the DSM-IV ADHD Behavior Checklist, Mr. and Mrs. Nichols and Sylvie concurred that Sylvie exhibits all nine of the inattention symptoms but only one of the hyperactivity–impulsivity symptoms. On the Brown ADD Scales, Sylvie's total score of 98 was far above the cutoff of 50, consistent with ADHD; on the subscales, she reported significant clinical elevations for activating to tasks, sustaining attention, maintaining effort, and working memory (but not managing affect). Both her mother and father rated her in the clinical range for Learning Problems on the Conners Parent Rating Scale but not for Conduct Problems, Impulsive–Hyperactive, or the Hyperactivity Index. Her mother rated Sylvie as clinically distressed on the Child Behavior Checklist for School Problems, Attention Problems, Withdrawn, and Thought Problems (stares was the only item checked).

Five teachers completed the Child Attention Profile. Sylvie's French, algebra, and chemistry teachers reported that she displayed clinically significant degrees of inattention and associated difficulties completing assignments. Her English and history teachers did not report any such difficulties. None of the teachers noted any overactivity or impulsivity. The teachers also reported the percentage of Sylvie's assignments completed on time and similar data for the average student. Sylvie is getting considerably less done than her peers in French, algebra, and chemistry.

Although her performance on the Delay and Vigilance tasks of the GDS was in the normal range, her score for the number of correct responses was in the borderline range on the Distractibility Task, with increasing numbers of errors across successive blocks. Commission errors were within normal limits. These GDS findings suggest that when the demands for sustained attention are made more difficult by adding extraneous stimulation, Sylvie's performance deteriorates, and this deterioration worsens over time, but that there is no evidence for difficulties with impulse control.

Clinical interviewing with Sylvie corroborated the other measures. She reported that she feels "like my mind is a TV remote constantly changing channels" and that it has become very difficult to concentrate on reading a book, listening to a lecture, or buckling down to study for an exam. Sylvie indicated that she had always had difficulty with concentration, but she never really had to study or exert much effort academically until ninth grade. She often finds herself reading the same page of her chemistry textbook over and over again and has no idea what she just read. She also reported numerous examples of forgetfulness, is disorganized in how she keeps her clothes, CDs, and other things, and is chronically late.

Results of Cognitive Testing/Learning Disability

Sylvie related well to the examiner and was attentive during the testing situation, but become mentally fatigued and somewhat distractible toward the end. On the Wechsler Adult Intelligence Scale—Revised, she obtained a Full Scale IQ of 102, with a Verbal IQ of 99 and a Performance IQ of 104. These scores place her in the average overall range of intellectual ability, with average verbal and average performance abilities. In the verbal area, she received average scores on subtests of cultural information, short-term memory, word knowledge, and abstract reasoning, but low-average scores on subtests of mental arithmetic and commonsense reasoning. In the performance area, she received a high-average score on the subtest of part–whole assembly, average scores on the subtests of visual sequencing, nonverbal abstract reasoning, and motor speed and accuracy but a low-average score on the subtests of fine motor discrimination.

On the Wechsler Individual Achievement Test, she obtained average scores in Basic Reading, Spelling, Reading Comprehension, and Numerical Calculations, but a superior score in Math Reasoning. A discrepancy analysis of achievement predicted by Full Scale IQ and actual achievement, using the regression tables provided in the WIAT manual, revealed no significant differences. Thus, there is no evidence suggestive of a specific learning disability.

Differential Diagnosis

Extensive clinical interviewing did not reveal the current presence of any clinically significant mood, anxiety, or other psychiatric disorders. The depressive reaction which Sylvie had to the difficult circumstances at the beginning of 11th grade was explored in depth. Sylvie was appropriately sad about significant losses in her life. She was also frustrated and upset about her increasing inability to keep up in school. These events overwhelmed her at the time she ran away, and at that time she could be seen as having met the criteria for a Major Depressive Episode. However, her mood was no longer so severely depressed, although she probably could be seen as meeting the current criteria for a Sadness Problem in the DSM-PC, but not a DSM-IV Mood Disorder. In addition, the chronically increasing course of her organizational and attentional problems could not be explained on the basis of these episodes of depressive affect or any other psychiatric condition.

Conclusions and Recommendations

The results of this evaluation indicate that Sylvie Nichols meets the criteria for an Attention-Deficit/Hyperactivity Disorder, Predominantly Inattentive Subtype, with a recent past history of a Major Depressive Episode. Her chronic pattern of poor focus, poor task completion, poor organization, and forgetfulness cuts across situations but does not include any impulsivity, hyperactivity, or conduct problems. No other psychiatric syndromes could explain these findings, and cognitive testing further revealed that

Sylvie has average intellectual ability with commensurately average cumulative achievement. These ADHD symptoms are creating significant impairment, as judged from Sylvie's poor grades and low percentage of assignments completed, the running-away episode, and her emotional turmoil.

I made three recommendations to Sylvie and her parents:

Medical. Sylvie is highly likely to benefit from a trial on stimulant medication, dosed to help her with focus, attention, and concentration during school and when completing homework. She was referred to Dr. Howard Schubiner for medical treatment of ADHD.

Psychological. Continued therapy with Mrs. Snead is also essential for helping Sylvie learn to cope with the impact of ADHD on her life. Therapy should focus on (1) life management skills, such as the efficient use of a planner and lists; (2) stress and anger-management techniques; (3) self-esteem issues; and (4) family interaction.

Educational. Based on the teacher reports in three subjects of relatively low percentage of assignments completed, it is strongly suspected that Sylvie's ADHD is educationally handicapping her in school. It is therefore strongly recommended that the Bloomfield Hills Public Schools conduct an appropriate evaluation to determine the presence of such a handicapping condition, then develop a Section 504 plan to accommodate Sylvie's handicap. The following accommodations may be helpful to Sylvie: (1) being seated near the teacher, (2) teacher standing near her when giving directions, (3) adjusting the workload in selected subjects, (4) teacher giving her copies of overheads and teacher notes for lectures, (5) note-taking training, (6) redirecting her to the task if distracted, (7) breaking down long-term assignments into shorter units and monitoring her performance step by step, (8) permitting her to have extra time for examinations and to take them in a nondistracting environment, (9) regular meetings with a case manager who will help her plan and organize her approach to getting homework done and studying for examination, (10) instruction in efficient reading and study techniques, and (11) careful selection of courses and teachers.

Arthur L. Robin, PhD
Licensed Psychologist

Comment

It would have been easy to attribute Sylvie's current academic difficulties to the environmental stresses, which also accounted for her recent depression, rather than diagnosing ADHD. However, careful analysis of the rating scales and history indicated that the increasingly prevalent pattern of attentional and organizational difficulties has been occurring for some time. In addition, the borderline score on the Distractibility Task of the GDS was a tip-off as depression is not associated with any abnormalities on CPTs. In fact, when the therapist noted that these school difficulties persisted despite Sylvie's rebound from depression, she referred Sylvie for an ADHD evaluation. Sylvie presented the way most girls diagnosed as ADHD present: without excessive hyperactivity and impulsivity but with some associated internalizing behavioral problem features. Because the girls do not disrupt their classrooms or families, they do not get referred for evaluation until ADHD clearly impairs their academic or later vocational functioning. Many suffer silently through their adolescents and even into adulthood, with terrible self-esteem, not understanding why they cannot meet the expectations put upon them. Readers interested in a thorough clinical account of the lifelong course of ADHD, Inattentive Type, in women might consult *Women with Attention Deficit Disorder* (Solden, 1995).

CASE 2: ODD; TEACHERS AND PARENTS SHOPPING FOR AN ADHD DIAGNOSIS

ADHD Consultation Report

Name: Mark Bergen
Date of Evaluation: 12/6/95
Date of Birth: 12/12/83; Age: 12 years, 11 months
Parents: John and Ann Bergen
Examiner: Arthur L. Robin, PhD

Referral Question

Mark Bergen was referred for an evaluation of ADHD and possible learning disabilities by his therapist, Dr. Katz, after his teachers suggested that Mark "has an ADHD profile."

Background Information

Mark presented as a 12 years, 11-month-old sixth-grader at Crestwood Middle School in Dearborn, Michigan, who is displaying significant behavioral and academic problems primarily in school. Mark's primary academic teacher, Mrs. Jones, complains that he disrupts the class by talking out of turn, teasing other youngsters, or responding in a sarcastic manner when called on to answer a question. Further, she complains that he does not keep his place in the materials, does not follow her directions, and fails to complete his in-class or homework assignments in a timely manner. She indicated that Mark is a "strong, take-charge personality" who is extremely popular with his peers, independent, and a leader. Sometimes, he incites his peers to pick on weaker children, and they follow his leadership, for better or worse. He does not easily take "no" for an answer, even from adults, whose authority he frequently challenges. In one recent episode, for example, when told not to take his shoes off in class, he purposely took them off and threw them across the room into the trash. Mrs. Jones has an ADHD child of her own and felt that Mark displays "the profile of an ADHD child." On that basis, she suggested to his parents that they have him evaluated.

Mark was certified as learning disabled (LD) in speech and language during his kindergarten year and received resource room services and speech/language intervention from kindergarten through sixth grade. He was recently decertified as no longer formally meeting LD criteria in fourth grade but was offered one class period per day continued help in a resource room.

Mark resides with his natural parents and 14-year-old brother. His father is a physician and his mother is a nurse. At home his parents deal with Mark's strong personality by not placing a great deal of structure or demands on him. They do report some difficulties with defiant behavior but appear to minimize the extent of these problems compared to the teachers. They reframe much of their son's defiant behavior as "independence," which they encourage. They view their son's teachers as "repressive" of his freedom of expression. Both Mr. and Mrs. Bergen have a history of having been very liberal and leaders in the Students for a Democratic Society movement during the 1970s, which may have colored their attitudes toward defiant behavior.

Mark's birth and early developmental history were unexceptional. He walked at 11 months, spoke single words at 13 months, spoke sentences at 23 months, and was toilet trained by 30 months. He cried a great deal as a baby and was not easily adaptable to change. Mark's medical history was significant for severe asthma, first diagnosed at age 3. He has been hospitalized on six occasions for asthma attacks, and has 5 to 10 visits to the emergency room per year for asthma. The chronic illness has caused his parents to be very worried about his health and to be somewhat lenient in their discipline, tolerating relatively high levels of defiance. Fortunately, his asthma has improved in the past 2 years, and he rarely has a bad attack now.

Family psychiatric history was significant for maternal depression, severe paternal dyslexia, and a maternal uncle with schizophrenia and substance abuse who committed suicide, in 1985. No close relatives had ADHD.

Measures Administered (See Table 6.3)

Wechsler Intelligence Scale for Children—III (WISC-III)
Woodcock–Johnson Psycho-Educational Battery—Revised (administered by schools)
Gordon Diagnostic System (GDS)
DSM-IV ADHD Behavior Checklist (Parents, Teachers, Teen)
Brown Attention Deficit Disorder Scales
ADHD History Grid
Conners Parent Rating Scale
Child Behavior Checklist
Teacher Report Form
Child Attention Profile
Conflict Behavior Questionnaire
Issues Checklist

ADHD Symptoms

On the DSM-IV ADHD Behavior Checklist, Mr. Bergen reported that Mark exhibits 3 inattention symptoms and Mrs. Bergen reported three inattention symptoms. Neither reported any Hyperactivity–Impulsivity symptoms. They also reported that Mark exhibits two ODD symptoms. Mrs. Jones reported that Mark exhibits seven Inattention and eight Hyperactivity–Impulsivity symptoms, along with six ODD symptoms. Mrs. Shirsky, Mark's resource room teacher, reports that he exhibits three Inattention, two Hyperactivity–Impulsivity, and five ODD symptoms. Mark reported only one Inattention, two Hyperactivity–Impulsivity, and zero ODD symptoms.

On the Conners Parent Rating Scale, Mr. and Mrs. Bergen indicated that Mark displays clinically significant levels of Conduct Problems, but no other significant elevations. On the Child Behavior Checklist, Mrs. Bergen's scores included significantly low functioning on the School scale and significant elevations for Aggressive Behavior but not for Attention Problems.

By contrast, Mrs. Jones reported significant problems on the Teacher Report Form for Social Problems, Thought Problems, Attention Problems, Delinquent Behavior, and Aggressive Behavior; Mrs. Shirsky reported similar scores for Social Problems, Delinquent Behavior, and Aggressive Behavior. Similarly, on the Child Attention Profile, Mrs. Jones reported high levels of Inattention and Overactivity whereas Mrs. Shirsky did not. Mrs. Jones reported that in all his subjects, Mark has completed a mean of 50% less schoolwork than the average student in her class.

Mark did not report any problems at all. All his scores on the Brown ADD Scales were within the normal range.

Interviews were consistent with the pattern emerging from the rating

TABLE 6.3. Psychological Test Scores

Name Mark Bergen	Date of Evaluation 12/6/95
Date of Birth 12/12/83	Parents John and Ann Bergen
Age 12-11	Examiner Arthur L. Robin, PhD

WISC-III

Full Scale IQ	80	Low Average
Verbal IQ	85	Low Average
Performance IQ	78	Borderline

Verbal Scaled Scores		Performance Scaled Scores	
Information	8	Picture Completion	5
Similarities	6	Picture Arrangement	5
Arithmetic	11	Block Design	6
Vocabulary	7	Object Assembly	8
Comprehension	5	Coding	8
Digit Span	9		

Woodcock–Johnson Psycho-Educational Battery—Revised
(completed by teacher consultant in schools)

Subtest	SS (age)	SS (grade)
Broad Reading	97	109
Broad Mathematics	95	113
Broad Written Language	87	95
Broad Knowledge	89	95

Peabody Picture Vocabulary Test—Revised Form M (School Administered)

Standard Score—95	Percentile—37

CELF-R—Clinical Evaluation of Language Fundamentals—Revised
(School Administered)

Receptive Language Standard Score	85
Expressive Language Standard Score	95
Total Language Score	89

Gordon Diagnostic System (GDS)

Delay Task	Efficiency Ratio	.86 (>.83 is normal)
Vigilance Task	Correct Responses	44 Normal
	Commission Errors	1 Normal
Distractibility Task	Correct Responses	40 Normal
	Commission Errors	3 Normal

DSM-IV ADHD Behavior Checklist

	Teen	Mom	Dad	Teacher 1	Teacher 2
Number of Inattention Items—2 or 3:	1	3	2	7*	3
Number of Hyperactivity–Impulsivity Items—2 or 3:	2	0	0	8*	2
Number of ODD Items—2 or 3:	0	2	2	6*	5*

(continued)

TABLE 6.3 *(continued)*

Brown Attention Deficit Disorder Scale—Adolescent Version

Total Raw Score: 43

Subscale *T*-Scores:		
	Activating to Tasks	51
	Sustaining Attention	50
	Sustaining Effort	57
	Managing Affect	53
	Working Memory	<50

Conners Parent Rating Scale (*T*-scores)

	Mother	Father
Conduct Problems	70*	70*
Learning Problems	57	66
Psychosomatic	43	43
Impulsive–Hyperactive	55	46
Anxiety	41	41
Hyperactivity Index	37	51

Child Behavior Checklist (*T*-scores)

		Teacher Report Form	
		Teacher 1	Teacher 2
Activities	46		
Social	55		
School	30*		
Withdrawn	58	58	55
Somatic Complaints	50	50	50
Anxious/Depressed	52	59	53
Social Problems	50	69*	63*
Thought Problems	50	65*	50
Attention Problems	54	65*	56
Delinquent Behavior	59	70*	68*
Aggressive Behavior	67*	77*	66*

Child Attention Profile

	Inattention	Overactivity	Comments
	(9 is cutoff)	(6 is cutoff)	
Mrs. Jones	10*	6*	Suggested ADHD evaluation
Mrs. Shirsky	5	0	Resource Room teacher
Mean Score	7.5	3	

Percentage Assignments Completed on Time

	Mark	Average student	Difference
Math	45	95	−55
English	50	90	−40
Social Studies	35	95	−60
Science	40	90	−50
Mean Score	43	93	−50

(continued)

TABLE 6.3 *(continued)*

ADHD History Grid

```
Paying attention—problem since kindergarten
Staying seated—problem only in kindergarten
Fighting—problem since 5th grade
Disturbing other children—problem since 5th grade
```

Conflict Behavior Questionnaire

```
Mother—5   Father—3   Mark with mother—1   Mark with father—3
```

Issues Checklist

Number of Issues	Mother—5	Father—4	Mark—1
Mean Anger/Intensity	Mother—1.6	Father—1.7	Mark—1.2

* Significant elevation.

scales (e.g., clear-cut ODD but not consistent ADHD). Mark exhibits a great deal of challenging, "in your face" defiant behavior but is not described as having many ADHD symptoms across situations. His parents report that at home he has an excellent attention span and is very well organized and rarely forgetful. He can, however, act very spoiled and oppositional, although his parents give him a great deal of leeway. His teacher reports ADHD and ODD symptoms.

Results of Cognitive Testing

Mark was attentive but bored during the testing. On the WISC-III, he obtained a Full Scale IQ of 80, with a Verbal IQ of 85 and a Performance IQ of 78. These scores place him in the below-average range of intellectual ability, with below-average verbal and borderline performance ability. In the verbal area, he received average scores on subtests of mental arithmetic, short-term memory, and cultural information; low-average scores on subtests of verbal abstract reasoning and word knowledge; and a borderline score on the subtest of commonsense reasoning. In the performance area, Mark received average scores on subtests of part–whole assembly and motor speed and accuracy, low-average scores on subtests of nonverbal abstract reasoning, and borderline scores on subtests of fine motor discrimination and visual sequencing.

These IQ scores are comparable to those obtained on the WISC-R when Mark was tested during his kindergarten years: Full Scale IQ = 85; Verbal IQ = 87; Performance IQ = 82.

Because the teacher consultant had recently administered the Woodcock–Johnson Psycho-Educational Battery—Revised, along with speech and language measures, this examiner did not give any achievement tests. On the Woodcock–Johnson, Mark obtained average scores on the Broad

Reading, Broad Mathematics, and Broad Knowledge clusters and a below-average score on the Broad Written Language cluster. On the Peabody Picture Vocabulary Test—Revised, Mark scored in the average range of receptive language, while on the Clinical Evaluation of Language Fundamentals—Revised, he received below-average scores on Receptive Language and an average score of 95 on Expressive Language. Comparison of Mark's achievement and ability scores indicated that in most areas, Mark was in fact achieving more than would be predicted by his ability. This finding corroborates the school's decision to declassify him as learning disabled.

Differential Diagnosis

Mark shows no current or past history of depression, anxiety, or other psychiatric symptoms, based on either the interview or the ratings scales. The major differential diagnosis in this case in Oppositional Defiant Disorder. Mark's parents and teachers report many examples of ODD, more severe at school than at home, but the difference between how adults in the two environments may react to him may influence the picture of severity. On the Issues Checklist and Conflict Behavior Questionnaire, Mark and his parents do not report negative communication, conflict, or specific disputes.

Conclusions and Recommendations

The results of this evaluation do not indicate that Mark Bergen meets the diagnostic criteria for Attention-Deficit/Hyperactivity Disorder at the present time. Even though Mark's teachers describe him as inattentive and inconsistent at following directions and completing assignments, this pattern is specific to the school situation rather than cross-situational. His parents do not report the same kinds of difficulties with organization, focus, concentration, and impulse control at home. More importantly, there are two, viable alternative explanations for Mark's academic difficulties in school: (1) low ability; and (2) ODD.

Mark's intellectual ability has been consistent in the below-average range over the course of his school career. The average child in his affluent, suburban school system has an IQ of approximately 115. He will in fact struggle academically given this disparity. The past history of speech and language difficulties probably further amplified his struggles. The fact that his achievement scores were basically in the average range is a testimony to the help and support he has received from his school and his parents. He is, in fact, doing the best he can academically with the abilities he has.

It is not uncommon for youngsters in such a predicament to get frustrated and engage in high levels of oppositional behavior in school. School has got to be academic agony for Mark, even though at his stage of early

adolescence, he cannot readily admit it. Acting-out behavior is a natural response to that frustration. Two additional factors are believed to have contributed to the defiant behavior pattern. First, Mark's severe asthma set the
stage for his parents to be more lenient with him, given how fragile he had
been medically and how special this makes him to his parents. Children
with chronic illness are often pampered in this manner. Second, his parents'
political beliefs and general antiauthority attitudes caused them to reinforce the developing repertoire of rebellious behavior that Mark has displayed.

Taken together, these factors have contributed to a clinically significant pattern of ODD, which is considered the primary diagnosis in this
case.

I made two recommendations to the family:

Psychological. Mark and his parents need to participate in a manage-
ment-oriented family therapy designed to address his oppositional behavior at school and at home, his underlying feelings and beliefs about his
ability structure, and self-esteem issues. His parents need to be taught how
to encourage independence without unduly infantilizing Mark or prompting and reinforcing rebellious behavior against school authorities. Mark
and his parents also need to be helped to develop realistic expectations for
Mark, given his cognitive structure. It appears that the family was looking
to the possibility that Mark had ADHD as an "easy answer" to a complex
situation. A combination of family problem-solving training, communication training, behavioral contracting, and cognitive restructuring would accomplish these goals.

Educational. Continued placement in a resource room is likely to be
helpful to Mark. The school needs to coordinate its effort with the family,
through the therapist, and develop a clear-cut set of consequences for oppositional behavior in the classroom. A home–school behavior contract
with weekly monitoring sheets sent home should be an intrinsic part of this
intervention.

Mark needs to be tracked in a prevocational direction and helped to
select courses he can handle given his ability structure.

Arthur L. Robin, PhD
Licensed Psychologist

Comment

I commonly encounter upper-middle-class families in affluent suburbs
searching for an ADHD diagnosis and medication recommendations when
their children are not doing well in school. It is easy these days for such
families to construct a clinical history consistent with ADHD and convince

the inexperienced practitioner who does not conduct a comprehensive evaluation that the youngster does in fact have ADHD. In this case, Mark's teacher's personal experience with her own son suggested to her that the pattern of behavior she saw in Mark was consistent with ADHD, and from her perspective without having the full picture, it may well have been a perfectly reasonable hypothesis. However, it became clear as the evaluation proceeded that Mark did not have the kind of cross-situational history of ADHD symptoms consistent with a positive ADHD diagnosis. The inconsistency between the parent and teacher rating scales and the normal scores on the GDS helped me to rule out ADHD in this case. The fact that the parent and teacher ratings concurred in the ODD area, together with the parents's liberal attitudes and their response to Mark's chronic asthma, helped clinch this diagnosis. Then, a careful history and testing revealed alternative explanations for Mark's problems. Youngsters with below-average ability who have ADHD typically get diagnosed before adolescence, because their below-average ability impairs their school functioning in early elementary school. This case also illustrated that when the schools have conducted ability or achievement testing within the past few months, the practitioner can save time and money by integrating the school's testing into the evaluation. The only time I redo the school testing is when I have reason to doubt its accuracy or the referral question specifically calls for a second opinion.

FEEDBACK AND RECOMMENDATIONS

After reaching a diagnostic decision, the practitioner completes the evaluation by giving the adolescent and the parents feedback and recommendations and in many cases writing a report such as those illustrated in the previous case examples. The process of giving feedback and recommendations blends into treatment, which is the topic of the remainder of this book. I discuss the details of giving feedback and recommendations in Chapter 7 (this volume), after I outline the treatment options and discuss how to educate families about ADHD.

SECTION THREE

○

TREATMENT

Introduction

This Introduction provides the practitioner with a framework for conceptualizing, organizing, planning, and selecting the appropriate elements of a comprehensive, multidimensional treatment program for the adolescent with ADHD. The chapters in Section III provide detailed guidance for implementing each of these elements. Because ADHD is a very broad umbrella term covering a family of related disorders whose subtypes, topology, and etiology are constantly evolving with the advent of new neurobiological, genetic, and environmental knowledge, treatment needs to be defined broadly. Traditionally, ADHD treatment has included medications, behavioral/psychological interventions, and educational interventions. Zeigler Dendy (1995) quite correctly pointed out that many other activities can be extremely therapeutic for adolescents, even though they are not traditionally considered "treatments," including succeeding at sports or hobbies, having a girlfriend or boyfriend who is a positive influence, doing fun things with parents or family, and generally maintaining positive relationships with friends. All such activities that have a positive therapeutic effect on the teenager and the family are considered here. The decision tree in this chapter helps guide the practitioner in tailoring these diverse elements to the unique characteristics and life circumstances of particular adolescents with ADHD and their families.

PHILOSOPHY OF INTERVENTION

Because ADHD is generally regarded as likely to last for a lifetime and is typically considered to be of neurobiological/genetic origin, it is appropriate to conceptualize treatment as designed to maximize *coping* rather than *curing* ADHD. Until we have methods for permanently altering the underlying neurochemical and/or neurophysiological substrates of ADHD, we will not be able to "cure" it. But, we must certainly help the adolescent and the family learn how to maximize the quality of daily life and minimize the damage wrought be ADHD symptoms.

Furthermore, to the extent that we subscribe to Barkley's (1997a) theory of impaired behavioral inhibition as explaining ADHD (see Chapter 1, this volume), we must keep in mind Barkley's point that the deficit of ADHD is not a lack of skill or knowledge but, rather, a failure of prepotent inhibitory responses to stop the adolescent from acting for a long enough time so that the four executive functions can guide behavior in a planful direction. Therefore, interventions that impart knowledge or teach skills in a clinic or office-based setting (e.g. cognitive behavior therapy and social skills training) *by themselves* are insufficient for influencing disinhibited responding in the natural environment. Instead, the most useful interventions are those put in place at the *point of performance* in the natural environment. For instance, training parents to respond by withdrawing a privilege when an adolescent provokes an argument would be predicted to be more effective than the therapist teaching the adolescent to self-instruct about why he should not provoke an argument. However, this does not mean that cognitive techniques are totally useless. The cognitive technique of self-instruction, for example, may prove adjunctively useful if the parent is trained to prompt and reinforce the adolescent to employ self-instruction in the natural environment when the parent issues a command that previously provoked an argument. The point is that these cognitive techniques operate less efficiently with individuals who have neurobiologically based impairments in self-control than they do with individuals without such impairments.

In fact, throughout Section III, I emphasize two cognitively oriented interventions: (1) problem-solving communication training and (2) cognitive restructuring. This emphasis requires some justification, in light of my belief in Barkley's theory of ADHD.

I conceptualize problem-solving communication training as a "point-of-performance intervention." I teach families how to follow the steps of problem solving to resolve disputes and how to identify and correct their negative communication during office-based therapy sessions. However, I do not expect them to successfully employ these techniques without contingencies in the natural environment. I give families specific assignments to employ problem solving and communication training at home during regular family meetings and daily interactions and coach them in carrying out these assignments. Thus, I present problem solving and communication as behavioral strategies to carry out when a conflict occurs in the natural environment, not as cognitive techniques taught in the therapy session and expected to generalize on their own to the natural environment.

Cognitive restructuring is employed more during the therapy sessions to address attitudinal problems that are manifest during the patient–therapist interaction. These attitudinal problems typically interfere with family members' implementation of point-of-performance interventions and must be addressed before the family can be expected to carry out such interventions. Thus, direct change in attitudes during the therapy session is the target of cognitive restructuring interventions.

In essence, a treatment philosophy similar to that used with patients with permanent prefrontal lobe injuries will prove effective (1) to teach some symptomatic management of the impairments in adaptive functioning; (2) to arrange a prosthetic environment, including external structure such as prompts, cues, and consequences within the natural environment; (3) to provide greater supervision and external management of the adolescent's daily needs by others; (4) to reduce the demands placed on the adolescent for normal levels of selected adaptive functioning and productivity; and (5) to program the maintenance of these adjustments and environmental structures for extended periods of time if not indefinitely. Stimulant medication, behavior modification interventions, and selected school-based accommodations illustrate the principles of effective intervention outlined by Barkley and have in fact proved most helpful in treating adolescents with ADHD.

LENGTH OF TREATMENT

In this era of managed care, accountability, and short-term treatment, the notion of designing lifelong prosthetic environments to accommodate the needs of developmentally handicapped ADHD individuals may seem impractical. However, such programming does not necessarily mean that frequent, continuous, and costly face-to-face therapy sessions are needed for effective treatment of ADHD adolescents. In reality, we have found that the majority of ADHD adolescents and their families benefit strongly from an intensive burst of intervention at the point of diagnosis and/or referral to the mental health professional. Such interventions typically consist of anywhere from 10 to 20 1-hour sessions spaced over several months, at first at weekly intervals and later at increasingly longer intervals. Afterward, the patient needs regular follow-up several times per year to help ensure maintenance of new routines, environmental changes, and interventions set in place during the initial intensive burst of treatment. Periodically, typically at major developmental transition points (e.g., entry into high school or college, leaving home, and entering the job market) or family crises (divorce, death, etc.), the adolescent and the family may again need another burst of intensive intervention.

We call such an approach the "dental checkup" model of ADHD follow-up care. Most people go to the dentist once or twice per year and have a checkup and cleaning. The cleaning helps maintain the condition of their teeth and prevents erosion or decay. The checkup may uncover some cavities or other problems; then, the individual returns for more intensive dental treatment. Analogously, teenagers with ADHD and their parents need to have "regular checkups" with the therapist who conducted the initial burst of intervention. At these checkups, the therapist reviews their implementation of the techniques they learned during therapy and looks for the early warning signs of any new problems. If any new problems are uncovered, the family can return for more intensive therapy. Otherwise, they return several months later for another checkup.

Good oral hygiene is a partnership between the patient and the dentist. Between checkups, the patient must brush his teeth, floss, and generally maintain appropriate oral hygiene. Analogously, coping with ADHD is a partnership between the mental health care professional and the family. Between checkups, the adolescent and the family must apply what they learned from therapy, and often the adolescent must take his or her medicine. Individuals who do not go to the dentist for checkups eventually are likely to have problems with their teeth; repairing the subsequent damage could be costly and painful. If families with ADHD teenagers do not go to follow-up checkups with a therapist or professional, problems are likely to arise. If untreated, such problems can eventually lead to negative outcomes, including substance abuse, delinquency, school dropout, poor self-esteem, and excessive family conflict.

The dental checkup model is consistent with the emphasis on short-term intervention and Barkley's theory of impaired response inhibition, which points to the need to ensure indefinite maintenance of prosthetic environments. In the following discussion of treatment sequencing, we assume that the practitioner is starting at the point of diagnosis and/or referral, and wishes to conduct this initial burst of 10 to 20 1-hour sessions.

PRIORITIZING TREATMENT GOALS

At the point of diagnosis and/or referral, most adolescents with ADHD are (1) experiencing difficulty completing their schoolwork and making satisfactory academic progress and (2) getting into frequent conflict with their parents not only about their poor school performance but also about a variety of compliance-related issues such as chores, curfew, dating, bedtime, fighting with siblings, negative voice tone, and general disrespect. Some also are having significant difficulties with peer relationships and behavior in the community, as well as low self-esteem, depression, anxiety, and other comorbid conditions. A minority are actively antisocial, aggressive, in trouble with the legal authorities, and/or abusing marijuana, alcohol, or other substances. To make matters worse, many of the younger adolescents, ages 12–15, vehemently deny that there is anything wrong with them and strongly resist taking medication or participating in any other interventions. All these problems appear to have a high priority for treatment. The practitioner needs a systematic approach to prioritizing treatment goals and sequencing treatment components. Because there has not been any research evaluating the optimal sequencing of components in a multi-modal treatment, the suggestions given here are based primarily upon clinical experience and logic. Figure III.1 provides a comprehensive flowchart for decision making and prioritizing treatment goals.

The practitioner first needs to decide whether the adolescent is out of control in an antisocial, aggressive, and/or substance-abusing manner (e.g., comorbid diagnosis of CD or Substance Use Disorder). If either or both of these conditions apply, they become the highest-priority treatment goals. In the case of substance abuse, I decide whether the severity of the problem merits immediate referral to a substance abuse specialist or whether I can proceed with my treatment program while guiding the parents to monitor the adolescent for signs of substance use. If the adolescent is using marijuana or alcohol on a recreational basis on weekends or even once or twice a week, and she or he will make a genuine commitment to work toward curtailing drug use, I usually keep the case but help the parents develop a plan to monitor whether the adolescent is using substances. Such a plan might involve periodic unannounced searches of the adolescent's room, backpack, car, or other personal spaces; careful inspection for signs of intoxication; home breathalyzer tests for alcohol; or even arrangements for random urine testing.

More frequent marijuana or alcohol use or any use of cocaine, heroine, hallucinogens, or other drugs are cause for an immediate referral to a substance abuse specialist, who triages the patient to either an inpatient or outpatient substance abuse program. Practitioners who do have substance abuse training might provide these intervention services directly.

Some emerging evidence suggests that aggressive medical treatment of ADHD in young adults with comorbid substance addictions may increase their resistance to relapses and make recovery from substances easier (Schubiner et al., 1995). Schubiner (1996) is currently conducting a double-blind, placebo trial of Ritalin (methylphenidate) and Cylert (pemoline), together with a comprehensive cognitive/behavioral substance abuse intervention, in treating cocaine addicts who also have ADHD. In selected clinical cases prior to the study, they found that treating the ADHD with stimulants makes it easier for their patients to recover from substances. No such studies have been reported yet with adolescents, but the results of the controlled trial will clearly have implications for the sequencing of treatments in dual-diagnosis cases in the future.

Parents should also be advised to regard tobacco use as a significant form of substance abuse with major health implications. Adolescents and adults with ADHD smoke cigarettes at 2 to 2.4 times the rates of non-ADHD individuals, are significantly more likely to begin smoking earlier than are non-ADHD individuals, and are much more prone to become addicted to nicotine than are non-ADHD individuals (Downey, Pomerleau, & Pomerleau, 1996; Milberger, Biederman, Faraone, Chen, & Jones, 1997; Pomerleau, Downey, Stelson & Pomerleau, 1995). In one study,

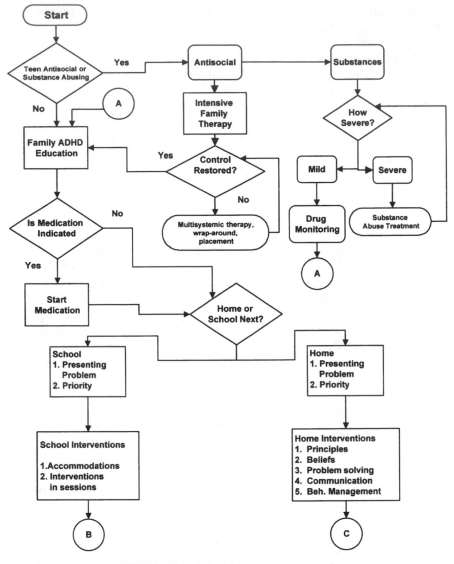

FIGURE III.1. Prioritizing treatment goals.

25% of ADHD teens began smoking before age 15, 46% between age 15 and 16, and 29% at age 17 or older (Milberger et al., 1997); these authors also found that the odds of having other drug abuse problems in the teens who smoked was five times greater than in individuals who did not. Although cigarette smoking by itself may not be cause for a substance abuse referral, it is clearly a cause for concern amidst ADHD individuals. The

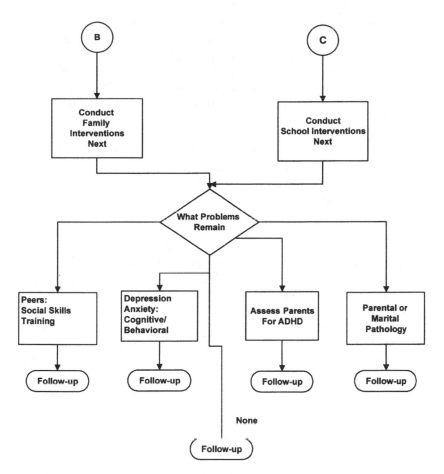

FIGURE III.1 *(continued)*

therapist and the parents should have a serious discussion about smoking with the adolescent and try to develop a plan when feasible to reduce, eliminate, or prevent tobacco use.

In the case of conduct-disordered, out-of-control behavior, the practitioner should begin intensive outpatient family treatment designed to restore reasonable parental controls through the use of strategic/structural family interventions. Chapter 12 describes this type of intervention. If several months of intensive outpatient family therapy fails to restore parental controls, the practitioner should consider intensive in-home programs (e.g., Henggeler's multisystemic therapy; Henggeler & Borduin, 1990; Smith & Stern, 1997), community mental health wraparound programs, or specialized day-treatment programs (e.g., Pelham's intensive summer treatment program; Pelham & Hoza, 1996). Some empirical evidence is available that supports the effectiveness of these interventions. As a last resort, the practitioner should turn to out-of-home placements, such as inpatient psychiatric hospitalization, therapeutic foster care, residential treatment, or even military school in certain cases. There is no solid empirical evidence, however, that these programs restore parental control upon the adolescent's return home, only that they change the adolescent's behavior while he or she is in the residential environment.

Upon the adolescent's return from such intensive placements, the practitioner should continue with the normal course of outpatient treatment for adolescent ADHD, modifying it as necessary if certain components were implemented during the placement.

In the majority of cases, the practitioner will proceed down the left-hand column of the flowchart in Figure III.1. The adolescent and his or her family are next provided with comprehensive ADHD education, designed to instill the coping attitudes and expectations necessary to benefit from the remainder of the interventions. Because the natural developmental changes of adolescents render many youngsters highly resistant to acceptance of chronic conditions such as ADHD and their treatments, ADHD education assumes a very important role. Such education takes place over several weeks through direct discussions in family and individual sessions, bibliotherapy, videotapes, referrals to local and national support groups, and putting the adolescent in touch with peers who have ADHD, who can serve as positive role models. Of course, like many facets of a comprehensive intervention, ADHD education continues for a long time beyond the initial efforts made by the practitioner. Chapter 7 discusses family ADHD education in detail.

Starting medication is the next phase of intervention. If medication is to be prescribed, it is important to begin it early in the overall intervention to help break the cycle of past failure and conflict abruptly and to have time to adequately titrate the dose and maximize the synergistic potential of medication plus educational and behavioral/psychological interventions. However, starting medication *after* family ADHD education is crucial; a common error is to start medication immediately upon diagnosis, without taking adequate time to make sure the adolescent understands and accepts medication. Such an error is likely to result in premature rejection of or resistance to medication, sometimes leading the adolescent to feel that the practitioner is not truly interested in him or her as a person but, rather, only interested in pleasing the parents by drugging the adolescent into compliance. Chapter 8 considers in detail how to decide whether medication is indicated and how to intervene with medication.

Whether to target school performance or home conflict next is an intriguing question which the therapist must decide in every case. If the family initially contacted me because of school performance problems, I usually target school problems first; if the family initially contacted me because of home conflict, I target this area first. Most times, both school and home issues were presenting problems, and I make a decision together with the family to prioritize targets. Most families choose school problems as higher priority than home conflict, and other things being equal, this is the preferred sequence. In cases of pure ADHD without comorbid ODD, most home-based conflicts are related to school issues such as homework or low grades; targeting school performance first is a parsimonious approach because improvement in this area typically results in amelioration of home conflict, reducing the need for lengthy interventions focused on parent–teen conflict. More important, failure at school may have more irreversible, devastating consequences for the adolescent than continued home conflict for another few weeks. Although the practitioner could conceivably target both areas simultaneously, devoting part of each session to each area, this approach tends to dilutes the effectiveness of the interventions and is less preferred. Chapter 9 discusses interventions for school success; Chapters 10–12 detail approaches to parenting the ADHD adolescent and resolving family conflict.

School- and home-based interventions comprise the real meat of the initial burst of treatment for adolescents with ADHD and often take 75% of the therapy sessions (15 out of 20) to complete. In cases of comorbid ODD, the parenting/home conflict interventions may take additional time. As the adolescent begins to experience success at school and the family begins to integrate solution-oriented communication and effective parenting principles into their natural response styles, the therapist assesses the need to address any residual problems. Such residual problems often include peer relationship issues, anxiety or depression, possible ADHD in the parents or siblings, or parental marital and/or personal problems. Individual cognitive-behavioral and supportive interventions are helpful for addressing adolescent or parent anxiety, depression, or related issues. Social skills group interventions may be used for peer relationship problems as long as the practitioner keeps in mind the lack of evidence for the generalizability and builds in procedures to spur generalization. Conjoint marital therapy is sometimes needed for the parents' marital conflicts. Most commonly, either a family member or the therapist suspects that one of the parents or a sibling also has ADHD and conducts an appropriate diagnostic workup. Following a positive diagnosis of ADHD in a parent, not only might a series of medical and behavioral interventions for adult ADHD be undertaken but the skillful therapist might address ADHD at the family systems level through family interventions. Readers interested in information about the diagnosis and treatment of ADHD in adults should consult Nadeau (1995) and Goldstein (1997).

In the last few sessions of the initial burst of intervention, the therapist lengthens the interval between sessions to 3 and then 4 weeks, helps the family consolidate the gains they have made, and shifts into the dental checkup model of follow-up care. Most families enthusiastically appreciate

TABLE III.1. Twenty-Session Intervention for ADHD Adolescents

- Family ADHD education—Sessions 1 and 2
- Starting medication—Session 3
- School success interventions—Sessions 4–9
- Home/parenting/family conflict interventions—Sessions 10–15
- Other issues/fading back to "dental checkup" follow-up model—Sessions 16–20

the idea of periodic ADHD checkups several times a year. Chapter 13 provides more information about the structure of these periodic follow-up sessions.

Table III.1 illustrates the allocation of the content areas to 1-hour therapy sessions in a 20-session, comprehensive intervention for the average ADHD adolescent following diagnosis and/or referral to the mental health professional. This outline assumes that the practitioner did not need to start with a module of treatment for extremely out-of-control aggressive behavior, which requires additional time. This outline also does not include any marital or individual therapy, which may be needed for the parents. Clearly, the exact number of sessions required for each phase of treatment depends on the severity of the problems in that area and the presence of comorbidity and parental psychiatric problems. I have generally found that this outline is a realistic projection of what is needed, and I have used it with case managers who require such information. I refer back to this outline throughout Chapters 7–13, as I discuss the sequencing for each module of the intervention in more detail.

CHAPTER SEVEN

○

Educating Families about ADHD

How does the clinician give feedback to the adolescent and the parents about the diagnosis of ADHD and the associated learning problems and comorbid psychiatric conditions? Then, how does the clinician involve the family in discussing and making decisions about the kinds of recommendations for treatment outlined earlier, and how does the clinician educate parents and adolescents about ADHD?

Adolescents and their parents react in a variety of ways to the news that the teenager has ADHD and its associated conditions. These reactions may include denial, resentment, anger, grief, confusion, self-doubt, guilt, worry, feelings of isolation and sadness, silence, indifference, bargaining, relief, acceptance, and any combination of these feelings. Researchers have not yet delineated empirically the developmental progression of reactions to the ADHD diagnosis, but clinical experience suggests that adolescents, ages 12 to 15, progress from denial, anger, and resentment, and indifference to grief, sadness, relief, and finally by acceptance ages 16 to 20. This progression parallels the accomplishment of adolescent developmental tasks and is similar to adolescent reactions to any chronic illness (e.g., diabetes, asthma, or renal disease). In early adolescence, when teenagers are just beginning to individuate from their parents and are very unsure of their identify, they have a great need to be omnipotent and perfect, have nothing wrong with them, and be similar to their peers but very different from their parents. A diagnosis of ADHD may suggest that something is wrong with them, challenging their fragile egos, and may be hard for them to accept. Hence, they resent and resist such a diagnosis and everything that goes along with it. Later in adolescence, as the youngsters are beginning to form an identify and have stronger ego strength, they can more easily tolerate a diagnosis of ADHD without personalizing it as a injury to their ego.

Parents more commonly react to the diagnosis of ADHD in their adolescent offspring with relief and acceptance. They have known for many years that something is different about their adolescent, but they have been unable to figure out what it is. The diagnosis comes as a natural explanation for a lifetime of difficulty and helps relieve their worries that their poor parenting caused the adolescent's problems. At least they now have a cognitive framework within which to understand and cope with their adolescent's academic, behavioral, and social problems. Because of the publicity about ADHD in recent years, parents bringing their adolescents for evaluation expect to hear a positive diagnosis. Unfortunately, uninformed parents sometimes look to a diagnosis of ADHD as a seemingly simple solution to a complex life problem (Armstrong, 1995). Ironically, it is therefore becoming more difficult to tell middle- and upper-middle-class parents that their youngster does not have ADHD than to tell them that he or she does have it. It may be tempting to equivocate or hesitate when faced with such pressures from parents, but it is crucial that the practitioner call it as he or she sees it.

As we give feedback and develop therapeutic recommendations, we educate families about ADHD. The goal of family ADHD education is to deal with the full spectrum of reactions to the ADHD diagnosis, spur understanding and acceptance of the ADHD diagnosis, and develop in the adolescent and his or her family the kind of coping, positive attitudes compatible with active participation in the multifaceted treatments discussed in this book. Typically, this is more challenging with the adolescent than with the parent. The practitioner begins this process at the feedback session where the results of the diagnostic evaluation are conveyed to the adolescent and the parents and continues it over the course of the first few therapy sessions. Of course, emotional acceptance takes time, so ADHD education becomes on ongoing issue throughout the entire course of therapy. First, I discuss the parental portion of this phase and then the adolescent portion.

PARENTAL FEEDBACK AND ADHD EDUCATION

In the case of a positive ADHD diagnosis, I make a clear statement to the parents of the diagnosis, assess their reactions, and then outline the treatment options. Let's join my discussion with Mr. and Mrs. Jones, parents of 15-year-old Bill Jones, recently diagnosed as having ADHD plus ODD, as I give them the feedback:

DR. ROBIN: I have now had a chance to talk to the two of you and Bill, to finish and score all of the testing, and to review all of the questionnaires. All of the information lead me to the same conclusion: Bill meets the criteria for Attention-Deficit/Hyperactivity Disorder, Combined subtype. The chronic difficulties he has been having with getting schoolwork done, his impulsive actions, his mental restlessness—they all add up to ADHD. I find no other feasible explanation for them. You have also given me many heartbreaking examples of the very unpleasant arguments and conflicts you each have with Bill, and how much he defies you at home. In addition to ADHD, I am diagnosing Bill as having Oppositional Defiant Disorder. This is really a fancy psychiatric term for arguing and defiance way beyond what even most adolescents do. And finally, the IQ tests indicated that Bill has above-average ability with above-average achievement test scores. So his poor grades are not the result of a learning disability, but more a result of ADHD. Before I go any further, what questions do you have?

MRS. JONES: This Oppositional Defiant Disorder thing. Is there a medication for that too?

DR. ROBIN: Not really. ADHD is thought to have a genetic/biological basis, but Oppositional Defiant Disorder is really good old learned bad habits. We will work together to try to teach Bill new ways of interacting with you, and two of you new ways of interacting with him.

MR. JONES: Doc, what is the bottom line here? What do we do now?

DR. ROBIN: I'm glad you asked. Let me tell you the general options, so you can think about how you would like to proceed. Then we'll get to the specifics. The single most important thing is learning everything you can about ADHD, and helping Bill to learn about it and accept it. Power comes from knowledge. There are three general areas of intervention: (1) medical, (2) behavioral/psychological, and (3) educational. Medical intervention, usually with stimulant medications such as Ritalin, is designed to supply the chemicals to the brain which aren't there where and when they are needed, so Bill can stop, think, look, listen, and concentrate, rather than acting on a whim or impulse. Without the right chemicals, other things won't work. But medicine alone is rarely sufficient. Behavioral/psychological interventions are designed to teach him new habits, in the family, school, and the community. This is also designed to address his beliefs and feelings about himself and the world around him. Educational interventions—some done by me and some by the school—are designed to accommodate his needs in school, as a youngster who has ADHD, which may handicap him educationally.

MRS. JONES: Will the school really help him if he doesn't have a learning disability?

DR. ROBIN: ADHD is getting in the way of Bill's getting his assignments done. His productivity is very poor, despite above-average ability. Most of the other kids without ADHD are getting their assignments done on time. This constitutes a handicap under federal law called

Section 504. We will ask the school to declare Bill handicapped under Section 504, and to plan some accommodations for him.

MR. JONES: I doubt those teachers will lift a finger. They do as little as they can.

DR. ROBIN: I understand how you feel. In my experience, most of the teachers in Bill's district are trying very hard to meet the needs of students with ADHD, but they are overworked and don't have enough backup. It may seem like they don't want to help, but this usually isn't true. If Bill qualifies for accommodations under Section 504, the school will have no choice but to meet his needs. I will help you with developing an appropriate plan which helps you to work collaboratively with the school and gets Bill the services he needs at school.

MR. JONES: But our insurance only covers five sessions of therapy, and with a 50% copay. Won't medication be enough?

DR. ROBIN: Bill made it clear to me that there was absolutely no way he was going to agree to take medication at this point. I imagine he has mentioned this to you.

MRS. JONES: Yes, he has.

DR. ROBIN: That's a pretty natural reaction for someone his age. I understand. But it points out, Mr. Jones, why medication isn't the whole answer for adolescents with ADHD. We first have to help him understand and accept what is going on with him, and then he may hopefully come to see the rationale for medication as part of an overall intervention. Honestly, I don't think medication alone will be enough to help Bill. Even if he would take it today, it wouldn't by itself address the family conflict. Mr. and Mrs. Jones, I completely understand the insurance situation. In fact, your insurance company won't even authorize any treatment if I use ADHD as the diagnosis. I have to use ODD as the diagnosis to obtain authorization for the five sessions.

MRS. JONES: Really. What good is the insurance then?

DR. ROBIN: This is a big problem with managed care these days. They see ADHD as the school's responsibility, yet the school's aren't able to deal with it alone. Mr. Jones, you may want to talk to you union about getting better mental health coverage when the new contract is negotiated next August. In the meantime, I will do the best I can to help the three of you, if you want my help. I have worked with that insurance company before.

MR. JONES: We definitely want your help. I'm glad you know how to handle the insurance company. We will do what we can.

This interchange shows how I summarize the diagnostic feedback and begin to discuss the treatment options. The reader can see how issues such as insurance coverage quickly enter into the discussion in these days of preauthorization, managed care, and limited benefits. The practitioner must be prepared to deal with this issues up front, as the parents raise them. Of course, I go into more detail about the diagnosis, particularly the results of the cognitive testing.

In Bill's case, some individual therapy focused on ADHD education needs to come before any other intervention, because he is not ready to accept medication. Next, I define the specific treatment goals together with the Jones family.

DR. ROBIN: OK. Next, we need to agree with each other about our treatment goals. Generally, we want to help Bill do better in school and get along better with you at home, but I want us to be more specific.

MRS. JONES: Bill needs to do all of his homework every night.

DR. ROBIN: I agree. Getting homework done regularly is clearly one of our goals.

MR. JONES: I don't want any more lip from him. He needs to treat me with respect.

DR. ROBIN: Respectful communication with parents in another. But communication is a two-way street. Would you agree that "positive parent–teen communication" should be our goal here?

MR. AND MRS. JONES: Yes,

DR. ROBIN: Also, I would say that "effective resolution of disagreements without arguments" is an important goal.

MR. AND MRS. JONES: Yes.

MRS. JONES: And stopping teasing his sister too.

DR. ROBIN: Coming to understand and accept ADHD and the need for medication is certainly the first goal. . . .

The therapist continues to give the parents feedback and develop specific goals for change, until all the goals have been specified and agreed on, and all the parents' concerns have been addressed.

It is also useful to review some basic information about the nature of adolescent development with parents at this point in the education process, although we typically go into more detail later when we deal with parenting issues (e.g., Chapter 10, this volume). The therapist might review the following points with the parents:

1. The major developmental task of adolescence is for teenagers to become independent of parents.

2. To become independent, teenagers must push away from their parents. Some conflict is normal during this process. Such conflict is most common from ages 12 to 14. Teenagers typically give their mothers a more difficult time than their fathers during this process.
3. As teenagers individuate from their parents, they discover who they are and what they stand for (e.g., define their identity).
4. It is normal for teenagers in the process of defining their identify to reject their parents' ideas, opinions, and values in favor of their friends' ideas, opinions, and values.
5. Another developmental task of adolescence is increasing the capacity for closer peer relationships and intimacy with peers. It is therefore normal that teenagers want to spend as much time with their friends as possible and as little time with their parents as possible.
6. Teenagers feel fragile inside as they are searching for their identity, but they do not want to show any weakness to their peers (e.g., they need to appear omnipotent). Therefore, they are likely to reject the presentation of any disability such as ADHD and not to want to accept that this is their problem. This also explains why they turn away from treatments such as medication for ADHD (such a response is not specific to ADHD; adolescents reject treatment for any common chronic illness).
7. Keeping this information in mind, parents need to develop reasonable expectations and pick their battles wisely. In general, teenagers are more likely to do what their parents want if they think it was their own idea and the parents give clear reasons for their rules.
8. Teenagers with ADHD are going through the same drastic changes in body and mind as are other teenagers. However, they have poorer inhibitory control. Their minds are behind their bodies in development. They have the same desires for independence, peer affiliation, and sexuality as their peers, but they may be less mature and less ready for independence. This creates a dilemma for parents, and the parents must keep it in mind as they deal with their adolescent's problems.

ADOLESCENT FEEDBACK AND ADHD EDUCATION

After educating the parents about ADHD, the therapist turns to the feedback and education session with the adolescent. I find it helpful to divide the discussion of ADHD with the adolescent into five components: (1) give the facts about ADHD; (2) listen to the adolescent's reaction to the facts; (3) use cognitive restructuring to correct myths and false beliefs and instill positive, coping attitudes toward ADHD; (4) assign homework to build on cognitive restructuring in changing attitudes; and (5) collaboratively develop treatment goals with the adolescent.

Give the Facts

I usually start by making a clear statement that ADHD applies to the adolescent, giving a brief definition of ADHD, discussing its neurobiological/genetic etiology with the aid of concrete information such as a photograph of the PET scans from Zimetkin's study (Zimetkin et al., 1990), and highlighting how ADHD impairs the quality of their life in practical ways to which teenagers can relate. I talk in short, simple sentences which teenagers can understand, incorporate things the teenagers previously told me into my explanations, and pause often to check for understanding and questions. If the adolescent does not spontaneously bring up the most common myths about ADHD and its treatment, I bring them up and debunk them.

The practitioner needs to cover the following points, made here in the language used with teenagers, throughout this presentation, although not necessarily all in one meeting or in the order given here:

1. ADHD is a disorder involving difficulty paying attention, controlling the urge to act before thinking, and feeling or acting restless.
2. You are not crazy or sick if you have ADHD. It is a mild, but invisible disability that represents the extremes of traits or characteristics that all people exhibit to greater or lesser degrees.
3. ADHD usually lasts a lifetime but changes as you mature and grow older. In particular, the restlessness changes from more physical to more mental, but the inattention and impulsivity remain.
4. ADHD affects all areas of your life, not just school. It may influence how you get along with other people, how you relate in intimate interpersonal situations, how organized you are at home, how you do in sports and hobbies, how easily you fall asleep and wake up, how you feel about yourself, and how you do on the job in the future.
5. ADHD is not your fault, your parents' fault, or anyone's fault. It is a physical disorder, usually inherited, and is caused by a mild chemical imbalance in the brain.
6. Chemicals called neurotransmitting chemicals, which pass signals for self-control throughout the brain, aren't operating efficiently in ADHD people. It would be like having too little brake fluid in your car; when you press the brake pedal, you can't stop. When an idea to do something pops into the ADHD person's mind, he can't stop and think whether it is good or bad before he does it, because the chemicals which help the brain stop and think aren't working properly.
7. Because ADHD usually is inherited, it is possible that your parents, brothers or sisters, or other relatives also have ADHD, even if they don't know it. If you have kids some day, they may also have ADHD. This could make family life like a real roller coaster!

8. ADHD is also influenced by your environment, e.g. your parents, your school, your friends. A good family, a good school, and good friends can make life a lot easier for the ADHD person.

9. ADHD is a challenge, not an excuse. You are still responsible for your actions, even though you have a physical disorder which makes it harder for you to control your actions.

10. ADHD is influenced by your physical health. It will be easier to deal with ADHD if you take proper care of yourself (e.g., get enough sleep, maintain good nutrition, don't smoke or put drugs or alcohol in your body, and exercise regularly).

11. Because ADHD is inherited and physical, we can't totally cure or eliminate it. Instead, we can help you learn to cope so life goes well for you. There are three general methods for learning to cope: (1) medical, (2) behavioral/psychological, and (3) educational. We will talk about these in detail as time goes on.

I use Bill Jones, a 15-year-old male adolescent I recently diagnosed and treated, as an example, to illustrate how to give the facts, as well as the later stages of family ADHD education. Bill and his parents have completed the full evaluation discussed earlier in the book, and I am now meeting individually with Bill to tell him my diagnosis and educate him about it.

DR. ROBIN: You know how you told me that you zone out during football practice when the coach is talking strategy and then he gets really mad at you for not listening?

BILL: Yeah.

DR. ROBIN: And you told me you absolutely go nuts with restlessness sitting through boring algebra class.

BILL: You bet.

DR. ROBIN: And remember last July 4 how you heard "God Bless America" on the radio as you saw a red spray paint can in the garage. That spray paint somehow just popped into your hand as you suddenly thought it would be a neat idea to spray paint "God Bless America" on the outside of the garage door?

BILL: My parents made me spend hours cleaning that one up!

DR. ROBIN: These things all make sense to me now that we've done all this testing, forms, and talking. Trouble paying attention, feeling restless, and acting before thinking all fit together to make Attention Deficit Disorder, or ADD. ADD is definitely you. What do you think, could this be you, a nice guy with ADD who just happens to get in hot water, not on purpose, but it just somehow happens?

BILL: Well, I don't know, maybe. . . .

DR. ROBIN: By the way, ADD is not your fault, your parents' fault or anyone's fault. It's the way you are born, the way your brain works. There is something different about the way some chemicals in the brain work that make it hard for ADD people to pay attention and control themselves. Stuff just happens and they act; then it is too late. Look at this picture *(shows Zimetkin's [Zimetkin et al., 1990] PET scan picture)*. What do you see?

BILL: Looks like some weird kind of X ray.

DR. ROBIN: Exactly. It's called a PET scan, a kind of computer picture of the brain. The dude on the left has ADD. See how the colors are different than the dude on the right, who doesn't have ADD. The difference in color show us that the dude on the left has less brain activity than the dude on the right and isn't paying attention as well.

BILL: So what's the big deal? Who cares?

DR. ROBIN: No big deal. This just goes to prove there is something physically different about the brains of people with ADD and people without it. It's not in their imagination, they are not crazy or mentally ill; it's a physical difference in how the chemicals in their brains work that is inherited.

Notice how the explanation of ADHD is interwoven with Bill's life experiences and presented in a lively, interactive format. Toward the end of the interaction, several common myths are brought up and debunked (ADD people are mentally ill, crazy).

Listen to the Reactions to the Presentation

After presenting the facts, the practitioner listens carefully to the adolescent's reactions, using active listening to clarify how he or she is feeling but not challenging or being confrontational. It is very important for adolescents to feel that they have been listened to and understood and their opinions have been taken seriously, because in the past their ideas may have often been discounted or put down by adults. Let's continue with the example of Bill:

BILL: So does this mean I am dumb and have a bad brain? Great news, Doc!

DR. ROBIN: You're feeling like having ADD means your stupid.

BILL: All the retards on the special education bus go to the office to get their pills at lunch. The whole football team whips their butts at gym.

DR. ROBIN: You would be very embarrassed if you had to go to the office and take a pill at lunch. It would make you feel like a retard, and you think your friends on the football team would give you a hard time about it.

BILL: Yeah, this is the kiss of death for me. My parents are going to freak out and take me to a million doctors, tutors, and shrinks. I'll probably miss football practice and get kicked off the team! And they will make me take medicine that will make me weird.

DR. ROBIN: So ADHD is going to mess up your whole life, take away all your free time and fun, and make you into a zombie?

BILL: Yeah, and just when Jennifer was starting to like me too. Now Mike will get her for sure.

DR. ROBIN: You will also strike out with girls? This all sounds like a nightmare.

BILL: Yeah.

As Bill voices his fears and anxieties about peer ridicule, feeling stupid, having to go to a lot of doctors, getting kicked off the football team, losing his freedom and never having a girlfriend, I empathetically clarify them but do not yet deal with them. Many adolescents might be thinking what Bill verbalized, but it could take many sessions before they become comfortable confiding their worries in the therapist, although an advantage to working with impulsive people is that they often blurt out their worries despite their desire to hide them.

Deal with Reactions: Application of Cognitive Restructuring

Cognitive restructuring and reattributional techniques, two of the mainstays of cognitive behavior therapy (Braswell & Bloomquist, 1991), are applicable techniques for dealing with adolescents' negative reactions to the ADHD diagnosis. Typically, one or more of the following types of distorted beliefs underlies the negative reaction:

1. ADHD is a life sentence; my life is over. I'll never amount to anything.
2. This means I am a really dumb, stupid, crazy, or bad person. All the bad things my parents and teachers have said about me are really true.
3. I'll never have any friends anymore; they will all think I'm a total nerd.
4. I'll never have any fun because I will have to spend all my time with tutors, doctors, and therapists.
5. Medication will change my personality in bad ways. I like being wild, loud, and crazy. This is me, who I am, and no one is going to change me.

6. I'm different from my friends and I'll never be normal.
7. I've really messed up now. It's all my fault.
8. This whole ADHD thing is bull; it's just one more way my parents are trying to control my life.

These beliefs are really variations on the underlying extreme belief themes of ruination, autonomy, and perfectionism, to which adolescents commonly adhere (Robin & Foster, 1989): (1) ruination—this ADHD diagnosis is going to ruin my life, fun, and friends; (2) autonomy—having ADHD will take away or limit my freedom; or (3) perfectionism—now the world will know I'm less than a perfect person and that's terrible. I revisit these beliefs within the context of parenting and family conflict in Chapter 10.

In cognitive restructuring with adolescents, the therapist tactfully collaborates with the patient to (1) identify the distorted belief, (2) provide a logical challenge to it, (3) suggest a more reasonable belief, and (4) help the patient discover based on collection of evidence that the reasonable belief is more valid than the unreasonable belief (Robin & Foster, 1989). Often, the clinician reframes negatively valenced ideas or thoughts to more positive motives or connotations along with cognitive restructuring.

Through actively listening to the adolescent's negative reactions to the ADHD diagnosis, the therapist has already identified a number of Bill's distorted beliefs in the case example. Let's see how cognitive restructuring might proceed:

DR. ROBIN: I understand how you feel that ADD will mess up your whole life, but before we jump to any quick conclusions, let's look at the evidence.

BILL: What evidence? I'm done, finished, all washed up!

DR. ROBIN: Start with the idea that you are dumb. On the IQ test I just gave you, you received a score of 115, which is above average. You may feel like you are dumb, but in fact you are smart. ADD has nothing to do with being smart or dumb.

BILL: If I'm so smart, why do I do dumb things like spray paint on the garage?

DR. ROBIN: Good question. Your brain is like an expensive sports car without any brake fluid. The sports car is beautiful, powerful, and fast, but without any brake fluid it is going to crash when the driver tries to stop. Your brain is smart and gets all kinds of neat ideas, but if you act on them all without thinking about the consequences, you will crash into many brick walls. The brake fluid in the car allows it to stop; certain chemicals in your brain allow you to think about your neat ideas before you act on them. People without ADD press the brake pedal and it works; they don't act on all of their ideas. People with ADD press the brake pedal and nothing happens. That just keep on acting. This has nothing to do with IQ.

Let's take your worry about having to go to the office to take pills and your friends teasing you. First of all, not everyone with ADD takes medication. You would only take medication if you agree to, after you fully understand it. But let's say you did agree. We now have medicines which you take once in the morning and they last all day, so the only way your friends will know about it is if you tell them.

BILL: Great! Those drugs would make me into a weird zombie all day then.

DR. ROBIN: The truth is, most people don't feel any different on medicine for ADD, except they are not as hungry while it is in their body. Are any of your good friends on medicine for ADD?

BILL: You wouldn't catch me hanging out with those retards.

DR. ROBIN: Do you know a kid named Danny Selby? [Danny gave the therapist written permission to disclose his name to other adolescents for motivational purposes.]

BILL: Danny Selby? Sure. The whole school knows him. He is captain of the football team, Mr. Cool. Every girl in school goes nuts over him. But he is really a great guy. .

DR. ROBIN: He has ADD and takes medicine for it every morning.

BILL: No way. Not Danny. He's too cool. Doc, you're kidding, right?

DR. ROBIN: Nope. Don't take my word for it. Ask him. He is glad to talk about it privately, but he has no reason to announce it on the overhead speaker system in school. And don't forget to ask him whether medicine makes him feel weird.

The steps of cognitive restructuring flowed together in this case example. The discussion of the IQ test illustrates challenging a distorted belief with the introduction of a more reasonable alternative and clear-cut evidence to back it up.

Positive Peer Models

The introduction of a highly regarded positive peer model who happens to have ADD is the most potent type of evidence for changing beliefs about ADHD because peers are such an important part of teenagers' lives. It behooves every clinician who plans to work with adolescents to develop a referral list of such positive ADHD peer models. Of course, as in Danny's case, these peer models need to sign a written release form permitting the therapist to disclose their names. Clinical experience strongly suggests that adolescents will be more convinced to accept and cope with ADHD by their peers than by adults. The use of credible peers to help ADHD adolescents change negative attitudes toward ADHD is an application of the social psychological principle of appealing to a credible higher authority figure to help a person stuck in a rigid, opinionated stance (Robin & Foster, 1989). Adolescents are more credible authority figures than adults on many adolescent issues. Robin and Foster (1989) outlined how to apply this principle to mediating seemingly unresolvable conflicts between parents and adolescents.

To help clinicians plan to encourage adolescent acceptance of ADHD, I have organized examples of reasonable, alternative beliefs for each of the distorted positions mentioned earlier (see Table 7.1). Clinicians can use this material to help develop cognitive restructuring rationales and discussions with their adolescent patients.

Books and Audiovisual Materials

The use of books and audiovisual materials on ADHD written by adolescents for adolescents and the orchestration of teen forum group sessions directed by adolescents are additional techniques for fostering understanding and acceptance of ADHD. Antony Amen and Sharon Johnson, two college-age adolescents with ADHD, teamed up with Dr. Daniel Amen, Antony's stepfather and a well-known psychiatrist, to write A Teenager's Guide to ADD (1996), a guidebook to ADD for teenagers, accompanied by an audiocassette recording of a presentation they did at an adult ADD conference in Ann Arbor, Michigan (Amen & Amen, 1995). The book is written in easy-to-understand, colloquial language, chock full of anecdotes about how ADHD interfered with their lives in elementary, middle, and high school and how they overcame the many obstacles facing them. Adolescents can easily identify with such stories. In addition to conventional topics such as the definition of ADD, diagnosis, acceptance, medication, therapy, and education, Amen et al. (1996) give teenagers with ADHD frank advice on ADHD and its impact on love relationships, friends, driving, drugs and alcohol, overcoming anger and negative thinking patterns, and staying motivated and on their legal rights. The stories written by Michael and Chris in Chapter 14 of this volume, may also make useful reading for some adolescents.

Therapists may also find it useful to watch an appropriate videotape in the session together with their teenager clients. Viewing videotapes of adolescents discussing their ADHD with the teenage patient during the ADHD education session is a way to provide some peer contact in situations in which the practitioner does not have positive peer models readily accessible. One such videotape is *ADHD in Adolescents: Our Point of View* (Schubiner, 1995). In this 20-minute videotape, Dr. Schubiner interviews five adolescents with ADHD, discussing what ADHD is, how it af-

TABLE 7.1. Extreme and Reasonable Beliefs Concerning ADHD

Extreme belief	Reasonable belief
ADHD is a life sentence.	ADHD is a life style, not a life sentence. It is true that you have to do things to cope with ADHD, but it's not all that bad. ADHD people have high energy, are very creative, and often can accomplish more than others.
I'm dumb and stupid.	ADHD has nothing to do with IQ. You are at least as smart if not smarter than your peers. Some of the world's greatest geniuses—Einstein, Churchill, and others, probably had ADHD.
I'll lose all my friends because they will think I'm a nerd.	Your friends will only know if you tell them. They like you for whom you are. You've always had ADHD but didn't know it and they were your friends, so why would it change now? If they drop you, they aren't worth having anyway.
I'll spend all my life going to doctors, shrinks, and tutors.	Your parents would not want to pay for all that anyway. Look at most people dealing with ADHD. They see their doctor three or four times a year for 30 minutes. They may see a therapist for a number of weeks or a tutor, but you spend more time watching TV in a month than the average ADHD person spends in a year seeing doctors, tutors, and therapists. It's just not that bad.
Medication will change my personality in ways I don't like.	No one can really change your personality. Medicine is short-acting. It makes it easier for you to pay attention, think before you act, and feel less restless. It doesn't change personality.
I can never be a normal person.	Who is normal anyway? Everyone has their strange habits. You are not different than anyone else in this regard. ADHD is just a part of you, not all of you. It's an invisible disability so your friends won't see it.
This is all my fault.	ADHD is inherited and biologically based. You could not have caused it if you tried.
ADHD is just another way for my parents to control me and take away my freedom.	Actually, your parents are not controlling you at all. The issue is you controlling yourself, not others controlling you. ADHD means you are having trouble controlling yourself. We need to help you be in control of yourself.

Note. From *ADHD in Adolescents: Diagnosis and Treatment* by Arthur L. Robin. Copyright 1998 by The Guilford Press. Permission to photocopy this table is granted to purchasers of *ADHD in Adolescents* for personal use only (see copyright page for details).

fects their lives, how they learned about it, medication, school, psychological treatment, family relationships, and drugs and alcohol. At the end, each adolescent gives the audience key advice for coping. These adolescents come across as very spontaneous, caring, and normal in the tape. Most teenagers viewing this tape quickly realize that people with ADHD are not freaks, just normal teenagers like themselves. It would not be difficult for readers to make similar, educational videotapes with their patient populations, permitting them to tailor the material to their ethnic, geographic, or otherwise idiosyncratic patient situations.

Psychoeducational Groups/Teen Forums

Attending psychoeducational groups with other adolescents directed by adolescents is a powerful way of mobilizing positive peer pressure to increase understanding and acceptance of ADHD. I have helped to arrange and monitor such teen forums through Children and Adults with Attention Deficit Disorder (CH.A.D.D.) at the local chapter level and at the national conference level. Based on these experiences and feedback from the teenage participants, I specifically recommend the following to practitioners who wish to arrange such support groups through their own practices or local organizations:

1. Arrange to have a one-time teen forum lasting 1½ to 3 hours at maximum.
2. Limit enrollment at any one time to 20–30 teenagers per group. If you anticipate a larger enrollment, have several smaller sections.
3. Separate the groups by grade or age. Run separate sessions for middle school, high school, and college-age youngsters. They have separate issues which do not mix well.
4. Locate and train several teenager discussion leaders to run the groups. They need to be teenagers who "know the ropes" of ADHD, have been to the bottom of the pit and back, and have good leadership skills and are not afraid to speak their minds and self-disclose. The quality of the teen discussion leaders makes or breaks the meeting. Involve the teen discussion leaders in the planning of the session.
5. Decide on your exact purpose and plan the session activities accordingly. For example, at the CH.A.D.D. of Eastern Oakland County Teen Forum, our primarily purpose was to facilitate group interaction among the adolescents about coping with ADHD, not to provide specific educational content. Therefore, we chose to conduct a 90-minute evening meeting with two parts. First, the audience watched Dr. Schubiner's 20-minute videotape. Second, the teen leaders used the videotape as a springboard for an open-ended discussion about anything the audience wanted to discuss. At the first CH.A.D.D. National Teen Forum, the purpose was a combination of interaction and education about specific content. A curriculum with handouts was developed covering basic information about ADHD, medication, study strategies, dealing with family issues, and high-risk behaviors. Brief talks by adult experts were intertwined with group discussion led by adolescents.

6. Build in frequent breaks, especially if you are presenting education-al material. Breaks are needed every 20–30 minutes.
7. Allow plenty of opportunity for interacting and socializing, which may be the primary motivators for adolescents to participate.
8. Serve decaffeinated, low-sugar snacks.
9. When feasible, bring in a high-profile sports or entertainment fig-ure who has disclosed his or her ADHD to serve as a motivational speaker for the teenagers.

Many of the beliefs summarized in Table 7.1 spontaneously arise and are discussed during such a teen forum. The teen discussion leaders can also be trained to interject them strategically and spur discussion of them. Research on the effectiveness of such psychoeducational teen forums is sorely needed, and readers are urged to conduct such programs and collect data on their effectiveness in fostering knowledge about and acceptance of ADHD.

School-based peer coaching programs are another group-based pro-gram that may also prove effective in encouraging adolescents to accept and cope with ADHD while also teaching organizational skills. Peggy Bird (personal communication, January 27, 1997) described a middle and high school peer coaching program designed to train students to set long-term goals, establish daily priorities, and set an action plan. Students are as-signed partners and taught to use Hallowell's HOPE model. Taking turns being the coach and then the player, each member of the pair asks the ques-tions that the key words prompt: *H*ello, *O*bjectives, *P*lans, and *E*ncourage-ment. Student pairs meet daily in school. They set long-term and daily ob-jectives, but in each daily interaction, they focus on the three most important things they must do for that day. These things may be related to short- or long-term objectives. We need to evaluate the effectiveness of such coaching efforts.

The Role of Metaphors

Metaphors such as the story about brake fluid discussed earlier are invalu-able tools in helping adolescents understand and accept ADHD. The visual impairment and the television metaphors often prove useful for this pur-pose.

Visual Impairment Metaphor. Some people do not see clearly. They are born with the genes for poor vision. Visual problems are first apparent during childhood and change over time, but they generally continue over the course of a lifetime. A person who does not see clearly gets glasses; this helps them cope effectively. As they grow and mature, they may need a new prescription because their eyes change. Like visual impairment, people are born with the genes for ADHD. The ADHD person first has trouble paying attention and controlling impulses/restlessness during childhood. These difficulties may change as the person grows older, but they often last a lifetime, like visual impairment. The ADHD person can be helped too. Medication, accommodation in school, and psychological interventions are like glasses. When people put on their glasses, they see clearly. When medication is in their body, they attend well and control themselves efficiently. When they apply what they learn from therapy or educational accommodations, they manage their life effectively and have good interpersonal relationships and good academic achievement. There is no stigma to wearing glasses; there does not have to be any stigma to accepting and coping with ADHD.

Television Screen Metaphor. Sometimes a television is out of focus or the channel changer becomes stuck in scanning mode, continuously changing from one channel to another. When this happens, it is difficult to watch the television. It gets so frustrating that most people just turn off the set and do not even try. ADHD is similar to a stuck channel changer or a blurry TV screen. It may be difficult to focus the brain or to keep it on one channel or project. The brain keeps making the ADHD individual want to switch to another project or task, before he or she finishes the last one, and it is difficult to obtain a clear view of each task. Sometimes people with ADHD get so frustrated because they have been trying so hard that they just stop trying. We can understand why that happens because no matter how much the individual wants to accomplish, it is sometimes not possible for the individual to make his or her mind stay on one thing long enough. Treatment for ADHD can help focus the TV screen in the mind and keep the channels (e.g., thoughts) from changing so quickly. Medication, therapy, and educational accommodations are like adjusting the tracking on a VCR and the focus on the TV or getting the channel changer fixed.

Assign Homework and Plan Treatment

As in the case example described earlier, asking Bill to talk to another teenager with ADHD is one of the most common types of homework assignments designed to enhance positive attitudes toward the disorder. Attending support groups such as the teen forums outlined previously is a closely related method of helping teenagers understand and accept their ADHD. In addition to the book by Amen et al. (1996), there are a variety of other excellent books and videotapes available for educating adolescents about ADHD (see Quinn, 1995; Gordon, 1993; Parker, 1992; and Nadeau, 1994, for illustrative books written by adults along with a videotape by Goldstein, 1991).

If the practitioner does assign homework to collect evidence bearing on attitudes toward ADHD, it is important to review the homework at the beginning of the next session. Failure to review early homework assignments models inconsistent follow-through and decreases the chances of adolescent compliance with future homework assignments. Let's look in on the review of Bill's homework assignment to talk with Danny, the ADHD peer.

DR. ROBIN: So what happened when you talked to Danny about ADD?

BILL: I realized that if a neat kid like Danny has ADD, it's not that bad. I'm really OK with this ADD thing now, Doc. Do you think my teachers will let me out of homework if I tell them I've got bad genes? Or will my chemistry teacher give me a hall pass if I tell him that the chemicals in my brain are making me bored and restless?

DR. ROBIN: Do they let Danny out of homework and get hall passes for boredom?

BILL: Just kidding. Danny told me ADD is a challenge, not an excuse. I guess he was right about the challenge part. But you know the best thing of all?

DR. ROBIN: (*puzzled*) What's that?

BILL: Danny told Jennifer what a great kid I am. And now she is going to homecoming with me!

As soon as Danny, a credible higher authority figure on teenage issues because of his popularity in high school, sanctioned ADHD as an okay thing to have, Bill became comfortable with it, at least at an intellectual level. It will, nonetheless, take time to determine whether his superficial embracing of ADHD translates into hard effort and emotional acceptance. Quite typically, Bill then tested whether he could use ADHD as an excuse to avoid work. Not surprisingly, the most significant event for Bill was the fact that Danny helped him get Jennifer to be his girlfriend. Practitioners need to humbly realize that this kind of peer event probably has more impact on attitudes towards ADHD than anything done in a therapy session. If the homework assignment to talk with Danny had not had the intended impact, I would have continued with a cognitive restructuring discussion.

Typically, the process of developing coping attitudes toward ADHD takes some time for most adolescents. Most commonly, the teenager remains skeptical after one or two discussions of ADHD. The practitioner should reinforce healthy skepticism, congratulating adolescents on being wise consumers but urging them to continue collecting information to inform themselves about ADHD. Such a position is consistent with adolescent development and works much better than any authoritarian tactics.

The last phase of the family ADHD education process with the adolescent is treatment planning. Once Bill became more open to ADHD, I directly approached him about participating in treatment.

DR. ROBIN: We have one last thing to talk about—exactly what you are going to do and how your parents, teachers, and I am going to help you deal with ADHD. For one, are you now willing to consider medication as one way to deal with ADHD?

BILL: I guess so.

DR. ROBIN: I'm not asking you to take it for sure, but just to go talk to a friend of mine, Dr. Schubiner, who specializes in medicine for ADD teens. Agreed?

BILL: OK. What else?

DR. ROBIN: Do you want your parents off you case at home? And your teachers off your case at school?

BILL: Sure. How?

DR. ROBIN: You got to be willing to learn some new habits. I am willing to be like a coach and give you ideas and guide you, if you will come in several times, but you will have to do the work.

BILL: Will I have to come at this time? I'm missing one of my favorite TV shows?

DR. ROBIN: Absolutely not. We can find another time.

BILL: I'll try.

I continued to discuss and formulate the treatment goals with the adolescent, interacting in this informal manner. Once the therapist takes the time to listen to and deal with the adolescent's reactions, the teenager becomes more cooperative. Most of the time, this strategy works. But the practitioner needs to be prepared to be patient in those minority of cases in which the adolescent's resistance lasts a longer time. It is difficult to enlist some 12- to 14-year-old adolescents collaboratively in the treatment process. Occasionally, the only reasonable strategy to follow is to decide to treat the case as if the young teenager were an 8- or 9-year-old and work with the parents on a management approach without regularly involving the adolescent. Clearly the less preferred approach, this is nonetheless sometimes necessary.

CONCLUSION

This chapter outlined how practitioners should plan the treatment program and how they should explain it to the family and enlist their understanding and cooperation. Chapters 8 through 12 discuss the specific components of the treatment program in great detail.

CHAPTER EIGHT

———————— ◯ ————————

Medical Interventions

WITH HOWARD SCHUBINER, MD

After the clinician has conducted family ADHD education, he or she should consider medication before continuing with school and home-based interventions. For the majority of individuals coping with ADHD, medication is usually a necessary but insufficient treatment. Without the biological correction provided by medication, it is difficult for most adolescents with ADHD to pull their lives together and to succeed at school, get along with their families, feel good about themselves, and accomplish the developmental tasks of adolescence. To start with medication early in the overall treatment is helpful because the clinician can then find the residual difficulties with which the adolescent needs to learn to cope. Medication works synergistically with psychosocial and educational interventions, which means that the adolescent on medication will benefit more from these interventions—paying better attention and getting more out of the therapy sessions.

In this chapter we provide practical answers for the medical and nonmedical clinicians to the following questions about the use of medication in adolescents with ADHD:

1. What do we know about the effectiveness of medication in treating adolescents with ADHD?
2. How widespread is the use of medication for treating adolescents with ADHD?
3. When is medication indicated for the adolescent diagnosed as having ADHD?
4. How can we explain medication to the adolescent and the family, and how can we enlist their cooperation?
5. Which stimulant or nonstimulant medication should be started?

6. What are the common side effects for each medication, and how can we manage these side effects?
7. How can we titrate the dose of medication and monitor its effectiveness?

EFFECTIVENESS OF MEDICATION

No other treatment for ADHD has been subjected to as much empirical scrutiny as medication, particularly stimulant medication. The educated professional ought to become familiar with the strengths and weaknesses of this research literature (see the Appendix at the end of the book for a detailed review).

Research suggests that an average of 70% of 5,608 children and adolescents with ADHD and 160 adults with ADHD participating in 155 studies of methylphenidate, amphetamines, and pemoline responded positively (Spencer et al., 1996). Positive effects were obtained on measures of overactivity, impulsivity, and inattentiveness, as well as on-task behavior, academic performance, social functioning, family, and peer relationships.

However, only seven (4%) of these studies were done specifically with adolescents, and all of them evaluated methylphenidate (the first two studies with pemoline have just been completed but not yet published (J. Biderman, personal communication, May 12, 1998; B. Smith, personal communication, January 12, 1998). A critical analysis of these seven studies indicated a 50% positive response rate with adolescents, 20% lower than the 70% overall positive response rate averaged across age; some investigators have argued that methodological factors in these studies may account for this lower response rate with adolescents, and it would be premature to conclude that stimulant medication works less often with adolescents than with younger children (Smith, Pelham, Gnagy, & Yudell, 1998).

Research regarding nonstimulant medication shows that tricylic antidepressants (TCAs) can be effective with adolescents but the majority of these studies have been done with younger children (Spencer et al., 1996). There is also some evidence for the effectiveness of the bupropion and clonidine but little controlled research to date on the selective serotonin reuptake inhibitor (SSRI) antidepressants with ADHD children and adolescents.

Until recently, there were no well-controlled, carefully executed studies of the long-term effectiveness of stimulant medication. Then, Gillberg et al. (1997) published a randomized, double-blind placebo trial of amphetamine in which the children (ages 6–11) received active treatment for 15 months. Amphetamine was clearly superior to placebo in reducing inattention, hyperactivity, and other disruptive behavior problems; treatment failure rate was considerably lower and time to treatment failure was longer in the amphetamine group than the placebo group. It is hoped that more such studies will appear in the near future.

HOW WIDESPREAD IS THE USE OF STIMULANT MEDICATION?

The prescription rate of stimulant medication has increased exponentially in the United States in the past three decades, although there is disagreement about the reasons for this trend. To get the best available answers to these questions, we review the work of Dr. Donald Safer, who has been studying trends in stimulant medication since the 1970s (Safer, 1996; Safer & Krager, 1985, 1988, 1988, 1994; Safer, Zito, & Fine, 1996).

The Drug Enforcement Administration (DEA) production quotas for methylphenidate in the United States increased from 1,768 kg in 1990 to 10,410 kg in mid-1995 (DEA, 1995). Because 90% of methylphenidate is prescribed for child and adolescent ADHD, this sixfold increase in production quotas has been interpreted by many to mean that there has been a profound increase in stimulant medication treatment for ADHD. These figures have been widely quoted in the popular media and have given rise to a great deal of negative publicity about ADHD and its medical treatment, including sensationalized headlines about Ritalin (methylphenidate) as "Kiddie cocaine" and "teachers as drug pushers." Barkley (1996c) has nicely chronicled how the negative media campaign about methylphenidate in 1995 and 1996 developed, and why it bore no rational relationship to any scientific data that would raise concerns about stimulant medication.

Safer at al. (1996) point out that the DEA production quotas for methylphenidate reflect a gross estimate of future use based on a variety of factors such as Food and Drug Administration estimates of need, drug inventories on hand, exports, and industry sales expectations. *This production quota is not based at all on actual data concerning patient usage of methylphenidate, and therefore the sixfold increase in production quotas does not mean that six times more children and adolescents are taking methylphenidate.* The media have completely misinterpreted and distorted these production quotas. Safer et al. (1996) mention the simple example that the annual production quotas for methylphenidate did not increase at all between 1976 and 1986, although patient use of methylphenidate did increase during this period (Safer & Krager, 1988; Rappley, Gardiner, Jetton, & Houang, 1995).

To get a more accurate picture of the extent of methylphenidate usage for ADHD in the 1990s and how this may be changing, Safer et al. (1996) compiled data from the following sources: (1) population-based time trends from their own Baltimore County biennial surveys of public school children on medication, (2) Maryland Medicaid data of methylphenidate prescriptions, (3) pharmaceutical company usage data, and (4) single assessment prevalence data from studies in Michigan, New York, Oregon, and Washington. The compilation of these data sources provides a more precise picture of actual trends in methylphenidate use for ADHD than do the DEA production quotas.

Safer et al. (1996) found that these four data sources revealed an approximately two- to threefold increase, not a sixfold increase, in the prevalence of youths receiving methylphenidate prescriptions from 1990 to 1995. For example, the percentage of youth receiving methylphenidate rose from 2.5% in 1991 to 3.2 % in 1995 in Baltimore County, and from 1.95% in 1990 to 4.7% in 1994 for the Maryland Medicaid data. Adjusting these regional figures for family income, prescription payment sources, and rural versus urban and private versus public school differences, Safer et al. (1996) estimated that in mid-1995, between 3–4% of United States youth aged 5 to 14 and between 2.5–3% of youth ages 5 to 18 were receiving methylphenidate treatment for ADHD. They estimated that between 1.3 and 1.5 million youth in the United States received methylphenidate in mid-1995, twice the projection made for 1987.

Why has there been a two- to threefold increase in methylphenidate prescriptions for ADHD during this period? Safer et al. (1996) examined several possible reasons:

1. *More youths are staying on medication for ADHD into their adolescent years.* Safer et al.'s (1996) Baltimore County data support this hypothesis. The proportion of secondary school students on methylphenidate increased from 11% in 1975 to 31% in 1995. In middle schools the increase was sevenfold; in high schools the increase was sixfold.
2. *More students with ADHD, Predominantly Inattentive subtype are being placed on medicine than in the past.* Teacher rating data revealed that in the 1970s, 7% of the students prescribed methylphenidate had attention problems without hyperactivity, but this increased to 18% by the mid-1980s (Safer & Krager, 1989).
3. *More girls are being diagnosed with ADHD and treated with stimulant medication.* The ratio of females to males on methylphenidate in Baltimore County has increased, particularly in secondary schools. In 1981, 1983, and 1985, the female/male ADHD medication ratios were 1:12, 1:10, and 1:10; in 1991, 1993, and 1995, the ratios narrowed to 1:7, 1:6, and 1:5.
4. *The public image of medication for ADHD has improved and parents are more comfortable with it.* The lawsuits of the early 1990s were settled, and among the negative publicity about methylphenidate is also some positive publicity.
5. *More adults are being diagnosed and treated medically with stimulants for ADHD.* Again, Safer et al. (1996) did not have hard data on this point, but clinically it appears to be true.

Although these data help us understand some of the reasons why we have had a twofold increase in methylphenidate usage in the United States in recent years, they do not directly address the issue of whether ADHD is being overdiagnosed or whether methylphenidate is being inappropriately prescribed. A study by Rappley (1996; Rappley et al., 1995) partially addressed this issue. The study looked at the use of methylphenidate in Michigan, which has been among the states with the highest per capita consumption of methylphenidate for over a decade. The study was conducted by examining the triplicate prescription data for all methylphenidate prescriptions written in Michigan during the months of February and March 1992. This period was selected because it represented a stable time of the school year, free of holidays. The results were based on 52,590 prescriptions written for 32,608 individuals (two were labeled "canine"). The 2-month point prevalence for the use of methylphenidate for those birth to 19 years was 11 per 1,000 (1.1%), representing 1.9% of boys and 0.4% of girls in this age range. Boys ages 8 to 11 received the highest rates of prescriptions (45% of total). There was a wide range of prescription rates across counties, but a small number of physicians accounted for the majority of prescriptions (50% written by 5% of pediatricians; 25% written by 1%). Although it was difficult to determine the amount of methylphenidate used per day because the 60-day time frame allowed only 2 months to be examined and directions regarding weekend use were not available, Rappley estimated that the most common dose was 10 mg twice a day, and that doses higher than 60 mg a day were typically written by child psychiatrists.

The per capita use in children of 1.1% was less than the expected prevalence of ADHD (3–5%) in a state known to have one of the highest per capita consumptions of methylphenidate. The amount prescribed per child per day did not seem excessive. The finding that a small number of physicians write a majority of the prescriptions probably reflects referral patterns and specialization interests. One concern about the study is that the point prevalence appears to have been computed using the total population birth to age 19 as the denominator, yet as the author herself pointed out, most methylphenidate was prescribed for school-age males. Using the total population in the computation when those age 0–5 hardly ever are prescribed the drug may result in underestimating the true prevalence of stimulant prescriptions. Despite this concern, more studies of a similar nature are needed.

WHEN IS MEDICATION INDICATED?

Medication is generally indicated when the following conditions are met: (1) a clear-cut positive diagnosis of ADHD, (2) moderate to severe impairment in school and/or home functioning, (3) agreement of the adolescent to take medication and concurrence of the parents with the adolescent's decision to take medication, (4) no abuse of alcohol, marijuana, or other illegal substances by the adolescent, and (5) no present medical contraindications such as hypertension, cardiovascular problems, or chronic diseases which are aggravated by psychoactive medication.

The impairment criterion is not clear-cut. To meet the criterion of "moderate to severe impairment" first there has to be evidence of clinical impairment to make the diagnosis of ADHD. A minority of youngsters diagnosed with ADHD during adolescence do not have any comorbid conditions, have difficulty with organization and follow-through in school, and generally have above-average intellectual ability and positive family environments. Such youngsters often respond well to a few well-orchestrated school-based accommodations and organizational aids, and may not need medication to cope successfully with the relatively mild impairment created by their ADHD. However, practitioners need to follow-up with such youngsters regularly because some will begin to have more serious impairments in college or adulthood and then might benefit from medication.

Unfortunately, there is no research yet with this group to back up the clinical impression that they may cope adequately without medication. The vast majority of adolescents with ADHD—either diagnosed during childhood or adolescence—do not fall into this category of mild impairment. In essence, these criteria mean that the vast majority of adolescents diagnosed with ADHD should be tried on medication, as long as they agree to it.

There is an unfortunate tendency among some professionals and families to look upon medication as a last resort or as a desperate intervention to be tried only when all other psychosocial and educational interventions fail to prove sufficient. Such professionals typically prescribe too low and infrequent doses of medication, setting up the adolescent for failure. If side effects occur, they readily abandon the medication rather than conduct a thorough trial of several stimulant and nonstimulant drugs. These professionals may communicate this last-resort belief to families, not allowing them to give medication a fair chance. Such an attitude represents a serious impediment to the welfare and effective treatment of adolescents with ADHD. It fosters a lack of acceptance of medication among teenagers, creates fears and anxieties in parents about medication, and goes against all the evidence reviewed in this book and other sources (Barkley, 1998). The evidence concerning etiology clearly points to neurobiological and genetic factors in the majority of cases of ADHD (Zimetkin & Rapoport, 1987). The treatment outcome literature indicates that although a variety of psychosocial and educational interventions are useful, medication receives the greatest consistent support as today's single most effective treatment (Barkley, 1998).

However, we are not advocating medication for every adolescent who has problems getting school work done, and we are certainly not advocating, as some authors and journalists have suggested (Armstrong, 1995) that youngsters be medicated so teachers do not have to teach and parents do not have to parent. Readers need to be prepared to respond to those who make these accusations. We advocate the judicious use of medication for those with a diagnosis of ADHD to put adolescents in control of themselves, not so that others can control them and make them docile. We also advocate medication together with other interventions because it is the most effective treatment we have when a thorough evaluation has resulted in a clear-cut diagnosis and the youngster is suffering from ADHD. Many cases of overmedicating are the result of a sloppy, incomplete diagnostic practice. Prescribing medication as a means of "confirming" the diagnosis of ADHD, for example, represents poor clinical practice and an error in logic.

EXPLAINING MEDICATION TO ADOLESCENTS AND THEIR FAMILIES

The following types of physicians are likely to understand how to explain the medication to the adolescent, and prescribe and monitor it: adolescent medicine specialists, developmental and behavioral pediatricians, child and adolescent psychiatrists, and some pediatricians or family physicians. If psychologists, social workers, or educators have difficulty locating a physician experienced in working with adolescents with ADHD in their region, they might contact the national office of either the Society for Adolescent Medicine (816-224-8010), the Society for Developmental and Behavioral Pediatrics (215-248-9168), or a local chapter of Children and Adults with Attention Deficit Disorder (CH.A.D.D.) listed in the yellow pages or located through the World Wide Web (http://www.chadd.org). The nonmedical mental health provider can also provide such an explanation and/or help educate the local physicians about what is needed.

Medication should never be forced on adolescents, instead the physician should talk to them about medicine, without the presence of parents, and give a clear explanation of ADHD as a neurobiological disorder, which can be explained to adolescents as "a mild chemical imbalance in the brain." It should be pointed out that the role of medication is not to change the person but to correct the chemical imbalance in the brain to allow the adolescent to maximize his or her potential in life. It can be explained that stimulant medication provides the missing chemicals allowing the adolescent to concentrate and thus accomplish tasks properly and to be in control of his or her life. The physician should explain medication to the adolescent in such a manner that the adolescent will be likely to attribute his or her successes while taking medication primarily to his or her own efforts (i.e., internal attributions) rather than to the medication alone (i.e., external attributions). Many of the suggestions made in Chapter 7 (this volume) regarding family ADHD education are also applicable to explaining medication to adolescents and their families. The visual metaphor and the television metaphor, along with photographs from the PET scan studies are useful in explaining medication. Zeigler Dendy (1995) also provides an excellent discussion of how to explain medication to adolescents.

Following the approach outlined in Chapter 7, after presenting some brief information about medication, the physician then needs to listen carefully to the adolescent's concerns about medication. They are likely to be issues such as fear of peer ridicule, embarrassment about having to take a pill at lunch, fear that medicine will permanently change their personality and make them feel "weird" or get them addicted or hooked, and/or concern about medicine as an extension of adult control over them. Bowen, Fenton, and Rappaport (1990) in fact assessed children's and adolescents' perceptions of stimulant medication and found that two variables influenced whether the children wanted to continue taking their medication: (1) the perception that the medication makes them feel as if something is wrong with them and (2) feelings of embarrassment about receiving the medication.

It is important for teenagers to feel that the physician is genuinely hearing their concerns and taking them seriously because many teenagers are used to having their concerns dismissed by their parents as not legitimate. As the teenager expresses his or her concerns, it may be helpful to develop a written list of the advantages and the disadvantages of taking medication. Sensitive physicians also know that the teenagers need to feel in control of the decision to start and continue medication, so they often tell the adolescent up front that he or she has veto power over all decisions about medication, and that it will not be started or continued without his or her agreement.

After the physician compiles the list of the advantages and disadvantages of medicine, he or she can review it along with the adolescent and decide whether the advantages outweigh the disadvantages. The physician can also provide medical input about ways to deal with some of the perceived disadvantages. For example, if an adolescent is concerned that he or she will be too mellowed out while on stimulant medication, the physician can point out that there are many different types of medication, and the dose and type can be fine-tuned to minimize this problem. If the adolescent is concerned about the effect of medication on growth, the physician can point out that growth will be monitored regularly and if there is any slowing, medication will be changed or stopped. The physician should also point out that a "trial" on medication means that the adolescent will be trying the medication to see if it is helpful, and if it is not, the physician will develop another plan.

When a skilled physician takes the time to talk to adolescents in this way about medication, most agree to try it. There will, however, still be a minority of adolescents, mostly those ages 12 to 14, who adamantly refuse to try medication. The physician can propose a contract whereby the adolescent agrees to bring up his or her grades and change specific behaviors over the next few months; if this works, the discussion of medication will be dropped. If the adolescent is unable to bring up his or her grades, then medication will be discussed again. For adolescents approaching driving age, it may help to point out the positive effect of medication on driving and that the clinician would be willing to advocate for the teen to take driver's training if the teen agrees to try medication. Introducing the adolescent to other teenagers who have had positive experiences with medication can also be a powerful strategy. Clinicians might contact local chapters of CH.A.D.D. to locate positive adolescent role models. In those few cases in which the adolescent refuses to consider medication, despite all these strategies, the topic should be dropped for the time being and brought up again if significant difficulties related to ADHD persist.

SELECTING AND STARTING MEDICATION

Stimulants are the first-line medications, as they appear to be the most effective and safe agents. They have been shown to be effective in ameliorating the core symptoms of ADHD, as well as improving academic productivity and social interactions. Although the exact mechanism of action of the stimulants on the brain is not known with certainty, research to date suggests that their ability to increase the availability of the important neurotransmitters dopamine and norepinephrine in the synaptic cleft accounts for their clinical effects in ADHD (Zimetkin & Rapoport, 1987). They may increase the availability of these neurotransmitters by blocking their reuptake in the presynaptic neuron and increasing their release into the extra neuronal space (Wilens & Biederman, 1992). Certain regions of the brain, such as the frontal and prefrontal cortex, which are responsible for inhibitory functions, are rich in dopamine and norepinephrine receptors and are thought to be the sites mediating the effects of stimulants on the central nervous system.

The physician has a choice of two short-acting stimulants (methylphenidate tablets or dextroamphetamine tablets) or four longer-acting stimulants (methylphenidate sustained release [SR], dextroamphetamine spansule, Adderall, or pemoline). Combinations of the short-acting and SR preparations of a given drug may also be used (e.g., Ritalin SR + Ritalin tablets; Dexedrine [dextroamphetamine] spansules + Dexedrine tablets), although combinations of different stimulants are not commonly used at the same time. Any of these stimulants may be prescribed initially, although there are good reasons to start with either short-acting Ritalin or Dexedrine spansules. Table 8.1 summarizes information about the stimulants. Some of the suggestions given here are based on previous work by the authors (Schubiner, Robin, & Neinstein, 1996).

There are two approaches to conducting a trial on stimulant medica-

TABLE 8.1. Stimulant Medications

Generic name	Trade name	Available doses	Length of action	Absolute range per dose	Weight-based dose ranges per day
Methylphenidate	Ritalin	5, 10, 20 mg	3–4 hr	5–30 mg	0.3–2.0 mg/kg
SR methylphenidate	SR Ritalin	20 mg	5–6 hr	20–60 mg	0.3–2.0 mg/kg
Dextroamphetamine	Dexedrine	5 mg	4–5 hr	5–20 mg	0.3–1.0 mg/kg
Dextroamphetamine spansule	Dexedrine spansule	5, 10, 15 mg	6–8 hr	5–30 mg	0.3–1.0 mg/kg
Four amphetamines combined	Adderall	10, 20 mg	4–6 hr	5–30 mg	0.3–1.0 mg/kg
Pemoline	Cylert	18.75, 37.5, 75 mg	6–12 hr	18.75–112.5 mg	1.0–3.0 mg/kg

tion. The first, most common approach, is an open clinical trial. The adolescent is started on a low dose of medicine for 1–2 weeks, and the dose is gradually titrated upward over time, based on feedback from rating scales, interviews, and school performance data. The second approach is a double-blind, placebo cross-over trial. Barkley, Fischer, Newby, and Breen (1988) described how to implement such a trial in a clinical setting. The physician arranges with the pharmacy to prepare a placebo and several doses of the active drug in identical capsules; the pharmacy decides on the order of the placebo and active drug doses, with 1–2 weeks under each condition then crossing over to the next condition. Until the entire trial is over, only the pharmacy knows the order of conditions. Measures are taken after each condition and compared at the end of the double-blind trial after the blind has been broken.

The advantage of the double-blind approach is that the effectiveness of the medication at each dose can be definitively determined without any bias. Adolescents, parents, and school personnel greatly appreciate such an objective trial. It helps build genuine commitment to take medication known to be effective. The disadvantage of a double-blind trial is the extra time and effort involved in making the arrangements and monitoring the outcome. However, many adolescents with ADHD are concurrently attending therapy with psychologists who are familiar with such research protocols; the psychologist could help make the arrangements and monitor and interpret the results if the physician is unable or unwilling to do this him- or herself. We would strongly urge practitioners to consider double-blind placebo trials of medication whenever possible.

It should also be mentioned that many textbooks on psychopharmacology provide formulas for dosing stimulants precisely according to body weight (e.g., mg/kg). Although physicians working with adolescents adhere to the general principle of prescribing more medicine with higher body weights, there is no empirical research to indicate that such formulas will yield the optimal dose for a given adolescent. In one study, for example, body mass index failed to predict the optimal dose of methylphenidate or gains achieved at an optimal dose. It also failed to distinguish between drug responders and nonresponders (Rapport & Kenney, 1997). Also, no blood level tests for the stimulants have proven useful in clinical monitoring. The dose of medication needed varies with the individual's metabolism, the severity of the ADHD symptoms, the presence of comorbid conditions, the individual's other behavioral characteristics, and the nature of the adolescent's school and home environments. The formulas simply provide the guidelines for dosing the stimulants and have been included in Table 8.1. Trial-and-error experimentation with gradually increasing doses, given careful feedback and monitoring, is used to determine the actual dose. Dosing the stimulants is based on the artful use of case study methods, close collaboration with the family and school, and a trusting relationship with the adolescent.

Methylphenidate

Dosing

Methylphenidate is used most frequently and should be started at low doses before building up to the optimal dose. A typical titration method for short-acting methylphenidate is to start with 5 mg two or three times a day and increase by 5 mg per dose at weekly intervals up to 20 mg doses, checking weekly by telephone for positive effects and side effects, and having a follow-up office visit with the physician at the end of 1 month. Methylphenidate has a half-life of 2–3 hours, and a variable peak plasma concentration at 1–2 hours postingestion. The clinical onset of action takes about 30 minutes, and either two or three doses a day are given on schooldays. Methylphenidate can be given in the morning and before lunch if the primary reason for taking the medicine is concentration while in the classroom. However, it is rarely the case that this is the only time when the adolescent truly needs the help of medication to cope adequately with the symptoms of ADHD, even though many families and adolescents insist that medicine is not needed at other times. A third dose in the afternoon and some weekend doses should be considered for most adolescents. The schedule of weekend doses may be different or more flexible than the schoolday doses. ADHD affects the whole fabric of an adolescent's life, including after-school sports, recreational activities, relationships with family and friends, driving performance, and of course completion of homework in the evening. There is risk of injury from potentially inattentive or impulsive behavior while bicycling, skateboarding, roller blading, boating, driving, and so on. There are decision-making challenges concerning life style risks (e.g., temptations to use drugs or alcohol or to engage in sexual intercourse without contraception) which take place throughout the late afternoon, evening, and weekend, when the two school-day doses of methylphenidate have worn off or are absent. For all these reasons, as the adolescent matures, it makes sense to negotiate a treatment plan that provides coverage by medication throughout the day and on weekends.

Sustained-release methylphenidate can be a useful medication as long as clinicians understand that one dose may not last for the entire school-day. Although rated for durations of up to 8 hours, it lasts 5–6 hours for the majority of adolescents. It has a half-life of 2–6 hours with peak levels occurring from 1–4 hours and peak behavioral effect occurring within 2 hours. It only comes in a 20-mg preparation, which is supposed to be the equivalent of taking two doses of 10 mg apiece. Clinical experience suggests that 20-mg SR methylphenidate is the equivalent of taking two 7.5-mg short-acting tablets on separate occasions. It takes 45–60 minutes for SR methylphenidate to start acting. In addition, adolescents should never cut SR methylphenidate in half because that destroys its slow-release properties and may create unusual effects. SR methylphenidate is helpful for those patients who only require small doses or those who experience too many "ups and downs" with the short-acting preparation. A reasonable starting dose would be 20 mg SR once or twice a day, although some will require a doubling of this dose. Those adolescents with mild ADHD symptoms and most of their heavy academic classes clustered in the morning may make it through the school day with one dose, but most of them will need a second dose 5–6 hours after the first. It is common to add SR to short-acting methylphenidate to slightly lengthen and smooth out the overall effect of each dose. For example, if lunch is fifth period and short-acting methylphenidate wears off before fourth period, a combined dose may carry the adolescent until lunch.

There has been concern that tolerance might develop to the initial effects of methylphenidate such that the initial effects would be greater than any subsequent effects. In their review, Wilens and Biederman (1992) found that the need for increased doses over time was almost always accounted for by growth. In one large-scale study where children on methylphenidate were followed up over 4 years, only 3% of the children had a loss of effect attributable to tolerance (Wilens & Biederman, 1992). Clinically, tolerance rarely develops with adolescents, and drug "holidays" are not usually required (with the exception of a few adolescents who have a decrease in their growth velocity).

Clinical reports also show that the brand-name Ritalin is sometimes more potent than some generic forms of methylphenidate. There are many forms of generic methylphenidate which may differ slightly in their fillers, and the standards for the generic drugs allow 25% variability in the bioactive agent. There are no research studies comparing generic and brand-name methylphenidate. Therefore, it is difficult to evaluate the widespread belief that methylphenidate should be prescribed as DAW (dispensed as written). A reasonable approach is for the physician to remain open-minded, honor any personal preference the adolescent or the parents may express in this regard, and try both the generic and the brand-name drugs. The physician should expect that a slightly higher dose of the generic drug may be needed.

Side Effects

Serious side effects and relative contraindications for methylphenidate include the following:

1. Elevated blood pressure.
2. Arrhythmias (more likely when used in association with alcohol, caffeine, nicotine, or sympathomimetics). Teenagers often need to regulate caffeine while taking Ritalin, based on trial and error.
3. Development of acute psychotic reactions (rare, and they typically remit upon cessation of the stimulant).
4. Development of motor tics. Most patients who are going to develop tics do so prior to adolescence, but there are exceptions. Such patients may have underlying tic disorders such as Tourette's Disorder (comorbid to ADHD in 2–5% of cases) and should be managed by a primary care physician in conjunction with a neurologist.
5. Methylphenidate may lower the threshold for seizures in those predisposed to the development of seizures. Management by a neurologist is indicated in such cases.

Minor side effects of methylphenidate include appetite suppression often accompanied by mild weight loss; headaches; abdominal pain (usually in the first few days after starting the drug); dizziness; dry eyes or mouth; sweating; irritability, particularly when the medicine is wearing off; and insomnia (if the medication is taken too late in the evening, although some patients seem to have an easier time falling asleep while taking stimulants). For reasons that are yet completely understood, the negative effect of stimulants on sleep may occur a number of hours after the clinical effect of the drug has clearly worn off.

Persistent symptoms of nervousness or jitteriness and feeling either "spaced out" or "overfocused" are indications that the dose is too high. A few adolescents who are highly reactive to all types of medications may experience these symptoms even at low doses of methylphenidate. Ultimate height has been shown not to be compromised, and suppression of growth is rarely a problem in adolescence. Some adolescents develop "rebound" with symptoms of irritability, hyperemotionality, and acting out when the dose of methylphenidate is wearing off. If doses are spaced too far apart, they describe themselves as having "peaks and valleys." Methods to handle rebound medically include (1) making the doses closer together (3–3.5 hours); (2) making the last dose of the day lower than the earlier doses, easing the person off of medication; (3) switching to SR methylphenidate either alone or together with short-acting methylphenidate; and (4) switching to a different long-acting stimulant. Behaviorally, the adolescent can plan to "veg out" during the rebound period, if necessary.

If tics develop after the initiation of stimulant therapy, there are a few treatment options to consider. Initially, the stimulant should be stopped and if the tics resolve it can be restarted at a lower dose. If the tics persist on the least effective stimulant dose, a trial of clonidine or a tricyclic antidepressant may be given. Sometimes a low dose of a stimulant can be given if clonidine controls the tics. If none of these options provides an acceptable balance of control of tics and ADHD symptoms, a neurologist should be consulted.

When considering the significance of reported side effects, it is necessary to assess the base rate of the side effects in unmedicated groups of individuals with ADHD. Barkley, McMurray, Edelbrock, and Robbins (1990) compared parent and teacher reports of 17 common side effects in a controlled, placebo evaluation with 83 children ages 5–13 on placebo, lower dose (0.3 mg/kg), and higher dose (0.5 mg/kg) of methylphenidate. Using parent report, only 4 of the 17 side effects occurred significantly more often in the drug than the placebo conditions: decreased appetite, insomnia, stomachaches, and headaches. Fewer than half of the children experienced these side effects, and the mean severity ratings were in the mild range. Using teacher ratings, none of the side effects were greater during the medication than the placebo condition, and three of the side effects were significantly lower while taking the medication compared to the placebo condition: sadness, staring, and anxiety. Of course, teachers may not be in a position to observe the most common side-effects such as insomnia and loss of appetite. The percentage of subjects reporting common side effects under placebo was sometimes very high; that is, 40% of the parents reported insomnia under placebo, versus 62% and 68% under low and high doses of methylphenidate. This study points out how easy it would be to erroneously conclude that an adolescent has many side effects if the clinician failed to assess their occurrence prior to the onset of medication.

Practically, the adolescent's physician should ask the parents and the adolescent to complete the Barkley Stimulant Drug Side Effects Rating Scale before beginning medication and then at each follow-up visit. Table 8.2 presents this rating scale. It is important to understand the meaning of items endorsed positively on the side effects rating scale. For example, many parents check off "Tics or nervous movement," but upon further inquiry, they often misconstrue restlessness as "nervous movement." Some parents thought "tics" referred to tiny insects.

It is also important to realize that teenagers have different concerns

TABLE 8.2. Barkley Side Effects Rating Scale

Name_____   Date_____

Person Completing This Form_____

Instructions: Please rate each behavior from 0 (absent) to 9 (serious). Circle only one number beside each item. A zero means that you have not seen the behavior in this adolescent during the past week, and a 9 means that you have noticed it and believe it to be either serious or to occur frequently.

Behavior	Absent									Serious
Insomnia or trouble sleeping	0	1	2	3	4	5	6	7	8	9
Nightmares	0	1	2	3	4	5	6	7	8	9
Stares a lot or daydreams	0	1	2	3	4	5	6	7	8	9
Talks less with others	0	1	2	3	4	5	6	7	8	9
Uninterested in others	0	1	2	3	4	5	6	7	8	9
Decreased appetite	0	1	2	3	4	5	6	7	8	9
Irritable	0	1	2	3	4	5	6	7	8	9
Stomachaches	0	1	2	3	4	5	6	7	8	9
Headaches	0	1	2	3	4	5	6	7	8	9
Drowsiness	0	1	2	3	4	5	6	7	8	9
Sad/unhappy	0	1	2	3	4	5	6	7	8	9
Prone to crying	0	1	2	3	4	5	6	7	8	9
Anxious	0	1	2	3	4	5	6	7	8	9
Bites fingernails	0	1	2	3	4	5	6	7	8	9
Euphoric/ unusually happy	0	1	2	3	4	5	6	7	8	9
Dizziness	0	1	2	3	4	5	6	7	8	9
Tics or nervous movements	0	1	2	3	4	5	6	7	8	9

Note. From Barkley (1981). Copyright 1981 by The Guilford Press. Reprinted in *ADHD in Adolescents: Diagnosis and Treatment* by Arthur L. Robin. Permission to photocopy this table is granted to purchasers of *ADHD in Adolescents* for personal use only (see copyright page for details).

about side effects than do parents. Teens are often less concerned about appetite suppression, insomnia, or tics than they are about whether stimulants will make them feel different or change their personality. Sometimes, extroverted adolescents come to view their hyperactivity as part of their personality and when stimulant medication calms them, they conclude that it has changed their personality.

No potentially deleterious effects of methylphenidate have been found and there is no evidence that it can become addictive with normal oral administration, or that protracted use of it leads to later increased use of alcohol or illicit drugs. It has not been proven that methylphenidate is associated with depression, suicide, or violence, and there are no published cases of a suicide from an overdose of it. An adolescent who took an overdose would act bizarre or at worst, experience an acute psychotic reaction until it wore off.

Abuse

There have been some anecdotal reports of abuse of methylphenidate by adolescents and adults (Rosenberg, 1996). A national sample of adolescents is surveyed every year for the Monitoring the Future (MTF) Survey of the University of Michigan. Data from this study are critical to a determination of the magnitude of the problem of abuse by adolescents on methylphenidate. The most recent data (1995) reveal that amphetamines as a class of drugs are abused much less than other agents. For example, senior high school students reported that 75% used alcohol in the past year, with 64% using cigarettes, and 25% using marijuana or hashish. By comparison, 9% reported using any type of amphetamine without a physician's prescription in the past year. Cocaine, barbiturates, and hallucinogens were used by about 4% of seniors. During the two decades that this study was carried out, the proportion of seniors who report using methylphenidate without a physician's prescription has remained relatively stable. In 1976, 0.5% reported such use; corresponding figures for 1980, 1985, 1990, and 1995 are 0.6%, 0.4%, 0.5%, and 0.8%. Similarly, the National Household Survey on Drug Abuse found that the rate of nonmedical use of methylphenidate has been stable at 0.2% of the adolescent and adult population from 1988 to 1994. Even though methylphenidate is being abused by a small proportion of the population, its use does not seem to be rising significantly, and it is not the choice of stimulants among young people. For example, the MTF study found that 21% of seniors had used over-the-counter stimulants (legal products such as "stay awake" pills) in the past year.

Adolescents who abuse methylphenidate often crush the tablets and snort them intranasally. This method of administration is associated with relatively few dangerous medical effects. There are few reported cases of serious disorders from intranasal use, although seizures, sympathetic overactivity, hyperpyrexia and muscle breakdown can occur. There have been several case reports of adults who have used methylphenidate intravenously (often along with pentazocine).

It is our clinical impression that the patients prescribed methylphenidate are relatively unlikely to abuse it. They realize that its effects are calming and focusing rather than euphoric inducing. However, with the increased number of adolescents taking methylphenidate, it is likely that other teens will have access to it and will experiment with it as a stimulant. All adolescents who are taking methylphenidate (or other stimulants) should be counseled about the dangers of providing stimulants to peers.

Parents and professionals need to talk frankly with adolescents with ADHD about the problem of methylphenidate abuse (Rosenberg, 1996). Such a conversation should be held by the time the child reaches age 11 or 12. The topic might be brought up in conjunction with a television show or article about the issue of methylphenidate abuse. Perhaps, a parent might say, "Hey, I read something in a magazine or videotaped this TV show that seems important. Could you read it or view it, and then we could talk about it?" Parents should ask the teenager about his or her thoughts on the article or show, and whether he or she has encountered any situations with methylphenidate abuse in their school. Parents should ask how the adolescent would handle it if someone approached him or her and asked for the medicine. Listening to the adolescent on this topic is more important than lecturing. A possible responses for an adolescent might be, "No, this medicine is prescribed for me by my doctor, not for anyone else." In some cases, the therapist might role-play with the adolescent common scenarios concerning being asked to give away medicine, helping to prompt and reinforce assertive responses. The therapist should encourage adolescents to report any such situations to either their parents or the school authorities. Finally, parents should become aware of how their adolescent's school stores and dispenses medicine. They should not assume that all schools are aware of the problem and are taking adequate steps to store and dispense medicine appropriately.

Amphetamines

Dextroamphetamine

Dextroamphetamine spansules are effective, long-acting preparations which are tolerated well (often with fewer side effects than methylphenidate). It is the drug of choice when the adolescent objects to taking a noontime dose of medication. It comes in 5-, 10-, and 15-mg spansules and is generally considered to be twice as potent as methylphenidate. Therefore, few adolescents require more than 15–20 mg twice a day. The side effect profile is similar to methylphenidate, but if a second dose is prescribed, one has to make sure it does not have a negative impact on sleeping. A common initial regimen would be to start with 5 mg once a day and increase by 5 mg per dose at weekly intervals up to 15- to 20-mg doses, checking weekly by telephone for positive effects and side effects, and having a follow-up office visit with the physician at the end of 1 month. Coverage is typically provided for homework and after-school activities either by adding a second dose of the spansule or by adding a dose of short-acting dextroamphetamine tablets in equivalent milligrams to the spansule. The decision as to which afternoon dose to add depends on the length of coverage needed and the impact of the spansule on sleep. Sometimes, when afternoon and evening medication coverage is needed, a lower dose of the spansule will suffice. Short-acting dextroamphetamine tablets can also be used as a primary medication when needed. However, they have the disadvantages of being difficult to find and coming only in a 5-mg tablet, necessitating most adolescents to take a large number of tablets per day. Methylphenidate is therefore the drug of choice for a short-acting medication.

Many physicians are hesitant to prescribe dextroamphetamine because of concern about its abuse potential, the relatively greater difficulty finding it in most communities, and the fact that in some states it is more carefully regulated than methylphenidate. There are no data on the abuse of dextroamphetamine per se, although it is likely to occur to some degree. It is hoped that physicians working with adolescents will become more willing to prescribe dextroamphetamine spansules. Because of the long action of the spansule and the difficulty convincing many adolescents to take noon doses of medicine, dextroamphetamine spansules may often be the drug of choice. Another formulation of dextroamphetamine has been released recently under the brand name of Dextrostat.

Adderrall

Adderall is another amphetamine now available. It consists of a combination of four different amphetamine salts, including dextroamphetamine and amphetamine. Very little research has been done with Adderall, and the few completed studies have not focused on adolescents (Swanson et al., 1998). It comes in 10-mg and 20-mg tablets, which can be administered one to three times a day and lasts 5–6 hours per dose. Most adolescents need at least two doses a day. Clinical experience suggests that Adderall is generally as effective and Dexedrine and can be used interchangeably. Due to its slightly different formula, Adderall may be effective when other stimulants are not. The side effect profile is similar to methylphenidate.

Pemoline

Pemoline (Cylert) is a long-acting stimulant with an unknown mechanism of action different from those mentioned already. It comes in 18.75-mg, 37.5-mg, and 75-mg tablets, and is usually taken once a day, up to a maximum dose of 2–3 mg/kg. Clinical wisdom has held that pemoline needs to build up over time in the body (up to 4 weeks) before a clinical effect occurs, and then it must be maintained at a sufficient level to continue to exert a clinical effect; however, research cited later in this chapter suggests that some effects may be seen within 1 to 2 days. This question remains to be answered definitively. Because it is metabolized by the liver and could potentially cause liver damage, liver functions tests must be done every 3–6 months. Six controlled studies were performed with latency-age children (Wilens & Biederman, 1992). These studies found that a mean of 70% of the children had a positive response rate. Two double-blind placebo studies of pemoline with adolescents have recently been completed but have not yet been fully analyzed and reported (J. Biederman, personal communication, 1998; B. Smith, personal communication, 1998). Clinically, pemoline has been found to have a milder effect on adolescents than methyl-phenidate or dextroamphetamine.

A typical starting regimen of pemoline would be 37.5 mg once a day for a month (for a smaller adolescent, one might start at 18.75 mg), with a follow-up visit and then a dose increase to 75 mg if needed. Smith reports that the following, more rapid dosing schedule has also proven successful: 37.5 mg for two days, then move upward in 18.75-mg increments every 2 days to the target dose. Consider 56.25 mg of Cylert to be equivalent to 10 mg of methylphenidate and 112.5 mg of Cylert to be equivalent to 20 mg of methylphenidate. Unlike the other stimulants, pemoline has no cardio-vascular effects and a very low abuse potential, making it the drug of choice for adolescents recovering from substance abuse problems or ado-lescents living in substance-abusing families. Pemoline is also not as tightly controlled by the DEA as are the other stimulants.

In November, 1996, Abbott Laboratories issued a warning describing 13 cases of liver damage, 11 resulting in death or liver transplantation in children treated with Cylert. It was not clear that the periodic liver func-tion tests commonly conducted by physicians would be predictive of acute liver failure. On the basis of these finds, Abbott Laboratories recommend-ed that Cylert be downgraded as a treatment for ADHD and not be consid-ered as a first-line drug.

Comparison of Long-Acting Stimulants

There has been a single study published which systematically compared short-acting methylphenidate, SR methylphenidate, dextroamphetamine spansule, and pemoline in 22 boys with ADHD ages 8 to 13 attending a specialized summer camp for ADHD children (Pelham et al., 1990). It was a double-blind, placebo controlled evaluation in which each child received, in random order for 3 to 6 days apiece, comparable doses of the four drugs or placebo. Dependent measures included daily frequencies of five behav-iors (following rules, positive peer behaviors, noncompliance, conduct problems, negative verbalizations), standardized rating scales, a continu-ous performance task, and daily report cards.

All the drugs were superior to placebo, but there were few differences between the effectiveness of the one short-acting and the three long-acting medications. Dextroamphetamine spansule and pemoline tended to pro-duce the most consistent effects, with lower standard deviations on many measures than methylphenidate. An analysis revealed that all of the drugs had similar side effects. More subjects had side effects reported for dex-troamphetamine spansule than the others, but the differences were not sig-nificant.

At the end of the study, the staff reviewed all the available information and made recommendations for continuation of medication. Dextroam-phetamine spansule was recommended for six children; pemoline for four;

SR methylphenidate for four; short-acting methylphenidate for one; and no medication for seven who showed adverse reactions to medication. Thus, long-acting medications were recommended clinically for the majority of the youngsters.

An interesting aspect of the study related to the timing of the initial response to pemoline. The continuous performance test (CPT) measure was repeated five times on the first day of each drug administration (1, 2, 4, 6, and 9 hours), permitting the impact of the medications over these time intervals. All the drugs except short-acting methylphenidate showed a significant positive effect on omission errors on the CPT by the first hour; methylphenidate also showed an effect by the second hour. These results were particularly surprising in light of the clinical belief that it takes several weeks to see a positive effect of pemoline. Here a positive effect was seen on a CPT at 1 hour postingestion.

The authors of the study caution that their results apply to the short-term effects of these drugs administered over several days, and whether short-term positive effects reliably predict long-term effects is not known for sure. This study was also conducted with latency-age children, including a few young adolescents. There is every reason to assume that the results would generalize to older adolescents, but this is not certain.

Antidepressant Medications

Antidepressant medications are considered to be the second-line medications in the treatment of ADHD, and as noted earlier, research has primarily suggested the effectiveness of imipramine (Tofranil), desipramine (Norpramin), and nortriptyline (Pamelor). The TCAs are believed to work in ADHD by potentiating adrenergic synapses and by blocking the uptake of dopamine and norepinephrine at nerve endings and increasing dopamine levels. Clinical experience would suggest that they have less effect on concentration and executive functioning than the stimulants but equal effect on impulsive behavior and moodiness. Sometimes, in youngsters with mild ADHD and moderate to severe comorbid Mood or Anxiety Disorders, these TCAs may be the medication of choice because stimulants can increase anxiety and the Mood or Anxiety Disorder may be the primary problem needing medical treatment. Tricylic antidepressants can be given once a day (at bedtime if drowsiness is a problem), have a long duration of action, and have a very low abuse potential. An initial trial of 4–6 weeks is needed to begin to evaluate the full effects of these medicines. Doses can be gradually increased to the usual doses, and blood levels have proven useful at the higher dosage levels. Because of their cardiac effects and the few cases of sudden deaths, a baseline EKG and further EKGs after each dose change are prudent. The daily dosage is approximately 3–5 mg/kg of imipramine and desipramine and 1.5 to 2.0 mg/kg of nortriptyline. Common side effects include dry mouth, drowsiness, constipation, nausea, sweating, tremor, and postural hypotension. Rare but possible side effects also include seizures, an acute organic brain syndrome, and hypomania. Doses in excess of 3.5 mg/kg have been associated with mild diastolic hypertension, tachycardia, and electrocardiographic conduction anomalies.

The SSRIs have also been used extensively on a clinical basis with children and adolescents with ADHD, although as noted earlier, little research has been conducted with them. However, many adolescents with ADHD may benefit from the use of SSRIs in addition to stimulants because they are well tolerated and the common comorbidities of depression and anxiety disorders may respond to these agents. They do not appear to help the ADHD symptoms per se but can be safely used in conjunction with stimulants. They are typically given once a day, usually in the morning although sertraline (Zoloft) can be given at bedtime. Fluoxetine (Prozac), paroxetine (Paxil), and fluvoxamine (Luvox) are the other SSRIs commonly used.

Bupropion (Wellbutrin), an aminoketone antidepressant unrelated to other antidepressant agents, weakly blocks serotonin, norephinephrine, and dopamine uptake and has been reported to be superior to placebo in reducing ADHD symptoms in at least two double-blind placebo trials with children (Barrikman et al., 1995; Casat, Pleasants, Van Wyck, & Fleet, 1988). Spencer, Biederman, Steningard, and Wilens (1995) cautioned, however, that bupropion exacerbates tics in patients with ADHD and Tic Disorders and may also lower the seizure threshold in seizure patients; this decreases its utility in patients with these conditions. However, the development of seizures is minimal with single doses less than 150 mg. Bupropion generally seems to be less effective than the stimulants and therefore is another second-line agent. Usual doses range from 75 to 300 mg a day divided into two to three doses a day so that no single dose is higher than 100 mg. The initial dose should be 75 mg once daily or twice a day. Common side effects include agitation, gastrointestinal upset, tremor and headache.

Clonidine and Guanfacine

Clonidine stimulates alpha-adrenergic brain receptors reducing sympathetic outflow and is used as an antihypertensive. In the brain stem it may reduce the upward passage of data, making people with ADHD less distractible or impulsive. It can also reduce Tic Disorders and may be useful in cases of ADHD with comorbid Tic Disorders. Clonidine comes is tablets of 0.1, 0.2, and 0.3 mg and in transdermal patches of the same doses which last for up to 1 week. Although several controlled and uncontrolled studies have found clonidine to be effective with children diagnosed as ADHD (Spencer et al., 1996), none have systematically evaluated its effects with adolescents. We typically recommend it as a third-line medication when neither stimulants nor antidepressants can be used. In adolescents, clonidine is dosed as follows: Clonidine should be started with one half or one 0.1-mg tablet two to three times a day. This dose can be increased as tolerated (and if needed) to a maximum dose of 0.3 mg two to three times a day. Blood pressure needs to be monitored when using clonidine, which may also produce drowsiness. Because of the side effect of drowsiness, clonidine has also sometimes been prescribed as a bedtime medication for children and adolescents with ADHD who have a difficult time getting to sleep. When used for insomnia, the clonidine dose is usually 0.1–0.3 mg as a bedtime dose.

Guanfacine (Tenex) is a longer-acting alpha 2-adrenergic agonist which is less sedating than clonidine. It comes in 1- and 2-mg tablets and can be given once or twice a day with a maximum dose of 4 mg a day. To date, only open trials have been completed, but it appears to be a promising agent.

Combined Medications

Combinations of medication are commonly used in clinical practice for two reasons: (1) to more fully treat the symptom complex of ADHD and (2) to treat ADHD plus comorbid conditions. Most combinations involve the use of a stimulant and another agent. To improve control of the ADHD symptoms, clonidine may be added for those who are overly hyperactive. A tricylic antidepressant or bupropion may also improve the symptoms of ADHD, in conjunction with a stimulant. The treatment of comorbid disorders associated with ADHD is beyond the scope of this chapter. However, SSRIs with a stimulant are useful for individuals with ADHD and depression, anxiety disorders, or obsessive–compulsive disorders. Clonidine or a tricylic antidepressant can be used to aid adolescents with difficulty falling asleep. Clonidine, carbamazepine (Tegretol), or valproic acid (Depakene) can sometimes help adolescents, with aggressive behavior. Although combinations of medications such as a stimulant and an antidepressant or a stimulant and clonidine are more commonly used in practice with ADHD (Wilens, Spencer, Biederman, Wozniak, & Connor, 1995), only one controlled study has examined a combined regimen—desipramine and methylphenidate—in children (Pataki, Carlson, Kelly, Rapport, & Biancaniello, 1993). These authors found that each drug had separate but synergistic effects on normalizing cognitive deficits and were tolerated well without serious side effects. The degree of clinical experimentation with combinations of drugs is alarming given the scant research evidence for their effectiveness. Clearly, this is an area in which a great deal of research is needed.

MONITORING MEDICATION

Careful monitoring of the response to medication and titrating of the dose to help the adolescent cope most effectively with the symptoms of ADHD across time and settings is crucial to a successful outcome (Barkley, 1998). The adolescent should return for a follow-up visit with the prescribing physician 1 month after the initial prescription was given. There should be phone contact during the first month, if the adolescent is following a rapidly increasing dose schedule, or if any problems arise with a fixed dose schedule. There should be contact at any time if significant side effects occur. If any adjustments in dose are made at the 1-month follow-up, monthly follow-ups should continue until a stable medication regimen has been reached. Then, the adolescent should return for an office visit with the physician three to four times a year, on a quarterly basis. Monthly prescriptions can be mailed or picked up between follow-up visits, depending on the local legal requirements for dispensing controlled prescriptions.

We have found that in cases in which a stable medication regimen has been reached, if we reduce the frequency of follow-up visits to one every 6 months instead of once every 3 to 4 months, unanticipated problems often arise during the school year which go uncorrected for too long a time. When the adolescent is attending regular therapy sessions with a psychologist or other mental health professional and the therapist stays in touch with the physician, the frequency of physician follow-up visits can be lowered. In that case, the therapist should take an active role in assisting the family and physician to monitor the medication and can alert the physician if a problem arises. When the physician is the only professional conducting regular ADHD checkups, I believe that once a year, the physician should have a mental health colleague do a comprehensive review of the adolescent's functioning in the school, the family, and the community, as well as an updated screen for comorbidity. This is the essence of what we call "the dental checkup model of follow-up care." I discuss this model in more detail in Chapter 13.

An acceptable standard for monitoring medication at follow-up visits includes a brief clinical interview of positive effects and side effects, a height, weight, and blood-pressure check, and administration and review of psychometrically sound rating scales completed by the adolescent, the teachers, and the parents. I also review report cards, progress notes, and any other written correspondence from the school when available. Basing titration and long-term assessment solely on the adolescent or parents' subjective report can result in erroneous decisions and incorrect dosing. Because the response to stimulant medication in particular is often idiosyncratic and dose specific, the clinician should collect objective data regarding changes in the adolescent's school performance and behavior at home. When feasible, continuous performance measures can also be administered at medication follow-ups, as long as the practitioner does not rely solely on them (see discussion in Chapter 5).

When using rating scales to assess medication effects, the clinician needs to take into account the practice effects of completing the rating scales multiple times (Barkley, 1998). Scores always improve between the first and second administration. It is a good idea to have the rating scales completed twice before medication is started—once at the time of diagnosis and a second time just before medication is first prescribed.

Many of the rating scales reviewed in Chapter 3 can be used to monitor medication effects. The parent, the teachers, and the adolescent should each complete a rating scale. For parents, we use either the short form of the revised Conners Parent Questionnaire or the DSM-IV ADHD Behavior Checklist. For teachers, we use the Child Attention Profile or the Attention Problems Scale of the Teacher Report Form. For adolescents, we use the short form of the Conners and Wells Adolescent Self-Report Scale (Conners & Wells, 1997) or the Brown ADD Scales (Brown, 1996).

An advantage of using the Brown ADD Scales to assess treatment outcome derives from the fact that in his manual, Brown (1996) developed a psychometrically sound system for monitoring response to treatment. The system has two components that address the following: (1) the significance of the improvement and (2) the magnitude of the improvement. First, Brown computed a table of 90% confidence intervals around the true score at preassessment to control for measurement error and regression to the mean (i.e., the practice effect mentioned earlier). If the total score on the Brown ADD Scales after treatment has begun is lower than 90% confidence interval associated with the adolescent's pretreatment score, the change is clinically significant. Second, Dr. Brown has given us a system to rate the degree of clinical improvement from treatment. He examined the percentages of his nonclinical and pretreatment clinical normative samples of adolescents who received total scores below 50, between 50 and 60, between 60 and 69, and above 69. Then, he followed up ADHD adolescents treated with stimulant medication for 3 months and made independent ratings of the medication outcome as optimal, very favorable, positive but insufficient, equivocal, or negative. He examined the percentage of adolescents with each rating who scored below 50, 50–59, 60–69, and above 70. Based on this analysis, he made specific recommendations for rating the degree of improvement as optimal (below 50), very favorable (50–59), favorable (60–69), positive but insufficient (70 or greater), equivocal (within 90% confidence interval), or negative (above 90% confidence interval). A convenient treatment monitoring worksheet facilitates this treatment evaluation process. Ideally, developers of other rating scales will provide similar systems for quantitative analysis of the significance of treatment effects.

When we also want to monitor family interaction, we use the 20-item Conflict Behavior Questionnaire. The parent and the adolescent complete together the Barkley Stimulant Drug Side Effects Rating Scale. We give the family the rating scales for the next visit at the end of the previous visit, or, in cases of long follow-up intervals, we mail the questionnaires to the family 2 weeks before the follow-up visit. We ask each of the adolescent's teachers to complete the Child Attention Profile or the Teacher Report Format—Attention Problems Scale. All the rating scales are collected upon the family's arrival for the follow-up visit, scored, and reviewed briefly by the clinician before beginning the interview. When feasible, we keep either a graph or table in the chart with running totals of the most significant rating scale scores over time, for easy comparison across many follow-up visits over long periods.

A clinical decision to maintain or change the dose is made based on all the available evidence: The parent and the adolescent's reports in the interview of positive effects and side effects; the rating scales; and the weight, height, and blood pressure measurements. In the initial monitoring, we establish the optimal type of medication and dose range. Typically, two or three dose changes after the initial prescription are needed to achieve this goal if the adolescent responds positively to the first stimulant that is prescribed. In the subsequent monitoring, we often "fine tune" the medication by adjusting the timing to achieve optimal coverage throughout the schoolday and afterward, to eliminate any unwanted side effects, and to meet the needs of the adolescent's more flexible schedule on weekends and holidays.

A case example illustrates medication monitoring.

Case Example: Bubbly Sarah

In the Introduction to Section I, I introduced Sarah, a highly social 14-year-old eighth-grader diagnosed as having ADHD without any comorbid psychiatric conditions, and with associated low-average intellectual ability but no learning disabilities. Sarah was having difficulty getting her schoolwork done in class and at home, and she was becoming disorganized, forgetful, and overwhelmed. She did not have clinically significant conflicts with her parents and had excellent peer relationships. As part of a multidimensional treatment program, Sarah agreed to a trial of stimulant medication. Because there were no medical counterindications, Dr. Schubiner, her physician, prescribed an increasing dose schedule of 5, 10, 15, and 20 mg of Ritalin per dose over the first 4 weeks. Ritalin was prescribed to be taken at 7:30 A.M., 11:30 A.M., and 3:30 P.M. on weekdays. Sarah and her parents did not see a need for Ritalin on weekends unless she had homework. She agreed to take Ritalin on Sunday afternoon or on Saturday when she worked on her homework.

A brief telephone contact after the first week of 5 mg three times a day indicated that there were no side effects but no perceptible positive effects yet. Sarah returned with her mother for a 1-month follow-up visit. Sarah reported that she started to notice some effect of the Ritalin at the 10-mg dose, and at the 20-mg dose her mind felt much sharper and she was getting a lot more schoolwork done. She also mentioned, "It used to take me all day to clean up my room; now I can do it in one hour while I am on Ritalin." Her mother confirmed that Sarah was getting more schoolwork done, especially homework, without boredom or restlessness.

Table 8.3 presents the rating scale data at baseline at several follow-ups.

TABLE 8.3. Medication Monitoring Rating Data for Sarah

	Baseline	2/96	3/96	4/96	7/96	10/96	1/97
Ritalin dose		20, 20, 20[a]	20, 15, 15	15, 15, 15	17.5, 17.5, 15	20SR + 15, 15 20SR + 15, 15	20SR + 15, 15 20SR + 15, 15
Child Attention Profile							
Inattention							
(7 is 93rd percentile)							
Math	12	7	5	4	3	4	2
English	8	4	2	3	3	2	4
French I/II	5	3	1	0	2	0	3
Biology/Chemistry	13	8	5	6	5	10	7
History	9	5	4	5	4	8	5
Mean	9.4	5.4	3.4	3.6	3.4	4.8	4.2
Overactivity							
(5 is 93rd percentile)							
Math	3	2	0	1	2	2	3
English	2	3	1	2	2	1	3
French I/II	0	0	0	1	0	3	3
Biology/Chemistry	5	4	4	3	5	8	4
History	3	3	2	1	3	2	0
Mean	2.6	2.4	1.4	1.6	2.4	3.2	3.3
Brown ADD Scales							
(raw score for totals; *T*-scores for subscales)							
Total (raw score)	70	61	58	40	41	62	45
Activating to Tasks	69	62	62	51	51	73	56
Sustaining Attention	68	65	59	54	54	65	54
Sustaining Effort	70	66	66	<50	<50	<50	<50
Managing Affect	<50	<50	<50	<50	51	58	53
Working Memory	69	62	62	55	55	66	58
Conners Parent Questionnaire							
(*T*-scores)							
Conduct Problems	54	53	50	46	50	43	47
Learning Problems	96	76	74	68	57	68	51
Impulsive/ Hyperactive	70	69	64	55	55	51	55
Hyperactivity Index	61	62	59	53	53	50	50
Barkley Side Effects Rating Scale							
(0–9 scale)							
Insomnia	4	4	5	3	5	4	3
Talks less with others	0	9	7	5	5	4	4
Decreased appetite	1	6	5	5	4	5	5
Sad/unhappy	1	9	5	4	4	3	3

[a]Dose changed each week: week 1, 5 mg three times a day; week 2, 10 mg three times a day; week 3, 15 mg three times a day; week 4, 20 mg three times a day.

February 1996 Follow-Up

Inspection of Table 8.3 indicates that the rating scale data for the February 1996 follow-up supported Sarah and her mother's anecdotal reports. On the Brown ADD Scales, Sarah total score decreased from 70 to 61, which represents some improvement but is still within the 90% confidence interval (57–79) for her pretreatment score; inspection of subscales showed that the mild improvement was distributed across Activating to Tasks, Sustaining Attention, Sustaining Effort, and Working Memory (Managing Affect was never a problem). On the Parent Conners Questionnaire (old version), we need to examine primarily the Learning Problems factor score because in the case of adolescent girls without any comorbid conditions to ADHD, the other scores do not tend to be that high at baseline (with the revised Conners Parent Questionnaire, we would examine the Cognitive Problems and DSM-IV Inattentiveness Scores). Sarah's mother reported a large decrease on the Learning Problems score and a small decrease also on the Impulsive–Hyperactive score.

Five teachers completed the Child Attention Profile (CAP). All reported improvements on Inattention from baseline to the first follow-up. Three reported improvements which dropped below 7, the 93rd percentile cutoff for clinical significance. The low Overactivity scores at baseline and follow-up are typically found in girls such as Sarah. Inspection of the mean score shows how it is not representative of what is happening in each class and why the physician needs to look at the complete profile of teacher responses.

Although Sarah demonstrated moderate gains at the first follow-up, she complained strongly, "This medicine changed my personality; I'm no longer any fun to be around. I act withdrawn in school. My friends ask me what is wrong. This is getting me depressed." She also complained that the medicine was keeping her up at night. Her mother added that Sarah's appetite had decreased, which pleased Sarah because she was hoping it would help her lose weight. Table 8.3 shows the ratings for these four side effects on the Barkley Side Effects Rating Scale. The dramatic increase in scores from baseline to the February 1996 follow-up for "talks less with others" and "sad/unhappy" is a reflection of Sarah's degree of concern about how she feels Ritalin changed her personality. The fact that the baseline score for "insomnia or trouble sleeping" was about the same as the first follow-up suggests, as the therapist learned on further questioning, that getting to sleep has always been difficult for Sarah, and medication really has not changed that significantly.

Dr. Schubiner correctly surmised that he needed to attend seriously to Sarah's perception that Ritalin had dampened her personality. He attempted to explain to her that being extroverted and highly talkative in part reflected the form that hyperactivity–impulsivity took in Sarah. This point did not make sense to Sarah, who kept returning to the negative impact of this change on peer relationships. Dr. Schubiner decided to take the pragmatic approach to decrease the second and third doses of Ritalin to 15 mg, leaving the first dose at 20 mg. He explained that he would work with Sarah to find a dose and type of medicine with which she could be comfortable. She agreed to try the reduced dosage schedule.

March 1996 Follow-Up

When Sarah and her mother returned for the next follow-up in March 1996, Sarah reported that the decreased dose helped her feel more like herself in the afternoon and evenings while still permitting her to get her schoolwork and homework done. However, she still was upset by the change in her personality in the morning. Review of the rating scales in Table 8.3 reveals continued improvement on all of the measures, particularly the CAP Inattention Scale. A school progress report had also come home indicating that Sarah was making great improvements in getting her assignments in on time and was receiving C's or B's in all her classes. Dr. Schubiner suggested that Sarah reduce the initial dose of Ritalin to 15 mg and scheduled a 1-month follow-up.

April 1996 Follow-Up

At the next follow-up in April 1996, Sarah no longer reported that Ritalin was changing her personality but complained that she had to strain to concentrate in school in the mornings. The rating scales documented continued improvement, despite Sarah's comments. Dr. Schubiner pointed out to Sarah that she had a choice: Go back to the 20-mg dose of Ritalin and get used to feeling more mellow while in school, or stay at the 15-mg dose and experience some concentration problems with schoolwork. Sarah asked if she could cut the 5-mg tablet in half and take 17.5 mg in the morning and at noon. Dr. Schubiner agreed. Because the adjustment was relatively minor, he set the next follow-up in 3 months, asking Sarah to call in 1 month to report how things were going.

July 1996 Follow-Up

One month later, Sarah called and said that the 17.5-mg dose was ideal. When she returned in the summer for the 3-month follow-up, she proudly showed Dr. Schubiner her report card. She had received four B's and one A. Inspection of Table 8.3 shows that all the rating scales were still in the minimal problem range. Sarah asked to be off medication during the summer. Dr. Schubiner agreed. Because Sarah was switching schools and going into high school the next fall, Dr. Schubiner felt that it would be desirable to have the next follow-up approximately 1 month after the new school year began.

October 1996 Follow-Up

When Sarah returned in October of her ninth-grade year, she was experiencing problems in several classes. She had restarted Ritalin, 17.5, 17.5, and 15 mg, at 7:00 A.M., 11:30 A.M., and 3:30 P.M. when she entered ninth grade. Although the medication helped her concentrate, it did not last long enough and it was wearing off around 10:30 A.M. Inspection of the CAP scores for the history and chemistry teachers confirmed Sarah's impressions. A review of the Brown ADD Scale and the Parent Conners Questionnaire Learning Problems factor score also showed backsliding. Dr. Schubiner asked Sarah if she would consider taking a combination of slow-release and short-acting Ritalin, explaining how the SR Ritalin would take longer to kick in but would last longer too. He also pointed out that it would not last long enough to eliminate the noon dose. Sarah agreed and said that the noon dose was not a problem for her. Dr. Schubiner prescribed a combination of 20 mg of SR Ritalin and 15 mg of regular Ritalin twice, at 7:00 A.M. and 11:30 A.M. The 3:30 P.M. dose remained 15-mg short-acting Ritalin. Sarah asked why Dr. Schubiner did not further reduce the short-acting Ritalin dose. He explained that she had grown taller since the last school year and that 20 mg of SR Ritalin is the same as 7.5 mg of regular Ritalin taken twice. He set the next follow-up in 3 months, with a phone call in 1 month.

January 1997 Follow-Up

Sarah forgot to call in 1 month, but Dr. Schubiner contacted her mother. Sarah's mother said things were going well, and that the addition of SR Ritalin had solved the timing problem. At the next follow-up in January 1997, Sarah and her mother came in beaming, showing Dr. Schubiner her report card. Again, she had B's and A's. All the rating scales confirmed the anecdotal reports. When asked about her previous concerns about Ritalin changing her personality, Sarah said that was no longer a problem. She now had a boyfriend who liked her personality just as it is and she did not want it to change.

Comment

This case illustrates how the rating scales are interwoven with interviewing to monitor the effectiveness of methylphenidate in a relatively straightforward case of an adolescent girl without any comorbidity to ADHD. It was important for Dr. Schubiner to work with Sarah to help her feel comfortable with the medication, and to deal with her perception that it changed her personality. Failure to attend to her concerns may have resulted in her discontinuing the Ritalin. The fine tuning of the first dose to 17.5 mg may not have made a huge difference compared to 20 mg, but Sarah felt that it would be helpful, and there was every reason to support her reasonable suggestion. This enhanced her sense of control over the medication decision making. Inspection of Table 8.3 also illustrates how some measures change more rapidly than others. The teachers reported larger changes sooner than Sarah did. Only in April 1996 did Sarah's total score on the Brown decrease beyond the 90th percentile confidence interval. Finally, the long-term follow-up illustrates how new problems may arise at the beginning of a new school year, and how the physician may flexibly combine slow-release and short-acting medications to address timing issues.

SUMMARY

In this chapter we gave the reader some practical advice about when and how to use medication as part of an overall intervention plan for adolescents with ADHD. We pointed out that our research-based knowledge about using stimulant and non-stimulant medication with adolescents is limited. Practitioners often have to extrapolate from the studies done with younger children and apply these results to adolescents, taking developmental changes into account. We also discussed the special considerations a physician must take into account when approaching adolescents about medical treatment for ADHD. We would urge readers to review the Appendix at the end of the book to obtain a better insight into the specific research findings regarding medical treatment of ADHD in adolescence.

CHAPTER NINE

—————— ◯ ——————

Enhancing Academic Success

School is an educational endurance test for most adolescents with ADHD. Although they may selectively enjoy aspects of school in which they have particular strengths (creative studies, athletics, a favorite class), they generally do not look forward to the daily academic demands of secondary education. Adults can avoid or escape from most unpleasant endurance tests, but teenagers with ADHD have to face school every day. School is their full-time job. When they fail at their full-time job, the consequences are immense. Their self-esteem plummets, they get in trouble in the classroom, they feel depressed, and conflict escalates at home. For these reasons, as mentioned in the Introduction to Section III, I normally intervene first with school problems and later with home management problems. I wrote this chapter from the perspective of a practitioner who is working with the adolescent and his or her family in a clinic or an office-based practice rather than the perspective of the teacher or school-based personnel. Several excellent books about ADHD have been written from the perspective of school-based personnel (DuPaul & Stoner, 1994; Markel & Greenbaum, 1996). I review the common obstacles to school success that adolescents with ADHD encounter and then consider the role of the external consultant in helping the adolescent and his or her parents overcome these obstacles. Specific attention is devoted to homework, preparing for and taking tests, memorization techniques, reading comprehension strategies, listening and note taking, general organization, time management, and home/school note systems. I consider how the external consultant should work with the parents to approach the adolescent's school, what goals the consultant might reasonably accomplish at the school, and the types of accommodations that are helpful for secondary education students with ADHD.

My goal in this chapter is to guide the practitioner in identifying and intervening to change common school problems of adolescents with ADHD. I provide the practitioner with the basic information needed to accomplish these goals, keeping in mind that this is a chapter rather than an encyclopedia, and provide references to more detailed texts. Much of the material in this chapter is based on *Study Strategies Made Easy* (Davis, Sirotowitz, & Parker, 1996) and *Performance Breakthroughs for Adolescents with Learning Disabilities or ADD* (Markel & Greenbaum, 1996). Readers interested in book-length discussions of school interventions should consult these texts, as well as one by DuPaul and Stoner (1994).

TYPES OF SCHOOL PROBLEMS

Adolescents with ADHD commonly present with one or more of the following school difficulties:

- Failure to complete their homework
- Poor understanding of material
- Poor study habits
- Low test grades
- Coming to class unprepared
- Failing report card grades
- Poor classroom participation
- Failing to ask the teacher for help
- Sloppy handwriting
- Disrupting the class
- Arguing with teachers
- Getting in fights with peers
- Truancy

To understand how ADHD and associated learning problems lead to these 13 presenting problems, it is useful to place secondary education within the context of adolescent development. As youngsters make the transitions into middle and high school, secondary education places increased demands on students in eight particular areas (Mercer & Mercer, 1993):

1. Gaining information from printed materials.
2. Gaining information from lectures.
3. Demonstrating knowledge through tests.
4. Expressing information in writing.
5. Working independently.
6. Demonstrating a broad set of cognitive and metacognitive strategies.
7. Interacting appropriately with same and opposite-sex peers and adults.
8. Demonstrating motivation to learn.

The core symptoms of ADHD impair the adolescent's ability to meet these eight demands. The inattentive, distractible youngster may not pay attention to printed materials or lectures long enough to obtain useful information and will certainly have difficulty working independently and persisting at studying long enough to demonstrate knowledge through testing. For many, written expression is also a major problem, not to mention illegible handwriting. The impulsive/restless youngster rushes through academics in a careless, haphazard manner and also has trouble interacting appropriately with others. Impairments in verbal and nonverbal working memory, self-regulation of affect/motivation, and reconstitution render the development and utilization of higher-order cognitive skills less efficient in ADHD than in non-ADHD youngsters. Taken together, these ADHD symptoms set up the adolescent for failure, which in turn limits motivation to learn and leads to further acting out in school and, as follow-up studies have demonstrated, higher rates of grade retention, expulsion, and dropping out of school (Barkley, Fischer, et al., 1990).

Many adolescents with ADHD have associated learning problems with input, organization, memory, or output (Silver, 1992), which further complicate their difficulties in school. Those with input problems have deficits receiving information through listening, reading comprehension, or visual input. They may not understand information presented in a particular manner but could understand it if it were presented in an alternative manner. Those with organizational problems have deficits in sequencing and categorizing new information and relating new information to old information, relating details to the whole, and finding main ideas. Learning and retention, as well as the organizational aspects of listening and reading comprehension are difficult for these youngsters, who do not complete homework and come to class unprepared. Those with memory problems may participate well in class but do poorly on tests, forget things they just studied, and have particular difficulties with spelling, multiplication tables, and instructions. Those with output problems have trouble expressing themselves orally or in writing. In some cases, these adolescents qualify for services on the basis of a specific learning disability in one of seven areas: oral expression, listening comprehension, written expression, basic reading skills, reading comprehension, math calculation, or math reasoning.

In many cases, the youngsters did not have significant academic problems prior to middle or even high school. High intellectual ability, close parental monitoring, and mild to moderate severity of ADHD symptoms are often protective factors which prevent academic problems from emerging until the youngster encounters the increased demands of secondary education. In youngsters who are not hyperactive or do not display behavioral difficulties, the onset of these academic problems may often be insidious, and they may increase to crisis proportions before they are recognized. This is particularly true in teenage girls, who are less likely to display the kinds of externalizing behavioral difficulties in elementary school that cause boys to be referred for evaluation and treatment (Guab & Carlson, 1996; Solden, 1995) and may present to the practitioner with depression and school difficulties.

ROLE OF THE EXTERNAL CONSULTANT

From the school's viewpoint, the adolescent's therapist is an external consultant who may have useful ideas worth listening to but nonetheless does not have any direct control over the teachers, the administrators, and the school system. We must always remember that we are guests in another's home when we advocate for our patients in their schools, and we must try to act like guests. Some of our patients' school-related difficulties can be effectively addressed through our efforts in clinic-based individual and family sessions along with associated homework assignments. Other problems require intervention in the classroom and the school system. Some may be addressed in either setting. The therapist needs to learn to differentiate between these types of problems and handle each appropriately. For example, the therapist can be effective in teaching adolescents how to get their homework done and how to study differently for multiple-choice versus essay exams. On the other hand, the therapist may not be able to explain principles of physics or the finer points of Shakespeare to the adolescent; the teachers must take responsibility for helping the student understand basic concepts. Either the therapist or the content-area teachers could potentially teach the adolescent how to study more effectively for examinations; practical factors such as the availability and willingness of the teachers to provide direct test-taking instruction and the degree of rapport between the therapist and the adolescent might dictate who takes responsibility for this goal.

For those problems that require action in the school, the therapist must learn when and how to approach the school personnel; when to train the parents to make such an approach; what recommendations to make; how to build a collaborative relationship between the adolescent, the school, and the parents; and how to maneuver diplomatically with the broader school system. The therapist must also learn when things at the school system will not change, when to advise parents and adolescents to adjust to the status quo, and when to advise them to consider taking legal action against the school system. Throughout this chapter, I clarify the role of the therapist as an external consultant and provide answers to these questions.

STRUCTURING SCHOOL INTERVENTIONS

In this phase of treatment, the therapist meets with the adolescent and the family, conducts a detailed assessment of the reasons the adolescent is doing poorly in school, and establishes specific goals for change. Then, the therapist and family decide which goals can be addressed in the therapy sessions and which goals require action in the school. The therapist coaches the parents to approach the appropriate school officials to arrange for informal accommodations or set in motion either an evaluation for a Section 504 plan or a special education plan. The therapist backs up the parents' approach to the school by telephoning the principal and/or other school officials, and sending written reports and recommendations to the school. A school meeting is set up with the principal, the parents, the adolescent's teachers, any relevant support staff and the therapist. The adolescent is typically brought into the school meeting toward the end, when an agreement has been reached about the services to be provided and the school officials wish to explain it to the adolescent. In the case of Section 504 plans or special education plans, several meetings may take place before a plan of service is finalized.

Sessions 4 through 9 of the 20-session burst of treatment are typically devoted to school interventions. In Session 4, the therapist conducts the assessment and goal setting, and after Session 4, the parents approach the school. Parts of Sessions 5 through 9 are devoted to follow-up and coordination with the school. Meanwhile, in Sessions 5 through 9, the therapist intervenes in depth to address those academic problems that can be corrected primarily through individual and family therapy sessions. In the course of conducting such interventions, we usually uncover further accommodations which might be useful in school, and we communicate further with the teacher and principal to get these in place. If six sessions prove insufficient to begin to correct academic difficulties, this phase of intervention may be prolonged as necessary.

Clinicians vary in the extent to which they are comfortable playing an advocacy role in the schools. Some prefer to limit their involvement to activities that can take place in the office, with occasional phone or written communication with the school. Others regularly go to their clients' schools and assertively advocate for services for their clients. A minority are familiar enough with the relevant laws and special education rules to guide their clients through extreme adversarial situations such as due process hearings. Cases also vary with regard to the required amount of involvement with the school to obtain the desired services. For the majority of the adolescents I treat, coaching the parents to approach the school, coupled with a phone contact and written recommendations, is sufficient. In a significant minority of my cases, however, my attendance at strategically scheduled school meetings makes a world of difference in mediating parent–school disputes and facilitating obtaining services for my adolescent patients. Typically, I attend one meeting per case, and the average meeting lasts about 30–45 minutes. I charge for the meeting and travel time, which in my geographic area makes the cost of my average school visit $200.

When extremely adversarial situations arise involving due process hearings or major disagreements between parents and school authorities, I refer the parents to a professional advocate and/or a lawyer because I do not consider myself an expert at such matters. I continue to work with the family, the advocate, and the lawyer, but I know the limits of my knowledge and respect them.

A therapist can usually obtain the names of advocates and lawyers specializing in educational matters from local chapters of national support groups such as CH.A.D.D.

ASSESSING SCHOOL PROBLEMS AND ESTABLISHING GOALS

In Session 4, I pinpoint specific school problems the parents and adolescent present. I start by reviewing the most recent report card, discussing how things are going in each class. Which are the most difficult classes? Which are the easier classes? How much incomplete work does the teen have? How does the adolescent get along with the teachers in each class? Which teachers does the adolescent like and dislike, and why? What is the adolescent's ideal teacher? How willing is the adolescent to ask for help in class or after class? Is the adolescent making genuine efforts to succeed? Is the adolescent serious about school, or is he or she taking it all as one big joke?

Next, I review the Diagnostic Checklist for School Success (see Table 9.1). Systematically going through each item, I inquire about homework, organization, test preparation and test taking, note taking, reading comprehension, memorizing, and classroom participation and conduct. I get the parents' and the adolescent's perspectives on each item, explaining that my purpose is to identify problems and define goals for change.

Next, I review what the school is doing to help the adolescent. I ask the parents to bring in copies of any individualized education programs (IEPs), school notes, or testing reports. Is the adolescent receiving any special education or Section 504 services? To what extent does the accommodation match the areas of weakness identified on the checklist? Are the content-area teachers actually implementing the written IEP or Section 504 plan? Is there a case manager who monitors implementation of the plan, and are the teachers held accountable for whether they implement it?

I also inquire about the social scene for the adolescent. What is the peer culture at the school like? What messages are the adolescent's friends sending about the value of academic success? How are things going socially for the adolescent? Where in the popularity pecking order is the adolescent? Are there cliques, and is the adolescent part of one?

I assign each item on the checklist a rating on a 1 to 5 Likert scale, where higher numbers represent more positive ratings. I consider any

TABLE 9.1. Diagnostic Checklist for School Success

Name of Student_____ School_____ Grade_____

Date_____ Name of Therapist_____

The therapist should review each item on this checklist with the parents and adolescent, determining whether it applies. Most of the items refer to the behavior of the adolescent; some refer to the actions of the teachers and school personnel. Rate each item on a 1–5 scale:

1 = Never   3 = Sometimes   5 = Always
2 = A little   4 = Often

HOMEWORK
_____ 1. Uses an assignment book
_____ 2. Does homework in a nondistracting, quiet environment
_____ 3. Has a planful approach to the order for doing homework
_____ 4. Completes homework on time
_____ 5. Hands homework in on time
_____ 6. Spends sufficient time on homework
_____ 7. Keeps and follows a written plan with calender for long-term assignments
_____ 8. Is currently up-to-date on homework

ORGANIZATION
_____ 9. Comes to class prepared with materials
_____ 10. Keeps notebooks, papers, study area organized and accessible
_____ 11. Uses calender, schedule, planner to manage time
_____ 12. Keeps track of grades regularly/ knows grading criteria
_____ 13. Brings home materials needed for homework
_____ 14. Keeps locker and backpack organized

TEST PREPARATION AND TEST TAKING
_____ 15. Spends sufficient time studying (e.g., doesn't cram at last minute)
_____ 16. Matches study to the types of questions on exam
_____ 17. Uses old tests to help prepare for upcoming exams
_____ 18. Has an organized approach to studying (e.g., SQ4R)
_____ 19. Has an organized approach to taking tests
_____ 20. Reads and follows directions carefully and doesn't respond impulsively
_____ 21. Writes legibly or uses word processor
_____ 22. Pays attention adequately during tests
_____ 23. Receives passing or higher grades on tests
_____ 24. Does not cheat
_____ 25. Remembers information during the test
_____ 26. Finishes the test within the allotted time
_____ 27. Manages anxiety effectively during tests

NOTE TAKING
_____ 28. Takes notes during lectures
_____ 29. Gets main points in notes
_____ 30. Notes are legible
_____ 31. Uses notes for studying
_____ 32. Takes accurate notes

(continued)

TABLE 9.1. *(continued)*

READING COMPREHENSION

_____ 33. Uses organized method such as SQ4R
_____ 34. Can identify topics, main ideas, and details
_____ 35. Understands what has been read
_____ 36. Underlines text effectively
_____ 37. Can answer questions about text
_____ 38. Can summarize what was read
_____ 39. Has method for learning new vocabulary in readings
_____ 40. Can pay attention while reading

MEMORIZING

_____ 41. Plans strategies for memorization
_____ 42. Selects facts to memorize accurately from notes, books, handouts
_____ 43. Knows own learning style (auditory, visual, kinesthetic, combined)
_____ 44. Matches memorization techniques to learning style
_____ 45. Rehearses sufficiently to memorize material
_____ 46. Distributes rehearsal over time (e.g., doesn't cram)
_____ 47. Uses acrastrics (silly sentences)
_____ 48. Uses acronyms
_____ 49. Uses charting, graphing
_____ 50. Uses visualization
_____ 51. Uses word, sentence association techniques
_____ 52. Recalls information when needed

CLASSROOM PARTICIPATION AND CONDUCT

_____ 53. Attends all classes
_____ 54. Gets to class on time
_____ 55. Participates in discussion
_____ 56. Volunteers answers to questions
_____ 57. Is with the class when called on by the teacher
_____ 58. Cooperates with teacher
_____ 59. Raises hand and doesn't call out of turn
_____ 60. Follows classroom rules
_____ 61. Talks respectfully to teachers
_____ 62. Relates positively to peers
_____ 63. Asks for help when needed

UNDERSTANDING/ PROCESSING PROBLEMS

_____ 64. Understands material
_____ 65. Decodes accurately
_____ 66. Comprehends what is read
_____ 67. Has legible handwriting
_____ 68. Can express thoughts in writing
_____ 69. Can express thoughts orally
_____ 70. Understands mathematical concepts
_____ 71. Makes mathematical calculations accurately

(continued)

TABLE 9.1. *(continued)*

SCHOOL RESPONSIBILITIES

____ 72. IEP or 504 plan exists in writing
____ 73. Written plan meets needs outlined above
____ 74. Written plan is adequately implemented
____ 75. Content-area teachers are familiar with plan
____ 76. Case manager appointed to monitor plan
____ 77. Teachers are accountable for providing accommodations
____ 78. Informal accommodations (not in writing)
____ 79. Keeps parents informed of student progress

SOCIAL SCENE

____ 80. Adolescent has close friends at school
____ 81. Friends encourage academic success and prosocial behavior
____ 82. Student is happy with his or her social life

Note. From *ADHD in Adolescents: Diagnosis and Treatment* by Arthur L. Robin. Copyright 1998 by The Guilford Press. Permission to photocopy this table is granted to purchasers of *ADHD in Adolescents* for personal use only (see copyright page for details).

item rated 3 or less to be a potential goal for change. After reviewing the entire checklist, I highlight and read aloud to the family all the items rated 3 or less. I prioritize these items as goals for change, discuss approaches to achieving these goals, and divide up responsibility between myself, the adolescent, the parents, and the school for carrying out these goals.

APPROACHING THE SCHOOL

Who should be approached in the school and how should the approach be made? Answering such questions requires a basic understanding of school systems. Just as families are social systems, which have power hierarchies, subsystems, alignments, and degrees of cohesion, so are schools social systems, with hierarchies, subsystems, alignments, and cohesion issues. Just as families may have structural difficulties with cross-generational coalitions, triangulation, and disengagement, so too may school systems have structural anomalies which can become pitfalls when seeking help for our patients. It is extremely helpful for the clinician to conceptualize schools in family systems terms and to include the adolescent, the parents, and all external consultants in the broad-based conceptualization. A systems view makes it easier for the practitioner to decide who to approach to obtain services for a given adolescent, and how to understand the dynamics and reactions of various people in the school to the approach.

School Hierarchy

The principal is clearly in charge of the hierarchy in most school buildings. All general education teachers report to the principal, either directly or indirectly through department heads. General education support staff such as guidance counselors and advisers also typically report to the principal. However, special education staff may have dual reporting responsibilities. They may report by discipline (psychology, social work, teacher consultants, speech/language) to a districtwide director of special education and by assignment to a particular building, and they may also report to the principal. In some cases, they may report to an intermediate school district that services a number of local districts. Each of the adolescent's classrooms may also be conceptualized as its own minisystem, consisting of the teacher, the students, the physical space, the classroom environment, the materials, and the instructional process. The teacher is clearly in charge of the classroom systems. Beyond the school building, the principals usually answer to a central district administration, headed by a superintendent. The superintendent is responsible to the school board. State departments of education have some jurisdiction over local districts, as do federal agencies such as the Office of Civil Rights.

Most school systems have relatively clear boundaries by discipline and function, and respect for these boundaries makes life much easier when we seek services for our patients. For example, special education staff can typically be used to provide services for a student only when an IEP is in place, qualifying a student for special education services. Thus, teacher consultants are not usually able to implement Section 504 plans, which come under general education. On the other hands, some principals overrule this guideline and use special education staff for Section 504 plans anyway. Most schools have set procedures ultimately governed by state and federal law for seeking services for students with ADHD suspected of being handicapped educationally because of their ADHD.

We have to help our patients' parents understand and first try to work within the hierarchy of the school system, trying to build positive and clear communication and collaboration. If the positive approach fails, we have to know what recourses are possible beyond the school system, within the state and federal regulations. In Chapter 5 (this volume), we discussed the legal obligations of the public schools and methods for determining educational impairment secondary to ADHD and deciding what type of certification to request from the school.

The Approach

Although the therapist could approach the principal directly, I prefer to teach the parents to make such an approach on their own so that they will be prepared to deal effectively with the school long after therapy has been faded out to the follow-up mode. The therapist should use instructions, modeling, role playing, and feedback to coach the parents in carrying out the approach to the school. First, the parents should call the principal and indicate that they (1) are seeking help for their adolescent, (2) have reviewed their adolescent's current status with the therapist and developed a proposal for school-based accommodations, (3) have signed a release of information form and the therapist is available to talk by phone with the principal and will be sending a report with written recommendations, and (4) would like to set up a meeting to review their proposal with the principal. Second, the therapist should forward the written report with recommendations to the principal. Third, the parents should meet with the principal and make their request either for informal accommodations or a formal intervention under Section 504 or The Individual with Disabilities Education Act (IDEA). If the principal agrees with the parents' proposal, a meeting should be scheduled with the adolescent's teachers, the parents, and the principal to work out the details; the therapist can attend this meeting. If the principal does not completely agree with the parents' proposal or refuses to consider it, the therapist should now become directly involved, talking to and meeting with the principal and any other relevant school personnel.

When a request for a Section 504 plan or a special education program is being made, the parents should submit a short, written statement which clearly indicates that they suspect that their youngster has a handicapping condition, and that they are requesting that the school conduct a full evaluation to determine the presence of a handicap as defined under the law and the need for appropriate services. The clock starts running on the federal requirement for the evaluation to be done within 30 days upon receipt of such a written request.

THE SCHOOL-BASED ACCOMMODATION RECOMMENDATIONS

Table 9.2 presents a checklist of accommodations for secondary education which I attach to my reports and which serves as the central organizing focus for my specific recommendations to the principal and the teachers. The checklist is divided into sections for homework, test taking, reading comprehension, lesson presentation/ note taking, general organization, motivational techniques, additional support, parent involvement, and input to external consultants. The items on the checklist are specific. Many of these categories and the rationales for their many of the specific items are referenced when I discuss these areas throughout the remainder of this chapter.

The educational recommendations section of my evaluation report references the checklist. It also includes a statement suggesting the need for the school to conduct an IDEA or a Section 504 evaluation, if warranted.

TABLE 9.2. Accommodations for Secondary Education

Student Name_____ Date_____

School_____ Grade_____

We have listed below many of the school-based interventions that have proven effective with youngsters with ADHD and related problems. We have checked off the accommodations we believe are most relevant to the student named above. We would appreciate your considering these suggestions in planning for this student.

HOMEWORK ACCOMMODATIONS

____ Shortening homework assignments
____ Supplying daily assignment book and reminding student to use it
____ Sending home a week/month's assignments in advance
____ Giving credit for late assignments
____ Grading on content, not appearance or spelling
____ Providing a second set of textbooks to keep at home
____ Making an organizational check of assignment sheet/materials in school
____ Assigning study buddy for each class
____ Assigning peer tutor who reminds student to write down assignment
____ Providing teacher consultant to assist with tracking homework

TEST-TAKING ACCOMMODATIONS

____ Direct training in SQ4R method for test preparation
____ Permit extra time during tests
____ Let student take test in nondistracting environment
____ Arrange for oral testing
____ Let student demonstrate competence through an alternative modality
____ Permit short breaks during tests
____ Use short, frequent quizzes instead of longer tests
____ Provide computer/word processor access during essay exams
____ Adjust grading criteria
____ Permit student to retake tests
____ Allow open book examinations
____ Allow take-home examinations
____ Allow approved notes as prompts for recall during test

READING COMPREHENSION

____ Providing books on tape
____ Providing student with written outline of the chapters
____ Cueing the student to remain on task during reading
____ Highlighting main ideas in the text
____ Substituting easier texts on the same topic
____ Teaching SQ4R method for reading
____ Providing reading specialist to tutor student

LESSON PRESENTATION/NOTE TAKING

____ Seat student near teacher
____ Assign student to a low-distraction work area
____ Slow down rate of presentation of lecture

(continued)

TABLE 9.2. *(continued)*

_____

LESSON PRESENTATION/NOTE TAKING *(continued)*

___ Pause frequently during lecture to give student chance to take notes
___ Repeat information often
___ Summarize information often
___ Verbally emphasize key points for note taking
___ Write key points on board
___ Make sure lecture is audible and visuals are visible
___ Give permission to tape-record lecture
___ Allow laptop computer for note taking
___ Give student copy of teacher outline/overheads
___ Have another student, TC takes notes for student
___ Allow student to attend class twice/audit before taking for credit
___ Give student feedback on his or her notes
___ Provide direct instruction in note taking
___ Stand near student when giving instructions
___ Break lecture into short segments
___ Ask student to repeat your instructions
___ Call on student often

GENERAL ORGANIZATION

___ Schedule last period study hall
___ Schedule A.M. checkin to organize for day
___ Schedule P.M. checkout to organize for homework
___ Give time to organize locker during school
___ Assist in organizing binder/notebook/backpack
___ Train in time management
___ Prompt students to use calendar, planner
___ Permit student to bring backpack to each class

MOTIVATIONAL TECHNIQUES

___ Increase frequency of feedback in the following classes_____
___ Send weekly progress note home
___ Institute behavioral contracting
___ Schedule regular meetings with student, parents, teachers, administrators
___ Schedule in-school suspension
___ Provide special activities in school (computers, internet, hobbies)

ADDITIONAL SUPPORT

___ Peer tutoring
___ Learning resource center (regular or special education)
___ Librarian assistance
___ Teacher consultant services
___ Meetings with teachers before or after school
___ Hand scheduling of courses
___ Case manager assigned to oversee plan

PARENT INVOLVEMENT

___ Parent conferences. Frequency_____
___ Parental involvement in selecting teachers for next year

(continued)

TABLE 9.2. *(continued)*

INPUT TO MEDICAL/THERAPEUTIC SUPPORT

___ Provide narrative log of significant events
___ Complete teacher ratings as follows_____
___ Look for following medication side effects_____
___ Administer medication as prescribed
___ Remind student to go to office to take medication
___ Check to see if medication is wearing off too soon

Thank you for your assistance.

Note. From *ADHD in Adolescents: Diagnosis and Treatment* by Arthur L. Robin. Copyright 1998 by The Guilford Press. Permission to photocopy this table is granted to purchasers of *ADHD in Adolescents* for personal use only (see copyright page for details).

There are differences of opinion in the field about how strongly worded such a statement should be in a report to the school. Consider the following examples of alternative recommendations:

> There is a large discrepancy between Jennifer's academic productivity and the academic productivity of her peers of similar IQ, due to her difficulties with inattention and distractibility.
>
> 1. Therefore, Jennifer is educationally impaired due to ADHD. The Podunc Public Schools should conduct an immediate Section 504 evaluation and provide Jennifer with the accommodations on the attached checklist.
> 2. This discrepancy raises strong suspicions of the possibility of a handicapping condition. It is recommended that the Podunc Public school conduct an evaluation to determine whether such a handicapping condition exists, and in doing so, consider the accommodations on the attached checklist as possible interventions.
> 3. A Section 504 plan consisting of the accommodations on the attached checklist should be implemented as soon as possible to prevent serious consequences from happening to Jennifer.

Advocates would prefer the third alternative, which is strongest. School systems typically prefer the second alternative, which gives them the most room to maneuver. Most commonly, I use a variation of the first wording, which is intermediate in strength between the other two. Normally, it is better for external consultants not to tell the schools how to do their job, but to identify problems and suggest that the school follow its normal procedures to solve these problems. However, in confrontational situations sometimes strong recommendations need to be made. One should always be prepared to substantiate such strong recommendations with testing and evaluation data.

FOLLOW-UP

Careful follow-up is essential for ensuring the success of cooperative interventions involving the school, the student, the parents, and the therapist.
School meetings and written home/school reports are two methods of conducting such follow-up.

School Meetings

Periodic school meetings have proven to be a potent approach to follow-up
for monitoring and fine-tuning educational interventions for adolescents
with ADHD. Such meetings help to maintain accountability for the interventions and keep the lines of communication open between the family, the
school, and the therapist. Usually, the adolescents, the parents, the therapist, the case manager or an administrator such as the principal, and the
teachers attend such meetings. Progress toward the goals of the intervention plan is assessed, as each teacher reports the student's current level of
academic and behavioral functioning in that class. Being accountable in
front of all these adults usually motivates the adolescent to try to do well
because he or she won't be able to play the school and the parents off
against each other, avoiding unpleasant work as a result. When the adolescent does well, hearing all the teachers praise him or her is a highly reinforcing experience. Being accountable to the parents keeps the teachers and
the administrators on task implementing the accommodations. The parents
feel that they are being kept informed, and miscommunications can be
averted or cleared up before they become confrontations.

At an initial informal meeting, IEP, or Section 504 meeting, I usually
suggest scheduling a follow-up meeting 4 to 8 weeks down the line, and at
the follow-up meeting, I suggest scheduling several such meetings spaced
out over time. The team establishes specific goals to be monitored. For example, the goals may include timely completion of homework, overall
grade point average, test performance, and punctuality and attendance.
When things are going well for several months, the frequency of meetings
is faded out.

Home–School Report Systems

Written home–school report systems are a second approach to following
up on an initial intervention plan. In accordance with the initial plan, the
therapist works with the teachers, parents, and adolescent to define a set of
target behaviors which need improving—typically a combination of completing academic assignments and following classroom rules. The teacher
completes a brief written report delineating the student's academic
progress and behavioral functioning, typically at weekly intervals (e.g., on
Fridays), which the student brings home and shows to his or her parents. It

is often desirable to have progress reports completed daily or every other day, but I find that it is difficult to convince teachers in secondary education to go along with this recommendation; when reports are needed more often than once a week, it is more feasible to arrange for a guidance counselor to collect the information orally from the teachers and talk by phone with the parent. The therapist coaches the parents and the student to write a behavioral contract specifying how the student earns and/or loses privileges depending on the accomplishment of school-related tasks evaluated on the weekly report. The report provides information to the parents and motivates the student to complete schoolwork and behave appropriately in the classroom. Such reports can be used for all classes or only for those classes in which the student is having problems. Extensive research with home–school reports has demonstrated that they are often effective in motivating improved school performance (Atkeson & Forehand, 1979; Kelley, 1990).

Several factors enhance the efficacy of home–school reports with ADHD adolescents (DuPaul & Stoner, 1994). First, it is helpful to state the target behaviors in a positive manner rather than as the absence of negative behaviors; it is preferable to specify "complete in-class assignments" rather than "stop off-task behavior." Second, it is often useful to include both academic and behavioral targets, unless, of course, there are no behavioral targets. Third, it is better to specify a small number of targets at one time rather than too many targets. Fourth, it is helpful to provide both a quantitative and a qualitative format for the teacher to give feedback. Fifth, it is important to involve adolescents in the planning of the home–school report system. Sixth, it is prudent to write out a contract specifying the privileges to be earned or lost and exactly what the criteria for success and failure are. Finally, it is important to work out the details of where the student is going to pick up the form, when the teachers will sign it, what will happen if a substitute is in one class on the day the sheet is to be signed, what will happen if the student does not bring the sheet home, and so on. Most commonly, the student picks up a blank form from the adviser or the first-period teacher and asks each teacher to fill it out at the end of a class period. In some cases, it is wise to arrange for the student to start taking the sheet around Thursday, because it may take 2 days to get all of the teachers' comments and signatures. Of course, if the student fails to bring the sheet home, by definition we assume that the student received the lowest possible ratings.

Kelley (1990) has exhaustively reviewed alternative forms for use in constructing home–school reports. Many schools have their own forms, and therapists are advised to use the school's forms whenever possible, because this is likely to enhance cooperation. Table 9.3 illustrates one common format for the home/school note form. This form is set up to elicit yes–no answers regarding several target behaviors, weekly grades, and anecdotal comments. Space limitations precluded putting in all of the sub-

TABLE 9.3. Sample School–Home Report

Name_____ Date_____

MATH:	Came prepared for class:	Yes	No	N.A.
	Handed in homework	Yes	No	N.A.
	Talked respectfully	Yes	No	N.A.

       Weekly grade: Homework_____   Tests_____

       Any incomplete assignments:

       Comments:

       Teacher signature:

ENGLISH:	Came prepared for class:	Yes	No	N.A.
	Handed in homework	Yes	No	N.A.
	Talked respectfully	Yes	No	N.A.

       Weekly grade: Homework_____   Tests_____

       Any incomplete assignments:

       Comments:

       Teacher signature:

FRENCH:	Came prepared for class:	Yes	No	N.A.
	Handed in homework	Yes	No	N.A.
	Talked respectfully	Yes	No	N.A.

       Weekly grade: Homework_____   Tests_____

       Any incomplete assignments:

       Comments:

       Teacher signature:

jects, but they would continue on a second page in a similar format to math, English, and French.

The following contract between Sally and her mother specifies simply and clearly how the contract in Table 9.3 works.

"I, Sally Welby, agree to pick up a blank school–home note in my first-period math teacher's class each Thursday morning, and to have each teacher fill it out and sign it by the end of school Friday. I agree to bring it home on Friday and show it to my mother. If I earn 80% positive ratings on the yes/no items and grades of C or better on tests and homework, my mother agrees to pay me ten dollars. My mother will also check the teacher signatures and accuracy of the ratings on a random basis. If I don't bring the sheet home, I have earned 0% positive ratings."

In the second edition of his book *Defiant Children,* Barkley (1997c) also provides an excellent description of how to implement home–school reports, along with several models for the forms.

SPECIFIC INTERVENTION TARGETS

As indicated earlier, after making specific recommendations to the school, the therapist works diligently in Sessions 5 through 9 on intervention strategies for homework, organization, test preparation and test taking, note taking, reading comprehension, memorizing, and classroom participation and conduct.

Homework

Every adolescent with ADHD whom I have ever treated has experienced at least some difficulty with getting homework done and turned in on time. The degree of difficulty varies drastically from case to case. Elaborating on the items in Table 9.1, the therapist should conduct a logical analysis of where in the homework process there is a breakdown and aim the interventions at these weak links. The therapist should engage the parents and the adolescent in a collaborative analysis of the following aspects of the homework process: (1) writing down the homework assignments in an assignment book, sheet, or some other organized medium; (2) bringing home from school the assignment book, textbooks, notebooks, and other materials needed to complete homework; (3) parental monitoring of the assignment book; (4) availability of a quiet, nondistracting, well-lit, and comfortable place in which to do the homework; (5) an agreed-on time for starting homework; (6) presence of a parent in the house when the adolescent is supposed to be doing homework; (7) an organized plan of attack to sequencing multiple homework assignments in one evening; (8) use of a calendar to track long-term projects and upcoming tests and to allocate time to short versus long-term tasks; and (9) steps taken after completing the assignment to make sure it will get to school and be handed in on time.

The therapist also should examine whether the parents and the adolescent have severe conflicts about homework, and whether homework has become a battleground for adolescent independence seeking.

Delineating Responsibilities

As the therapist analyses these issues, he or she clearly needs to delineate for the adolescent and the parents various people's roles in the homework process (Markel & Greenbaum, 1996). The purpose of delineating roles is twofold: (1) we want the teenager to know that he or she is not alone, and that there is a collaborative support system between the student, the family, the school, and the therapist to foster successful completion of homework; and (2) we want to establish appropriate boundaries and structure around the homework process to provide hope that change can take place and to facilitate an orderly change process. At minimum, the roles of the teachers, student, parent, and therapist need to be clearly demarcated. In some cases, the special education teacher consultant, private tutor, principal, and other school administrators have a role in homework too. The teacher's role is to give the student a rationale for doing homework, to base homework on skills that have already been learned and need reinforcement or practice (not to ask students to learn new skills on their own or ask parents to teach new skills), to clearly give the assignment and outline expectations for its completion, to grade the completed assignment and give feedback to the students about their homework in a timely manner, and to keep parents informed when students fall behind on homework for more than 2 or 3 days. In addition, secondary education teachers need to keep in mind that there is life after school and make the amount of homework realistic. When there is an accommodation plan, the teachers are also expected to implement the accommodations relevant to homework.

The student's role is certainly to complete the homework, but it goes beyond this. Students are expected to keep track of what homework is assigned, develop a homework plan with assistance from their parents, decide when and where to do their homework with input from their parents, follow the homework plan without being nagged, ask for help when they need it, complete their homework to the best of their ability, check it over for mistakes and legibility, and hand it in on time.

The parents' role is to stay involved in the structuring of their youngster's homework, even though they may be hearing that teenagers should take full responsibility for their own homework; this does not work when teenagers have ADHD. Specifically, parental involvement includes helping the student develop a homework plan; providing the student with a nondistracting, comfortable location for doing homework; providing the student with the basic materials; being in the house to monitor compliance with the homework plan when they expect homework to be done; helping the student analyze homework problems when the student asks for help; expecting the adolescent to adhere to the plan; administering any agreed-on positive or negative consequences for doing or not doing homework; and communicating regularly with the teachers to track whether homework has been completed and discuss any homework problems that arise.

The therapist's roles are to guide the adolescent and family in determining the locus of the breakdown in the homework process, to provide guidance and direct instruction for fixing the breakdown, and to help coordinate efforts between the school and family around homework issues.

In explaining each person's role to the family, the therapist answers any questions that arise, assesses the family's acceptance of these roles, and deals with any resistance that surfaces. The adolescent's teachers are not typically present for this discussion (although it sometimes is possible to have the discussion during a meeting at the school). If the therapist receives reports that one or more teachers are not carrying out aspects of their functions or specified accommodations with regard to homework, it is the therapist's role to help the adolescent and parents approach the teachers or principal to rectify the situation.

Developing a Homework Plan

After clarifying and answering questions about everyone's role in the homework process, the therapist collaboratively involves the adolescent and parents in developing a homework plan that addresses the particular problem areas that they identified. The contract may be long and detailed or may be relatively short and general, depending on the therapist's judgment of what is needed and the family's style. Table 9.4 presents an example of a detailed contract for Fred Adams, a 15-year-old with a variety of school problems.

This contract illustrates the phrasing that can be used for every type of homework problem. It specified how Fred is going to record his assignments; what the teacher is going to do to inform Fred's parents about the assignments; when, where, and under what conditions Fred will do his homework; the daily organizational plan for attacking homework and turning assignments in; timely feedback from the teachers; and reinforcement at home. I find it useful to have such a contract available as a template to show parents when developing shorter examples covering subsets of homework problems. Everyone involved in Fred's contract has signed it. Dr. Jones, the therapist, arranged for the school personnel to sign the contract at a school meeting which they all attended, along with Fred, his parents, and Dr. Jones. The public commitment to comply with the contract made in front of the teachers, guidance counselor, principal, and parents is a very powerful motivator, as are the telephone privileges.

Not all contracts need to be so comprehensive. Petulia Clark is a 16-year-old 11th-grader who has been having difficulty getting book reports completed on time in an advanced literature class where the students have to work relatively independently. She records the assignments accurately, reads the books, and starts the reports but does not reliably finish them, or

TABLE 9.4. The Homework Plan for Fred Adams

I, Fred Adams, together with my parents, teachers, my guidance counselor, and Dr. Jones, agree to carry out to the best of our ability, the following homework plan:

I. Keeping Track of Assignments

   A. My teachers will write the assignments on the board every day. They will also give a copy of all the assignments for the week to Mrs. Smith, my guidance counselor, each Monday. She will keep a copy and mail a copy home to my parents.

   B. I will write down the assignment from the board every day before I leave each class. I will write it on the back of the section divider for the section of my looseleaf binder for each class. I will read over what I have written down to make sure I understand it. I will ask the teacher to explain any assignment I do not understand.

   C. During my last period study hall, I will read over each assignment which I have written down and make sure I understand what I am being asked to do. I will make a list of all of the materials I need to bring home and gather them from my locker. My study hall teacher agrees to give me a hall pass to go to my locker and find any materials I need during last period.

II. Bringing Home Materials

   A. I will bring home all of the materials I have gathered and the binder in which I have written my assignments down.

   B. My mother agrees to ask me nicely one time without nagging to see my list of assignments. I agree to show it to her without a big hassle or an attitude.

   C. As a backup in case I forget to write the assignment down, I will pick a study buddy in each of my classes, get that person's phone number, and post those phone numbers on the refrigerator door.

III. Schedule and Setting for Doing Homework

   A. From Sunday through Thursday, I agree to work on homework from 6:00 P.M. to 8:00 P.M. If I finish early, I will show my completed work to a parent, and if they agree that it is completed, I can do whatever I want.

   B. I will do my homework at the big desk in the den. I can listen to soft music with headphones, but no loud rock. If I find myself getting distracted, I will take a short break, do something physical (not telephone), and start working again.

   C. My mother will remind me once without nagging to start on my homework at 6:00 P.M. I will start without an attitude.

IV. Daily Plan for Organizing Homework Completion

   A. With help from my mother, I will make an organized plan for each night's homework. This plan will guide me in what subject I will do first, second, etc. It will also divide up homework time between assignments due tomorrow and long-term assignments. My mother agrees to permit me to determine the order of doing homework.

(*continued*)

TABLE 9.4. *(continued)*

B. My plan will estimate the time needed to complete each assignment, as well as how I will check each assignment over for accuracy, completeness, and legibility.

C. The plan will specify how often I will take breaks during homework time, how long the breaks will be, and how large assignments will be divided into smaller units.

D. The plan will specify where I will put the completed assignments and how I will make sure I turn the work in.

V. Medication

I agree to take a dose of Ritalin at 5:00 P.M. on Sunday through Thursday, to help me concentrate on homework.

VI. Turning in Assignments

A. As I finish an assignment, I will put it in the section of my binder for that class.

B. I will do my best to remember to hand in each assignment.

VII. Feedback

My teachers agree to tell me how I did within 2 days after I hand in an assignment. They also agree to mail my parents feedback about how many of the last week's assignments were turned in on time when they send the next week's assignment list. The guidance counselor will collect these materials from the teachers and mail them out.

VIII. Rewards

My parents agree to let me make 20 minutes of long-distance phone calls to my girlfriend each night that I do my homework. If I do my homework for 5 nights in a row, they agree to let me make 45 minutes of long-distance phone calls on the weekend.

Signed, Fred Adams   Robert Adams   Barbara Adams
         Bill Jones, Principal   Brenda Smith, Guidance Counselor
         Millie Broadbent, Algebra   Tom Jones, English
         Darla Breeze, French   Willima Somona, Chemistry
         F.A.O. Schwarz, Gym   Neiman Marcus, History

finishes them and forgets to take them to school. The following homework plan was written for Petulia:

"I, Petulia Clark, together with my parents and Mrs. Broadbent, my literature teacher, agree that I will complete my book reports and turn them in on time. My parents will remind me to spend 30 minutes per night on each report for 4 nights before it is due, and I will put it in my binder whenever I'm not working on it. For each completed book report I turn in on time, my mother will take me shopping for up to ten dollars of cosmetics."

This plan covers only the elements of homework that are problematic for Petulia.

Accommodations

As can be seen from Fred's homework plan, school-based accommodations are often part of a comprehensive approach to improving completion of homework. We most commonly request the accommodations listed in the homework section of Table 9.2.

When the family has bloody homework wars consisting of endless arguments about getting homework done, the therapist needs to separate homework as an educational issue from homework as an independence-related struggle. The therapist calls a truce in the battles and helps the family arrange for someone other than the parents to supervise homework. This could be a tutor, an older sibling, a relative, or school-based personnel, but the key is disengaging the parents at least temporarily.

Preparing for and Taking Tests

Adolescents with ADHD may do poorly on tests and examinations for a variety of reasons, including (1) difficulty understanding the material covered, (2) insufficient time for studying or cramming at the last minute, (3) not knowing how to study for different types of tests, (4) poor use of memorization techniques, (5) reading and writing deficiencies, which interfere with understanding and responding to the test questions, (6) difficulty remembering and organizing the information and writing it down during the test, (7) slow reading rate or lethargic cognitive tempo, resulting in inability to complete the test within the allotted time period, (8) difficulty maintaining attention during the test, (9) impulsive tendency to rush through objective tests and pick the first answer that is read without thinking carefully, (10) careless mistakes resulting from failure to read the directions or overlooking important details such as responding in the correct box on scantron sheets, and (11) test anxiety. Students can be helped to overcome difficulties with test preparation and test taking through a combination of direct instruction and accommodation.

A therapist external to the school can teach the adolescent how to prepare for different types of tests, how to take different types of test efficiently and effectively, and how to manage test anxiety and can help the parents structure the study situation effectively for the adolescent. The teachers and school administrators need to be willing to make the accommodation that may be necessary and help the student with understanding the material; the therapist can help the adolescent and the family obtain the needed accommodations and services from the school regarding test taking. Markel and Greenbaum (1996) argue persuasively that general education content-area teachers can and should take responsibility, with the assistance of teacher consultants, for the entire process of direct instruction in test-taking skills, but in reality, the external consultant often needs to do some of the instruction and spur the school system to do the rest.

Careful analysis of the Diagnostic Checklist for School Success helps the practitioner determine which test preparation and test-taking problems apply to a particular adolescent. In addition, the practitioner needs to gauge the adolescent's receptivity to help in test taking and, in the case of adolescents who deny their test-taking problems, determine whether anything can be done to overcome their denial. For adolescents willing to commit to a genuine effort to improve test taking, I recommend that the therapist (1) teach the adolescent a flexible, generalized approach to preparing for tests, such as the modified SQ4R method discussed by Markel and Greenbaum (1996); (2) teach the adolescent specific skills for taking objective and essay exams; (3) teach the adolescent how to identify his or her learning style and use memorization techniques appropriate to his or her learning style; and (4) ask the content-area teachers and school support staff to make selected accommodations and give direct instruction in test taking tailored to each class. The student may also benefit from an error analysis of previous tests (i.e., reviewing previous exams with the teacher to determine what the student did correctly and what the student did incorrectly).

Preparation for Tests

Many adolescents with ADHD think that studying for a test means lightly reading over the book the night before the exam; they do not have the faintest clue about how to prepare effectively for exams. Table 9.5 presents the modified SQ4R approach to preparing for a test. Students are taught to survey, predict questions, read and reflect, recite, write, and review and edit, with the particular items on the checklist customized to their situations. First, in preparing for the test, the student is asked to *survey* the topics to be covered on the test to determine what material to study. This includes surveying any written materials about the test, the relevant textbooks, other readings, previous homework assignments, and class notes, culminating in identifying and listing the key topics and terms likely to be on the test. Second, the student attempts to predict the test *questions* for each of the topics surveyed, locating sample questions in the book or handouts and creating different types of questions for each topic. The student should determine whether the test will consist of multiple-choice, fill-in, matching, or essay questions by talking to the teacher, so that the remaining stages can be customized to the format of the test questions. The sample questions should be generated in the same format as the test ques-

TABLE 9.5. Student Checklist for Applying SQ4R When Preparing for and Taking Tests

SURVEY to identify topics to be covered on the test.

___ Survey the test assignment, previous homework assignments, and previous lecture and/or text notes.

___ Survey the text's study aids (e.g., table of contents, chapter objectives, introductions, summaries, glossary, and illustrations).

___ Make a list of the most important topics and key technical terms.

___ Identify topics that are most and least familiar to you.

QUESTION to focus attention and arouse curiosity.

___ Locate sample questions or problems that could be included on the tests. These may be at the end of a text chapter or from lectures, class discussions, or review sessions.

___ Create possible test questions by using lecture notes or headings from readings.

___ Create different types of questions for each topic. Include How? Why? and What difference does it make?

READ AND REFLECT to understand the information related to your questions.

___ Use your prepared questions to guide your reading and thinking.

___ Ask the teacher about possible topics and types of questions and locate portions of information to confirm or add to your answer.

___ Reread portions of the text and lecture notes, circling or highlighting key concepts and facts that answer your questions.

___ Sort out essential from nonessential facts, details, or examples.

___ Visualize the information, explaining to yourself particular aspects of your mental picture that answer your questions.

RECITE the answers to your questions.

___ Talk to yourself by restating or reexplaining answers to questions, relationships between topics, or steps to solve problems.

___ Allow time to elaborate on the answers, including several facts and/or examples.

___ Say the answers to the questions in your own words, without reference to your notes.

___ Add details or examples.

(W)RITE answers to your questions.

___ Write the answers in your own words.

___ Use key words, phrases, symbols, abbreviations, or sketches.

___ Organize the information and relate information from different sources or topics.

___ Create a "miniquiz" and practice by taking an old test.

(*continued*)

TABLE 9.5. *(continued)*

REVIEW AND EDIT your answers as soon as possible.

___ Review your questions and answers.

___ Check the accuracy and completeness of your answers.

___ Reread, recite, redraw, or rewrite answers so the information is used in an organized and efficient way.

___ List additional details and examples.

___ Identify topics that need further explanation. Raise questions. How? Why? So what?

___ Identify topics or sections to relearn.

Note. From *Performance Breakthroughs for Adolescents with Learning Disabilities or ADD* (pp. 216–217) by G. Markel & J. Greenbaum (1996). Copyright 1980 by the authors. Reprinted by permission. Reprinted in *ADHD in Adolescents: Diagnosis and Treatment* by Arthur L. Robin. Copyright 1998 by The Guilford Press. Permission to photocopy this table is granted to purchasers of *ADHD in Adolescents* for personal use only (see copyright page for details).

tions. Third, the student *reads and reflects* to locate and understand the information necessary to answer the sample questions, including tests, notes, handouts, and so on. At this stage the student needs to sort out essential from nonessential facts, details, or examples. Fourth, the student memorizes the necessary information by *reciting the answers to the questions,* allowing sufficient time and distribution of practice to effectively learn the material. Some students may benefit from reciting the answers or facts into a tape recording and listening to themselves talking; others may benefit from reciting the material to a parent or even a peer in a group study session, or following one of the memorization techniques discussed next. It is at this stage that the practitioner deals with time management (e.g., planning study over several days to avoid cramming, etc.). Closely aligned to reciting is *writing answers to the questions*; the student needs to write the responses in the format likely to occur on the test to be fully prepared. Taking old exams is helpful here. Writing is especially important with essay exams, where the student needs to practice outlining, organizing, and actually committing sample essays to paper. The student needs to learn how much recitation and writing is necessary to be fully prepared for each examination through experimentation and practice. Finally, the student *reviews and edits* his or her written answers to the questions (both study and sample test questions), practicing checking for accuracy and completeness, identifying topics in need of elaboration, and identifying areas to be studied further. Parents and/or study buddies can be helpful as this stage.

If the adolescent's school does not already have instruction in SQ4R, the practitioner can teach this approach by reviewing Table 9.5 with the adolescent and either taking the adolescent through the steps with a make-believe exam or with the actual material for an upcoming exam. Such instruction is best done with a parent present, so that the parents can assist the student at home. SQ4R can be customized to the learning style of the student. Visual learners, for example, might skip the reciting stage and emphasize learning by writing and reading over the written materials. Students who are effective at memorizing but are unable to decide what is important to study can be helped to emphasize the survey and question stages the most.

Memorization Techniques

Encoding and retaining information in immediate, short-term, and then long-term memory is a challenge for restless, impulsive youth who have deficits in verbal and nonverbal working memory (Barkley, 1997b). Inability to remember facts they studied is one of the most debilitating and frustrating experiences ADHD adolescents have, often leading them to erroneously conclude that they are dumb and stupid. The therapist can make an immediate impact in the area by teaching the adolescent one or more simple memorization techniques (Davis et al., 1996). Therapists should review the memorization section of the Diagnostic Checklist for School Success to determine whether the student currently utilizes any of these techniques, then, in a session with the adolescent and the parents in attendance, present and discuss the following five guidelines for effective memorization:

1. *Accept the need for repetition and planning for effective memorization.* The therapist should point out that no matter how the student plans to memorize material, it is going to take repetition over several days to really learn it; this is a necessary evil. In addition, there is no magic to memorizing things; for the inattentive, restless person, planning and structuring the memorization situation are essential.

2. *Learn to accurately select the essential information to be memorized.* It is impossible for the student to memorize the entire chapter and lecture notes. Smart students learn to predict what information is likely to be essential and learn that information. The SQ4R method reviewed earlier is one helpful approach to discriminating between what is essential and what is unessential. In addition, the therapist can point out that the student can review past examinations for that teacher, lecture notes, outlines or study guides from that teacher. Teachers often give oral reviews with hints several days before the test. Finally, the student could ask the teacher for help selecting what is essential to memorize.

3. *Know what kind of learner you are (e.g., auditory, visual, kinesthetic, or combined).* Adolescents with ADHD do not necessarily stop to think how they learn best. The therapist should prompt adolescents to consider whether they learn best from what they hear (e.g., auditory learner), from what they see (e.g., visual learner), from what they write down and

get a tangible feel for (e.g., kinesthetic learner), or from a combination of auditory, visual, and kinesthetic modes.

4. *Select one or more memorization techniques that match your learning style.* Table 9.6 lists a variety of memorization techniques keyed to auditory, visual, kinesthetic, or combined learning styles. The therapist should review each of these techniques with the adolescent and the parent and ask the adolescent to memorize several items in the session using visual, auditory, or kinesthetic techniques, to help determine experientially his or her predominant learning style. Davis et al. (1996) give exercises that help students understand and apply each of these techniques. I briefly define each with an example here.

Acrostics is a mnemonic technique that has the individual make up a sentence in which the first letter of each word refers to one of the items on the list of facts to be memorized. Acrostics works best if the sentence is silly or humorous, making it easier to remember. To memorize the planets in order from the sun (Mercury, Venus, Earth, Mars, Jupiter, Saturn, Uranus, Neptune, Pluto), for example, we might make up the following sentence: My Very Educated Martian Just Sawed Ugly New Pillows. An *acronym* is a shorter version of an acrostic where the first letter of each concept to be learned forms a single word. We might memorize the Great Lakes (Huron, Ontario, Michigan, Erie, Superior) by using the acronym *HOMES*.

Charting, visual emphasis, and visualization are particularly suited to visual learners. In charting and graphing, the student makes up tables, charts, or graphs which represent the concepts to be learned. Artistically inclined students may enjoy drawing pictures and making up graphs to facilitate memorization. Material can be given visual emphasis by highlighting it in the text or in one's notes in a different color. Visualization consists of closing one's eyes and imagining a picture of either the text to be memo-

TABLE 9.6. Memorization Techniques for Different Learning Styles

Technique	Learning styles		
	Auditory	Visual	Kinesthetic
1. Acrostics	××	××	××
2. Acronyms	××	××	××
3. Charting		××	××
4. Visual emphasis		××	××
5. Visualization		××	
6. Associations	××	××	
7. Recall questions	××	××	××
8. Rehearsal	××	××	××

Note. From Davis, Sirotowitz, & Parker (1996). Copyright 1996 by Specialty Press. Reprinted by permission.

rized, the chart, the graph, or the diagram. The student practices imagining all the details, placement, and colors of the material, using the picture to facilitate recall. Those who also have a kinesthetic learning style might benefit from adding motion to their visualization; they might imagine the material as a slide show or video of moving images, as they actually trace or draw the diagram in their mind. Actively drawing a diagram in imagination might also help combat inattention for visual learners using this technique.

A variety of *association* techniques may also be helpful, particularly for memorizing lists of unrelated facts. The list of facts can be associated or linked to a common theme, story, phrase, sentence, rhyme, or even picture. For example, if the student needs to memorize the last five Presidents of the United States (Ford, Carter, Reagan, Bush, Clinton), he or she might make up a story such as the following: *Ford* ate *Carter's* peanuts, but *Reagan* ate jelly beans; they got so *Bushed* that *Clinton* had to step in.

Finally, with regard to rehearsal, the therapist should help the adolescent gear rehearsal to learning modes. Auditory learners need to repeat aloud the information or use a tape recorder. Visual and kinesthetic learners need to write down the information, draw pictures, and/or visualize it. Kinesthetic learners may also find it useful to relate the information to common objects, which they hold and get the feel of while studying.

5. *Engage in sufficient repetition distributed over time (i.e., not cramming) applying the techniques you selected to memorize the material.* The adolescent should be asked to make a commitment to try to use several of these strategies, with parental guidance if needed, and report back to the therapist at the next session how they worked. The therapist might ask the adolescent to write a brief behavioral contract specifying how much time he or she will devote to studying which content material using selected memorization. It can be pointed out that only through experience can the exact amount of time needed for memorization be determined.

Having an adequate dose of stimulant medication on board while trying to memorize material usually makes learning much easier. The therapist should review the timing of the medication and suggest (with the consent of the physician prescribing the medication) that the adolescent be sure to time the medication so that it is in the body during heavy memorization sessions.

Even with the help of memorization techniques, planning, and medication, some students with ADHD still have persistent difficulties recalling information during examinations. I have found this to be the case particularly with older adolescents and young adults in business and science college courses and professional schools such as medical schools, where tremendous amounts of material and complicated formulae need to be recalled accurately during examinations. Such students might benefit greatly from accommodations like open-book examinations, take-home examinations, or permission to use selected notes approved by the teacher as prompts for recalling information. For example, having the first term of a formula or an outline of key terms may be helpful. Instructors sometimes view such accommodation as unfair, and it behooves the therapist to help them understand the nature of these students' disabilities and the very real need for memorization accommodations. Suggesting that the skeptical instructor orally interview the student to feel reassured that the student is not simply copying notes on the examination often helps in this situation. Alternatively, breaking the examination down into a series of short quizzes evenly spaced over time, which require less memorization per quiz, may be helpful.

Taking Tests

The practitioner should help the adolescent understand that we are not born instinctively knowing how to succeed on tests, and that certain skills need to be mastered. Most students with ADHD need help refraining from impulsively starting the test without carefully reading the instructions and items, planning effective use of their time, noting how much each item counts, and deciding on the order in which they will answer questions. Many also spend an inordinate amount of time on the first difficult item, instead of doing all of the easy items first, then gradually working through the more difficult items. With regard to essay exams, many students do not take sufficient time to plan, and do not leave any time to review their answers for accuracy or completeness. The practitioner might prompt the adolescent to develop a brief checklist of the steps to be taken during an exam. Such a checklist might include items such as the following:

1. Carefully read the directions and circle key items.
2. Read the entire exam to identify the difficult items.
3. Answer all the easy items first, then slowly work through the difficult items.
4. Watch the time, so you don't spend too much time on one item.

Markel and Greenbaum (1996) have samples of such checklists for objective and essay examinations.

It is best for the therapist and student to go through these steps by working on a made-up practice exam. The adolescent might enjoy making up a humorous exam covering some topic of interest (rock music, why school is a waste of time, sports, etc.).

Test-Taking Accommodations

The test-taking accommodations listed in Table 9.2 have proven useful and feasible for many secondary education students with ADHD. The therapist needs to decide which of these might be helpful to a particular adolescent and, following the guidelines given earlier in the chapter, help the family approach the school to request these accommodations.

In the case of anxiety interfering with test taking, the therapist can use a variety of relaxation, meditation, exposure based desensitization, and cognitive-behavioral techniques to help the adolescent combat debilitating test anxiety (Kendall & Treadwell, 1996).

Reading Comprehension

Adolescents with ADHD often report that they hate to read and rarely read for fun. Even those who do read for fun often have difficulty getting through their school textbooks. Reading is clearly a developmental process, and on further investigation, many adolescents with ADHD do not like to read because their reading skills are not at a grade-appropriate level, due either to comorbid learning disabilities or to inattention and distractibility. As a result, they do not get much out of reading except aggravation. As Markel and Greenbaum (1996) pointed out, by the end of elementary school, students are required to locate and understand words, main ideas, and supporting facts and examples, as well as to follow sequences of events and draw conclusions. At the secondary education level, students acquire more complex reading comprehension skills. They face increasing demands to organize ideas and the relationship between ideas, incorporating multiple views. They need to comprehend the meanings of words in context, synthesize meanings of strings of words to understand their message and problem-solve to find hidden or unstated meanings. They further need to make predictions, draw inferences, and provide interpretations, identifying the author's purpose, tone, and opinions. Moreover, they need to evaluate material and master in-depth content, learning how to adjust their reading approach to the particular type of material with which they are faced.

Identifying Specific Reading Problems

Those adolescents with concomitant learning disabilities have poor decoding skills, poor comprehension skills, or a slow reading rate. More often, distractibility and short attention spans lead them to lose their place, have trouble keeping what they read in short-term memory, and have to read the same paragraph repeatedly to get any meaning out of it. As a result, reading becomes mentally fatiguing. Since the students also tend to become easily frustrated and emotionally overreactive, they give up on reading easily. Given the increased demands for in-depth reading comprehension in middle and high school, academics of adolescents with ADHD and reading comprehension difficulties may suffer tremendously.

Reading difficulties often require the intervention of a trained reading specialist, through general education, special education, or private reading programs in the community. Most psychologists, physicians, and social workers are not trained reading specialists, and behavioral interventions are likely to be adjuncts to remedial education interventions. Before undertaking any behavioral interventions, the practitioner should help the adolescent obtain a thorough reading evaluation through the school system or a private learning disability center. Although the kind of standardized achievement testing done by psychologists is useful, diagnostic testing done for prescriptive purposes by a reading specialist is essential. Often, such evaluations result in identifying the need for specific remedial reading interventions, in or out of school.

Adjusting Medication

Many individuals with ADHD find that when an effective dose of stimulant medication is active in their body, they can read with in-depth comprehension for the first time in their life, an experience they often cannot believe is actually happening to them. In fact, I often recommend that ADHD adolescents use reading a textbook as a "benchmark" to test out the effects of various doses of stimulant medication. I ask the adolescent to try taking a dose of medication and then reading difficult or boring material about 1 hour later, comparing comprehension to reading without medication. I ask them to try the same experiment each time their dose of medication is changed. Those youngsters who normally take stimulant medication primarily during the schoolday may never experience its impact on reading textbooks at home. Sometimes, a higher dose of medication may be needed to comprehend more difficult material, and again working with the physician, this ought to be determined.

Using SQ4R

When the therapist and adolescent know the extent to which medication enhances reading comprehension, behavioral approaches can be used for residual difficulties. The SQ4R method discussed earlier for test preparation was originally developed to enhance reading comprehension (Markel & Greenbaum, 1996). This method gives the adolescent a set of prompts for specific cognitive tasks which structure the reading process, breaking it down into stages and making it easier to slow down and extract useful information. First, the adolescent previews the reading assignment through a survey to get its general flavor, to focus attention, to identify study aids, to predict the time needed to fully comprehend it, and to become aware of the topic and the main points and to anticipate any challenges. Second, the adolescent generates questions as tools for structuring what he or she will look for when reading the assignment. Titles, headings, subheadings, and illustrations are converted into questions that orient the student to the main points. Both factual and higher cognitive reasoning and interpretation questions are generated. Third, the adolescent reads with an eye toward answering the questions; most adolescents with ADHD just read with no goal in mind, resulting in minimal concentration and wasted time. The highly distractible student can be asked to read enough to answer only a few questions at a time, with breaks in between. Fourth, the student actively recites the answers to the questions, summarizing and paraphrasing in his or her own words. This recitation facilitates learning the material and putting it in terms the adolescent can understand and relate to. Fifth, the student writes down his or her answers, further reinforcing learning and providing notes for review for examinations or written assignments. Finally, a review process further reinforces learning and retention.

The therapist can teach the SQ4R method in the session using either a sample reading passage from the adolescent's textbook or a humorous passage from material of interest to the adolescent. When teaching the entire SQ4R approach is too heavy-handed or overwhelming, the therapist might alternatively wish to teach specific components of it. Davis et al. (1996), for example, provide very simple, short instruction and exercise sheets for reading to understand, paraphrasing, identifying signals in a reading passage, learning new vocabulary, and rereading the text to answer questions.

Accommodations

In addition to remedial reading, the therapist might help the student obtain one or more of the accommodations listed in the reading comprehension section of Table 9.2.

Listening and Note Taking

Listening and note taking in class are particularly taxing for adolescents with ADHD because they are unstructured activities that require good sustained concentration where students need to provide their own structure and need to get it right the first time, because they cannot rewind the tape or flip back to the previous page of the book. More important, the distractible student must simultaneously do two activities requiring complex coordination of auditory processing, executive functioning, and fine motor skills. The auditory, attentional, and working-memory problems of ADHD students make it difficult for them to take in and remember information long enough to record what the teacher is saying. Their executive functioning deficits make it difficult for the student to determine what is essential to record in his or her notes and where to put the information in space on the paper. The fine motor, spelling, and written expression difficulties make it difficult to keep up with the writing of the notes in a legible, comprehensible fashion. Hyperactivity may limit the student's ability to sit through lectures on less than interesting material, whereas distractibility renders the ADHD student highly susceptible to get off track because of noise, the movement of others in the classroom, uncomfortable seating, or visual distractors. Add to these factors the lethargic cognitive tempo of some adolescents with ADHD, Predominantly Inattentive Subtype and it is amazing than any note taking takes place.

Indeed, traditional lectures and note taking are the worst possible means of imparting information to individuals with ADHD. In this situation we are fitting round pegs into square holes, or, to use the metaphor of Hartmann (1993), we are educating our hunter children in farmers' schools. Adolescents with ADHD would be much better educated in small seminars, discussion classes, experiential laboratory settings, or individualized instructional systems such as Personalized Systems of Instruction (Robin, 1976). Although such classrooms are sometimes available, unfortunately, most therapists and parents are not in a position to reform the U.S. public school system. Thus, the question becomes how to help adolescents with ADHD survive and learn in lecture environments where important information must be gained through listening and note taking. This is an area in which aggressive efforts to obtain accommodation are central to success. Although we can and should teach adolescents more effective means of listening and taking notes, it may be unrealistic to expect them to compete on an even playing field to their non-ADHD peers without accommodation.

Accommodations for listening and note taking fall into several categories: (1) modifications in the lecture and classroom environment, (2) the use of technology to expedite note taking, and (3) providing the student with the information from the lecture in another fashion. Under the first category, the teacher can slow down the rate of presentation of material in a lecture, pause frequently and to give the students an opportunity to write down their notes, repeat information and give frequent examples and summarizations, or emphasize key points by prompting the students to put them in their notes, using key verbal signaling phrases or outlining them on the board. The teacher can make sure that everyone can hear the lecture and see any audiovisual aids and can seat the ADHD student close by. Technology may be useful in the form of permission to audiotape lectures, the availability of laptop computers to eliminate handwriting as a source of problems during note taking, or even videotaping of selected lectures. In many schools, the information is made available to the students in an alternative manner such as copies of the teacher's outlines, another student's notes, or notes taken by the teacher consultant. If another student's notes will be shared with the patient, it is best to make sure that a modal student is selected; the note taker could be given carbonless copy paper to avoid the inconvenience of finding a copy machine. Students can attend the lecture two times or even audit a course before formally enrolling in it, but these approaches are not really practical except in extreme cases.

When asked what characteristics in a teacher help them stay on task and take good notes, most ADHD students indicate that they prefer highly animated, humorous teachers who talk in many different voice tones, kid the class often, and actually move around the room a lot. They prefer least the teacher who dims the lights, puts up an overhead, and lectures from the overhead in a monotone; such teachers put them to sleep. Thus, when the time arrives for selecting the courses and teachers for the next year, the therapist should help the parents arrange for hand scheduling rather than computer scheduling and should meet with the student's adviser and/or principal to take into account teacher characteristics that will increase listening and effective note-taking behavior.

As long as appropriate accommodations are in place, efforts should also be made to teach better note taking. Ideally, these efforts should be made in the classroom by the content-area teachers, with the assistance where necessary of teacher consultants, because the external consultant is so removed from the setting that it is difficult to do too much that will generalize to the school.

Evans, Pelham, and Grudberg (1995) researched the effectiveness of Directed Notetaking Activity (DNA; Spires & Stone, 1989) with a sample of adolescents with ADHD attending their summer treatment program. The students attended a lecture followed by a study hall 5 days a week and had a quiz on the previous day's material at each class. The DNA involves lecturing to the students each day while teaching the note-taking process. Throughout the lecture, the teacher provides the students with a model of the notes as they should appear in their notebooks. Students are asked to divide their notes into main ideas and details in an outline format. The teacher explains the rationale for each note as he or she presents that point within the context of the lecture and prompts the adolescent to record the point in the notes. Over time, the teacher gradually reduces the number of prompts while monitoring the students' notes to make sure they maintain quality. In essence, this procedure is an application of behavioral shaping and fading procedures.

In their first, uncontrolled study, Evans et al. (1995) assessed the effectiveness of the DNA procedure for improving the quality of 16 adolescents' notes. They found improvements in ratings of the students' notes with regard to clarity, comprehensiveness, format, legibility, the use of abbreviations, and the fraction of the details present in the notes. There were no improvements in the fraction of main ideas in the notes.

In their second study, Evans et al. (1995) examined whether the process of taking notes would decrease disruptive behavior and increase on-task behavior in the classroom and whether the notes would lead to improved comprehension on classroom assignments and quizzes. Fourteen adolescents with ADHD enrolled in the summer treatment program received 3 weeks of DNA training followed by 5 weeks rotating equally through four conditions, representing a factorial crossing of taking versus not taking notes in class and having versus not having notes in study hall (they were not permitted to take the notes home in this study). Taking notes resulted in higher on-task behavior, while having notes resulted in improved performance on classroom assignments. However, disruptive behavior did not decrease, nor did scores on quizzes taken 24 hours after the notes were taken improve as a function of note taking. Of course, the students did not have the opportunity, because of the need for experimental control, to study at home from the notes in preparation for the quizzes.

Evans et al.'s (1995) study provides empirical evidence for the effectiveness of the DNA procedure, which might be recommended to general education teachers in secondary schools. It also points out the potential utility of note taking as a means to maintain students' attention and on-task behavior.

The therapist can help the student prepare for note taking and have a strategy in mind to get through particular note-taking situations. Preparation should involve previewing the material to be presented during the lecture by reading the textbook chapter the night before and following the SQ4R survey and question stages, formulating possible questions that might be addressed by the teacher during the lecture. Realistically, I have not had good luck getting my high school clients to preview chapters the night before, but this method has worked with college students. Even if they have not previewed the material, though, planning a note-taking strategy can be useful. The therapist should help the student decide on the format for organizing his or her notes on paper. Davis et al. (1996) illustrate several different formats; the simplest format is an outline form, where the student plans to record the main points and the details in two different physical spaces on the paper. For example, the student might divide a piece of looseleaf paper by drawing a vertical line down the page about 2 inches from the left side. On the left of the line the student would record only key words, questions, or brief phrases. On the right side the student would record details, in short phrases, one per line, skipping a line between points. The student should plan to use abbreviations as much as possible.

The therapist might also discuss how to avoid panic or giving up in frustration if the student falls behind or misses something. One simple strategy is simply to put a question mark in the left column the moment a point is missed, go on, and talk to the teacher about it later. Alternatively, the student could raise his or her hand and ask a question, which will slow the pace of the lecture, provide the needed information, and give the student an opportunity to regroup. Ideally, students ought to review their notes as soon as possible after the lecture to clarify ambiguous points before they forget about them. Realistically, I have known very few ADHD adolescents who are willing to do this. Alternatively, it is invaluable if the teacher is willing to periodically check the student's notes for accuracy and provide written feedback. Often, a teacher consultant can perform such an accuracy check.

GENERAL ORGANIZATION

Organization was a constant thread throughout the discussions of homework, tests, reading comprehension, listening, and note taking. As the adolescent grows up and enters the adult world, the need for effective self-management to organize and structure his or her life will increase, even though most teenagers live too much in the present to appreciate this fact. Whenever possible, the therapist should try to teach the adolescent some general organizational strategies that transcend specific topics such as homework or tests. Basically, the adolescent needs to learn how to organize space and time effectively, because he or she will continue to have these organizational needs for the rest of his or her life. Space includes physical locations such as the locker, the bedroom, the desk, and the backpack. Time includes the use of a calender, a to-do list, a planner, and the ability to estimate time and prioritize tasks. The therapist should assess the adolescent's current abilities to organize space and time and build on them in a graduated fashion, using behavioral shaping procedures. The therapist should break organizational skills down into their component parts and teach one skill at a time. He or she should make a judgment about the extent to which a particular adolescent can tolerate such training and gear it to the adolescent's current tolerance level and attention span (i.e., develop simple systems which are practical rather than comprehensive and complex). Therapists should exercise their creativity by finding ways to make organizational lessons fun and interesting—through multisensory techniques, games, and exercises and/or the use of electronic organizers, computers, the Internet, phone answering machines, and other modern technology. The last thing most adolescent patients want to do is hear another lecture on organization, so the therapist should not preach. "Act, don't yak" is the principle to remember. In addition to the organizational materials provided by Davis et al. (1996), many of the chapters and books written for ADHD adults provide practitioners with ideas to develop (Nadeau, 1995, 1996).

I provide some specific approaches here to organizing space and time, but these are by no means all-inclusive. With regard to organizing space, the adolescent must keep track of his or her books, papers, binders, and school supplies and, beyond school, his or her clothes, CDs, games, electronic equipment, sporting equipment, mail, and other possessions. In addition to knowing the whereabouts of these items, the teenager needs to have them conveniently placed in an accessible fashion when they are needed. Most parents would add "neatly placed" to this requirement. Most of these possessions are kept in his or her room, or, in some cases, in his or her locker in school. Most parents aim their primary organizational efforts at the adolescent's room. Teachers may focus on the locker.

Organizing the Backpack

I believe that undue emphasis on the room or the locker as the central organizational focus is misguided and misplaced. Adolescents do not spend most of the day in their room, and they hardly spend any time at their locker. They travel from home to school to friends' houses to part-time jobs, and in school they travel from class to class every 45–50 minutes. They really are like traveling salesmen. For the traveling salesman, his or her briefcase, display case, laptop computer, planner, and perhaps car represent central organizational foci. A perfectly organized home or office is helpful but not essential on an hour-to-hour basis for a traveling salesman. What travels with the adolescent all day? Where does the adolescent put books, papers, leftover food, notes, and everything else he or she carries around? Typically, his or her backpack. Many adolescents literally carry their life histories in their backpacks. I believe that therapists should make the backpack the central organizational focus for adolescents with ADHD. In addition, the therapist rarely has access to the adolescent's room or locker, precluding direct modeling, coaching, and feedback as training techniques. But the therapist can have complete access to the adolescent's backpack, opening up new and creative opportunities for direct instruction in organizational techniques. Finally, it makes sense for the adolescent to keep everything related to school that will fit in the backpack, even when the backpack is at home, so that it is easily accessible and does not have to be packed or unpacked, creating more opportunities for misplacing things, and decreasing efficiency. Because the backpack usually holds less than the locker or the room, it is also easier to get and keep organized—a benefit for inattentive and restless youth. Organizing the locker or room can follow adjunctively, as needed, from organizing the backpack.

The Big Dump

The therapist should begin the process of backpack organization by having "The Big Dump" in the session. The adolescent brings in his or her backpack, and dumps everything out on the table in front of the therapist. As long as the therapist makes this request in a lighthearted manner and explains that this is for learning better organization and not an invasion of privacy, most adolescents comply and might even have fun. The therapist explains that the goal is to find a simple, useful organizational scheme for keeping track of everything in the backpack, making it easily accessible when needed in school, not to have any loose papers or unnecessary items. Furthermore, a crucial principle regarding paperwork is, "Either act on the paper now, file it someplace, or trash it; do not pile it up or shove it back in the backpack." Together, the therapist and adolescent look at each item on the table, answering the following questions: Is it alive, moving, smelly, or rotting? If so, trash it outside the building. Is it a paper or book the adolescent no longer needs to carry to and from school? If yes, will he or she ever need it again? If no, trash it. If the adolescent might need it again, he or she should create a file for it and take the file home to put in his or her room. Is it a paper to give to his or her parents? If so, he or she put it in a section of the notebook labeled "Papers for Parents." Is it homework or a test returned by one of the adolescent's teachers? If so, he or she should put it in the appropriate section of the notebook. Is it homework completed but not yet turned in? He or she should put that in an appropriate section of the notebook.

The Notebook

Next, the therapist should ask the adolescent to show him or her how the notebook is organized. I recently asked a 13-year-old teenager who was having frequent conflicts with his mother about chores, taking his medicine at home, and a variety of other issues to dump his backpack and show me his notebook. This teenager's mother had been describing his room as a major disaster area and his completion of chores as woefully inadequate. He and his mother had been having endless conflicts about cleaning up his room and doing his chores for months. He had been hospitalized twice for violent outbursts and was very oppositional at home. Based on my past experience with this adolescent, I expected his notebook to be a disaster. I was surprised and humbled when he showed me the following simple but eloquent organizational scheme, which I would highly recommend. In his three-ring binder was an assignment book/calender entitled "My Agenda," eight colorful hole-punched folders which opened out to have a left- and right-sided pocket, and blank lined paper. The folders were ordered sequentially for his first- to seventh-period classes; the last folder was for miscellaneous items which did not fit anywhere else. Inside each folder on the righthand side were all the homework papers and tests returned by his teachers, with the most recent paper on top. On the lefthand side were the current homework assignments due in the next few days. He proudly pointed out how he also had written the name of each subject on the upper inside left-hand corner, so if he quickly opens the notebook to a folder, he can immediately determine which class it is for. Inside "My Agenda" was a section calender/planner page for each day of the month, where he had written down all his assignments. He crossed out each one as he did it, leaving the completed assignment on the lefthand side of the folder until he handed it in the next day in school. A page of "My Agenda" listed each subject and had a place for exam grades. He had all of exam grades neatly recorded in columns. The rest of the contents of his backpack included pens, pencils, and other school supplies in small pockets and no loose papers. He said that he always kept all his school things in the backpack at home, except when he was doing his homework.

Then, I asked him about his locker. He indicated that he only had 4 minutes between classes to go to his locker. He kept all his books except those he needed for a given night's homework in his locker at all times. He has the books organized on a shelf from left to right in order of his seven class periods. He volunteered that he had his clothes at home in his closet organized by school, play, and work clothes. Despite the fact that the overall appearance of this adolescent's room was a total disaster, in areas where it really mattered, he was indeed well organized. His mother did not even realize how well organized her son was regarding school materials. Naturally, I praised him for his efforts. Therapists should never underestimate their patients until they have fully assessed the situation. The therapist should ask the adolescent to agree to a weekly update time when the backpack will be dumped out at home and straightened up on a regular basis.

Time Management

The therapist can also teach time management skills by breaking them down into their component parts and using modeling, instructions, rehearsal, and feedback to teach each component. Effective time management may be broken down to include (1) planning and following a daily schedule; (2) planning a daily to-do list, prioritizing the items on it, and keeping track of them as they are completed; (3) tracking long-term events, commitments, and plans on weekly and monthly calenders, and transposing these events to the daily schedule and to-do list as they come due; (4) estimating the time needed to complete various tasks and adjusting the daily schedule in accordance with the actual time it takes; and (5) using a watch or clock to keep track of the time while engaged in various activities and when it is time to begin to engage in various activities. Although it may be desirable for content-area general education teachers to provide direct instruction in time management (Markel & Greenbaum, 1996), fortunately they are the kinds of skills a therapist can also teach.

To-Do Lists and Schedules

I ask my adolescent patients to make a simple weekly schedule and daily to-do list. Often, schedules and to-do lists are built into the student planner books supplied by the schools or commercially available at office supply lists. Creatively inclined students may prefer to design their own forms, and those who are into computers and technology may prefer to use one of the many commercially available time management software programs. One young adult patient came in every week with elaborate, computer-drawn but hand-colored graphics embedded in computer-generated weekly schedule. More commonly, the therapist is lucky to get the adolescent to take seriously even a basic schedule and to-do list. For the majority of students who carry a looseleaf binder or notebook, putting the schedule and to-do lists in a section of the binder is simple and practical.

The therapist should model and guide the adolescent in completing a simple to-do list for that day in the session. To increase involvement, the therapist might have the adolescent focus primarily on tasks of interest to him or her (call her best friend, watch his favorite TV show, etc.) as well as on homework and chores. Putting humorous items on the list (e.g., tease brother or nag mother) also helps build interest and motivation. For younger adolescents, the number of items on the list should be kept short—no more than five or six. When the list has been completed, the therapist should explain the importance of assigning priority ratings and ask the adolescent to assign a three-point priority rating:

A = Must do Today or I'm Dead Meat
B = Important, But Don't Touch it Until A's are Done
C = Will Probably Put Off Unless I'm Having A Great Day

The therapist then helps the adolescent understand that he or she should go through the list doing the items marked "A" first, then the items marked "B," and, only if time remains, the items marked "C." Each item can be checked off as it is completed.

After completing the to-do list, the therapist and the adolescent should turn to the schedule and block out the times to do the various items on the list. In addition, the adolescent should block out regular commitments with friends, family, sporting event, and other activities. At first, the therapist might ask the adolescent to use the schedule only for one or two categories of activities, such as homework or items on the to-do list, gradually extending its use as it becomes more habitual. In modeling and guiding the adolescent to make up the schedule, it is important to build in recreational breaks between onerous homework and chores, prompt the adolescent to realistically estimate how much time certain activities will take, and build in planning times. One of the last things the adolescent might do before going to bed, for example, is start the next day's to-do list.

Role of Technology

Keeping track of time and remembering to look at the schedule and list are also important skills to teach. The therapist should point out that individuals with ADHD naturally have difficulty with the passage of time and remembering to do things within a time frame, such as taking medication at prescribed times. External prompts are often necessary. The adolescent and the therapist can creatively brainstorm various options. Alarm wrist watches, which can be set to go off at multiple time intervals, are one readily available and inexpensive option. Electronic and voice-activated organizers can also be very helpful, but they cost more. The visual learner might prefer the electronic models where one types in information and sees messages on a screen; the auditory learner might prefer voice-activated models. I find a voice-activated personal organizer to be very useful; I have trained it to recognize my voice and can program in up to 100 reminders, set to go off once or daily at any time up to 12 months from the time of programming. When a reminder comes due, the organizer beeps, and when I press the play button, I hear the message in my own voice. If I do not respond to the beeping, it will stop but restart every 5 minutes until I do respond. In addition, it can hold 100 phone numbers and has a calculator and several other functions. The organizer looks like a pager and is very appealing to adolescents. Because I am a visual learner, I rely primarily on my planner book. However, the voice-activated organizer serves as a back-up tool and also provides the time-based prompts to look at the planner book. The voice-activated organizer is particularly useful when one is in the middle of doing something and receives information that has to be remembered and paper and pencil are not handy.

After going through the schedule and to-do list in the session, the therapist gives the adolescent a homework assignment to try the to-do list and schedule over the next week, and at the next session they go over the results. The therapist helps the adolescent modify the procedures based upon what works and what does not work, keeping in mind that it is more important to teach some basic time management skills than for patients to follow eloquent schedules and lists. Therapists should not worry too much if they make only limited progress on general time management skills with some of their adolescent clients. They are planting seeds for the future; the adolescents will be dealing with time management for the rest of their lives, and any start they make in middle and high school is helpful. Many of the books written for adults with ADHD include excellent discussions of time management (Kelly & Ramundo, 1993; Nadeau, 1995, 1996), as do two books written for adolescents (Nadeau, 1994; Quinn, 1995). Davis et al. (1996) have a number of worksheets for teaching adolescents time management skills. In Chapter 14, Chris Edney tells his poignant but humorous account of how he organizes his backpack and uses a planner; therapists might give this chapter to their adolescent patients to read.

CONCLUSION

This chapter outlined a systematic approach to assessing academic problems of adolescents with ADHD, deciding which can be handled by the therapist as an external consultant and which need school-based accommodations, approaching the school to obtain such accommodations for the adolescent, and providing the needed assistance in relevant areas such as homework and test preparation throughout the therapy. Using the checklists and outlines in the tables, therapists will be able to select, target, and intervene to change the subset of specific problems they confront in a particular case. The practitioner should keep in mind that enhancing school success is an ongoing process, and in the initial burst of 20 sessions following an ADHD diagnosis, the primary goal is to reverse the chronic course of academic slippage and provide some hope and skills that the adolescent can succeed in school. Many of the details for enhancing school success need to be worked on long after the 20 sessions have elapsed.

CHAPTER TEN

○

Parenting and Family Interventions

In Chapter 2, I reviewed the series of studies showing that the interactions between ADHD adolescents and their parents are characterized by conflict, negative communication, coercion, and rigid beliefs (Barkley, Anastopoulos, et al., 1992; Barkley, Fischer, et al., 1990, 1991). I developed an integrative theoretical model which postulates that parental pathology, the adolescent's striving for independence, adolescent ADHD symptoms, and comorbid adolescent conditions such as ODD, CD, or Mood Disorders disrupt the homeostatic balance of the family system and promote increased conflict between ADHD adolescents and their parents. Parents who react with poor problem solving, negative communication, distorted cognitions, depressed or hostile affect, and authoritarian control set in motion a cycle of ever-escalating coercive interactions. Over time, these coercive parent–adolescent interactions shape a repertoire of entrenched, oppositional behavior in the adolescent. By contrast, parents who react with effective problem solving, positive communication, flexible cognitions, neutral affect, and authoritative discipline get much more positive outcomes from their adolescents with ADHD, which does not mean that they have perfect relationships with their adolescents but that they avoid the pitfalls of extremely oppositional behavior.

This model has a number of practical implications which have guided the development of interventions for the home management of adolescents with ADHD: (1) before intervening, the clinician needs to carefully assess the presence of parental psychiatric problems and adolescent comorbid psychiatric problems; (2) any effective intervention needs to operate at multiple levels, educating parents about adolescent development and helping them develop an appropriate childrearing philosophy, addressing parents' beliefs and expectations, and providing parents with effective strategies for discipline; (3) interventions directly targeting parent–adolescent conflict need to be supplemented by interventions targeting parental pathology, parental ADHD when present, and marital stress; and (4) general parenting advice must be realistic and geared to the specific situations in which the parents find themselves.

ORGANIZATIONAL FRAMEWORK FOR FAMILY INTERVENTION

Figure 10.1 depicts the organizational framework of our approach to parenting and family interventions. I chose an inverted cone metaphor to convey how I begin with a wide-angle field of view on global abstractions and then gradually zoom in as I move down the cone toward a narrow field of view on specific issues. As outlined in the Introduction to Section III, the therapist devotes 6 to 8 sessions of a 20-session intervention to home management. Typically, this phase of treatment begins in Session 10. Corre-

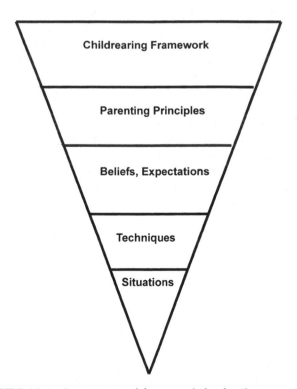

FIGURE 10.1. Organizational framework for family interventions.

sponding to the presentation of the inverted cone model are specific guidelines for the therapist to organize and conduct these sessions.

At the most global level of abstraction is an overriding philosophy and framework for parenting the ADHD adolescent. This philosophy, coupled with previous research on ADHD, leads us to a set of eight principles for parenting the adolescent with ADHD. To implement these principles effectively, parents must have a coping attitude and reasonable expectations. Thus, I next focus on beliefs and cognitive distortions. The clinician then translates these principles and beliefs into the family intervention techniques of problem-solving training, communication training, behavior management, and strategic/structural interventions. These techniques are applied to particular situations such as chores, curfew, and homework, which are problematic for a given family.

CHILDREARING/PARENTING FRAMEWORK

A parent's general approach to childrearing encompasses his or her philosophy, beliefs, expectations, and specific techniques for dealing with his or her children. To know what general approach to parenting works best with the adolescent diagnosed as ADHD, we first need a system for classifying parenting methods. Extensive research in child development, parent–child bonding, and the relationship of adult psychiatric disorders to parent–child bonding has suggested the utility and validity of a circumplex model with two orthogonal, bipolar dimensions illustrated in Figure 10.2: (1) affection and (2) control (Becker, 1964; Conger, 1977; Elder, 1962; Parker, 1979, 1983). The affection continuum ranges from warm and affectionate at one end to cold, hostile, and rejecting at the other end.

The control continuum ranges from highly controlling, authoritarian, overprotective, and dominating at one end to permissive, laissez-faire, and allowing complete autonomy at the other end. Any given parent's style of childrearing can be classified in one of the four quadrants shown in Figure 10.2. Using this model, the relationship of particular parenting approaches to adolescent and adult psychopathology can be studied through prospective and/or retrospective research. Parker, Tupling, and Brown (1979) developed the Parent Bonding Instrument (PBI), a 25-item questionnaire which adolescents or adults complete, retrospectively rating their mother or father over the first 16 years of the rater's life. The PBI has been used extensively in retrospective research. In the typical study, adolescents or adults complete the PBI, and groups with particular types of pathologies are compared to control groups on their retrospections of their parents' childrearing styles. The PBI was found to be a reliable and valid measure and has been used extensively in studies relating adult psychiatric disorders to retrospectively recalled parenting styles (Parker, 1990).

These studies have led Parker (1983) to conclude that in most cases,

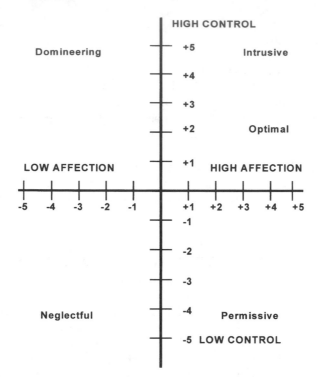

FIGURE 10.2. Circumplex model handout. From *ADHD in Adolescents: Diagnosis and Treatment* by Arthur L. Robin. Copyright 1998 by The Guilford Press. Permission to photocopy this figure is granted to purchasers of *ADHD in Adolescents* for personal use only (see copyright page for details).

the high-affection low-control parenting style is optimal, which means that it is associated with the least likelihood of adolescent or adult psychopathology. The other three less optimal quadrants have been labeled as follows: (1) affectionate constraint (high affection, high control); (2) affectionless control (low affection, high control); and (3) neglectful parenting (low affection, low control). These quadrants have each been associated, in retrospective research, with various adult psychiatric disturbances (Parker, 1990). Although no studies have directly addressed ADHD, Rey and Plapp (1990) examined the relationship between perceived parenting style and the development of ODD and CD by comparing the PBI ratings of 62 adolescents diagnosed with ODD, 49 diagnosed with CD, and 62 normal controls. The ODD and CD adolescents did not differ from each other, but both of these clinical groups retrospectively rated their parents as more controlling and less affectionate than the controls.

In her book for parents of adolescents with ADHD, Alexander-Roberts (1995) described four types of parenting styles and their impact on adolescents, which are consistent with the findings of research on the circumplex model

1. *Dominating or overly controlling parents* have high expectations for obedience and perfectionism from their children and do not give any explanations for their unilateral rules; their teenagers may become angry and aggressive, rebellious and disrespectful of authority.
2. *Neglectful parents* are usually not capable of emotionally supporting their children and have little control over them, putting their own needs first; their adolescents are likely to turn out insecure, with low self-esteem and rebellious behavior, hampering their emotional growth and development.
3. *Lenient parents* fail to establish rules and consequences, believing that teenagers will learn to live in society through choice and experience; such parents rarely discipline because they have disdain for authority. Their adolescents have trouble abiding by society's rules because they have no rules at home.
4. *Firm and loving parents* establish rules that involve the adolescents in decision making, provide reasons for rules, and give unconditional positive regard and focused time to their adolescents. This style is seen as most beneficial for adolescents in general, and for adolescents with ADHD in particular, because it fosters independence, provides adequate parental guidance and monitoring, and builds positive self-esteem.

The optimal parenting approaches might also shift with the child's age and developmental needs. For example, young children need a high degree of affection and a high degree of control, because they are not yet able to make their own decisions about many facets of their lives. Achieving independence is the major developmental task of adolescence (Conger, 1977). Child development research has repeatedly indicated that democratic childrearing practices (low control, high affection) lead to less conflict and better acquisition of responsible independent behavior by normal adolescents than do either the extremes of authoritarian or permissive approaches (Becker, 1964; Conger, 1977; Grotevant & Cooper, 1983). In democratic childrearing, the adolescent participates meaningfully in decisions regarding his or her life and the parent legitimizes rules through frequent explanations, but the parent retains the ultimate decision about many issues; that is, the adolescent has input, but it is not a truly egalitarian approach because the adolescent has not yet completely matured to adulthood. A behavioral analysis of democratic childrearing would suggest it is best suited to normal adolescents because it (1) makes available structured learning trials for independence behaviors; (2) provides positive parental modeling of competent independence behaviors; and (3) encourages parents to gradually shape independent behaviors, giving freedoms in exchange for responsible behavior.

Adolescents with ADHD are going through the same developmental changes and desire the same degree of independence as do normal adolescents, but their neurobiological disorder which impairs their decision making and causes them to act and look younger than their chronological age. As with many other learning tasks, to acquire independent decision-making behaviors, by comparison to non-ADHD teens, ADHD teens would be expected to need the following (1) more frequent and highly structured learning trials; (2) more frequent and salient parental modeling of independence behaviors; and (3) a breakdown of the shaping steps into smaller units with more frequent and salient reinforcement for accomplishing each step. Therefore, with regard to the circumplex model, we would suggest that the degree of control needs to be stepped up several notches relative to normal adolescents, and that optimal parenting style for the teenager with ADHD is in the high affection, moderate control range of Figure 10.2.

Introducing Childrearing Frameworks

The therapist discusses philosophies of childrearing and principles of parenting in approximately Session 10. This psychoeducational session is best conducted with only the parents because the adolescent will find the material boring and his or her presence would detract from the therapist's ability to devote undivided attention to helping the parents understand the material.

At the beginning of the session, I distribute copies of Figure 10.2. Then, I give the following rationale:

> "We are now entering the phase of treatment where we are going to work extensively on home management issues—how you get along with your adolescent, the conflicts that come up, the extent to which your adolescent does what you say, and how to improve this situation, etc. But first we need to talk a bit about the big picture, that is, your philosophy of childrearing. Researchers who have studied extensively how adolescents grow and develop have found that certain approaches to childrearing work better than others to get through adolescence with the least bumps and bruises. ADHD researchers have further found that there are certain principles which, if parents follow them, will make it easier for families with adolescents diagnosed as ADHD to have positive experiences during this admittedly difficult stage of family life. Any questions so far?"

Next, the therapist reviews the circumplex model, defining the two dimensions of control and affection, and describing the range of parenting styles along with each dimension and in each quadrant. In Figure 10.2, I have placed each dimension on an 11-point Likert scale, going from –5 at the lowest point to +5 at the highest point; this creates 111 points on the graph. Each point represents one combination of control and affection. The therapist can use this figure as a visual aid to help the parents understand the material and quantify their own style and to easily compare it to a variety of alternatives.

During the review of the model, the therapist first describes the four extremes of dominating parenting, neglectful parenting, meddling/intrusive parenting, and permissive parenting, locating them on the graph. Then, the therapist asks the parents to rate their own approach to parenting and assign it a point in the graph. It is also useful to ask each parent to rate the spouse's approach, so that perceived differences can be addressed. The therapist draws a line connecting the mother's and father's parenting points, emphasizing any differences between them. This usually leads to a discussion of similarities and differences between each parent's approach.

After discussing the parents' own approaches, the therapist characterizes a high degree of affection and a moderate degree of control as the optimal approach to parenting the adolescent with ADHD, citing child development and ADHD research. The discussion culminates in the therapist asking the parents to consider restructuring their approach to move more toward the optimal point and offering to assist them in this process throughout the remainder of the therapy sessions. I cannot overemphasize the importance of approaching this discussion in a nonblaming way which further engages, rather than disengages, the parents in a collaborative therapy effort aimed at resolving conflict and improving parenting skills. Most parents feel defensive about their approach to parenting, because they would not be coming to a therapist for help if they felt it was working.

To illustrate the therapist's presentation and a typical parental reaction, let us join Dr. Brown as she discusses childrearing approaches with Mr. and Mrs. Santana, parents of 14-year-old Stephanie, who has been diagnosed as having ADHD plus ODD:

DR. BROWN: In the figure, we have a line representing Control and a line representing Affection. Based on many years of study, these are the two most important aspects of how we parent, the ones that make the biggest difference in how our children turn out, whether or not they have any problems like ADHD. By Control, I mean, whether you dictate to your children without asking for their input, whether you treat them as equal partners in decision making, or whether you let them make their own decisions and are permissive; this is a continuum, with every possible point in-between total control and total lack of control. I've put this on a numbered scale, with +5 standing for highly controlling parenting, 0 standing for total equality in parent–child decision making, and –5 standing for the teenager being highly controlling and the parents having little or no control. Now, I'd like each of you to place a point on the graph where you would place yourself with regard to control and affection. (*Mr. Santana rates himself +4 for control and +1 for affection; Mrs. Santana rates herself as 0 for control and +5 for affection.*)

MRS. SANTANA: But last night I treated Stephanie as an equal when it came to deciding where we were going for ice cream, while last week I needed to read her the riot act about getting her homework done. I'm not always the same with her. Where do I fit in?

DR. BROWN: Excellent point. As a smart parent, you use good common sense about when to be more or less controlling. I'm not talking about your every day-to-day decisions here. All parents vary on degree of control in that regard. I'm looking at the big picture, your overall feelings and philosophy about how you treat her. If we took an average of all your decision making, it would tend toward one point on the continuum. Let me go on. The other line or dimension represents affection—from very warm and loving at +5 to very cold, hostile, and noncaring at –5. These two dimensions intersect, and you can see from the grid, that we could have any combination of Control and Affection, 111 combinations in all. Let's talk about the four extreme combinations and how they affect teens with ADHD.

MR. SANTANA: Stephanie would rate me at a +5 and her mother at a –3 for Control!

MRS. SANTANA: Honey, please . . .

DR. BROWN: That's OK, Mrs. Santana. Your husband has made two very astute points. My daughter would rate my husband higher than me on Control too. Dads usually get higher ratings. That's natural. ADHD teens—girls as well as boys—give their moms a harder time than their dads and typically perceive their dads as more controlling. It's also natural, and I'm glad you brought it up, that any two parents won't see eye to eye on this. You are two unique individuals, who came from unique families of origin, and you are entitled to your own opinions. We'll come back to how to deal with differences between parents a little later, when we talk about consistency. First, let's discuss the Dominating Parent, bossing a teenager around all the time and doing it in a nasty way. How do you think this is going affect the teenager?

MRS. SANTANA: A lot of disobedience and rebellion. And lots of anger, fighting, and yelling.

DR. BROWN: Right. And it's even worse when teens have ADHD because they blow up more easily and have a lot of energy to keep up the rebellion for a long time. That's how biology interacts with parenting style.

MR. SANTANA: Have you been spying at our house? That's Stephanie.

DR. BROWN: OK, I'll come right back to that, Mr. Santana. Now, the meddling and intrusive parent is also controlling, but does it with a great deal of affection and love, smothering the kid so much that it drives them crazy. Smiling and friendly, but always checking up on them and trying to get them to do things. The kids may not yell and scream that much, but they definitely don't confide in their parents and avoid them as much as possible. The kids often have a lot of guilt and anxiety. I bet you can guess what the neglectful parent is like.

MRS. SANTANA: Stephanie's friend Jennifer's mother, Mrs. Jones, fits that. She's never home, never checking up on Jennifer, never around for her. She is either out working, or running around with a different man each night, ever since she got divorced. And when she is home, she practically ignores Jennifer. Jennifer can do whatever she wants. Fortunately, Jennifer is a good kid. Jennifer spends more time at our house than at her own house. Poor darling!

DR. BROWN: Excellent description. You are clearly a very caring person, isn't she, Mr. Santana? [Therapist takes the opportunity to build further rapport with each parent and get the dad to compliment his wife.]

MR. SANTANA: (*smiling*) My wife is great!

DR. BROWN: You are a neat couple. A neglectful parent is emotionally unavailable and physically absent. The child ends up feeling insecure, unloved, and often turns to friends to get the needs met that the parents fail to meet. If the friends are into sex, drugs, alcohol, or crime, this could easily mean trouble for the teen, especially since the parent isn't keeping a close eye on things. Fortunately, Mrs. Santana, you and your daughter are a positive influence on Jennifer. [Therapist incidentally but purposefully points out a positive quality of Stephanie to her mother. This strikes a positive note in the dad.]

MR. SANTANA: Stephanie may be a pain in the butt to us sometimes, but when it comes to her friends, she is very loyal and tries to help them out.

DR. BROWN: She must have learned that from the two of you. I can see you are high on the affection scale. Next, we have the permissive parent, loving and kind, but letting the kids do whatever they want. Often, such parents had very dominating parents themselves, and somehow want to make it up with their own kids. This points out how our experiences as a child influence how we parent as an adult. Unfortunately, permissive parenting is a prescription for disaster with teens who have ADHD. If you let them do whatever they want, they don't do any schoolwork and may get in big trouble in the community. That brings us to the question of what works best. For teens in general, a high degree of affection, let's say a +3 or greater, coupled with about a 0 on control, that is, shared or democratic decision making, works well. Of course, Stephanie is special, and she has ADHD. So with ADHD youngsters, we find it's best to step up the control a notch or two, to around a +2. As you will see when we get to principles of parenting, ADHD teens like decision making power, but need structure longer than other teens. Thus, I put the point for optimal parenting of an ADHD teen at +4 for Affection and +2 for Control.

The discussion of parenting styles culminates in an "invitation" from the therapist to help the parents move in the direction of the style found to be most effective with ADHD adolescents. The therapist "invites" rather than "tells" the parents to change in order to: (1) model democratic decision making, (2) defuse resistance in case of rigidity, and (3) build motivation by requiring the parents to accept an invitation and ask for the therapist's assistance in carrying it out. If one or both parents decline the invitation, the therapist indicates that the issues of home management can still be worked on, but the parents need to understand and accept the possibility that the outcomes will be less effective; thus, the therapist has set up a rationale for explaining later failure if inappropriate parental attitudes persist. The discussion of childrearing philosophy transitions naturally into the next topic, presentation of principles for parenting the ADHD adolescent.

PRINCIPLES FOR PARENTING
THE ADHD ADOLESCENT

Is it better to teach parents general principles of effective parenting first and then help them apply the principles to specific situations, or to help parents solve everyday problems in raising their adolescents first, and then inductively move toward general principles? Behaviorally oriented clinicians have been debating and researching this question since the 1970s (O'Dell, 1974), with no definitive answer. Barkley (1995c) argues strongly for teaching the general principles first because these principles help keep parents on a straight course through a labyrinthine childrearing journey and help them act based on reason rather than react based on impulse. Having guidelines to prevent impulsive parenting is particularly important with a genetically based disorder such as ADHD because many parents may have impulsive tendencies similar to their children. Our solution to this dilemma is a combined approach. In the course of discussing alternative philosophies of childrearing, I briefly introduce parents to a set of principles for raising the adolescent with ADHD. Table 10.1 summarizes these principles. They represent a combination of principles outlined by Barkley (1995c) and several of my own ideas regarding adolescents. Then,

TABLE 10.1. Principles for Parenting the Adolescent with ADHD

1. Facilitate appropriate independence seeking.
2. Maintain adequate structure and supervision.
3. Establish bottom-line rules for living in your home and enforce them consistently.
4. Negotiate all other issues which are not bottom lines with your adolescent.
5. Use consequences wisely to influence your adolescent's behavior.
6. Maintain good communication.
7. Keep a disability perspective and practice forgiveness.
8. Focus on the positive.

Note. From *ADHD in Adolescents: Diagnosis and Treatment* by Arthur L. Robin. Copyright 1998 by The Guilford Press. Permission to photocopy this table is granted to purchasers of *ADHD in Adolescents* for personal use only (see copyright page for details).

I rapidly begin to translate these principles into specific techniques for surviving on a day-to-day basis with their ADHD teenager. As I go over specific issues, I frequently refer to the list of principles, teaching parents to deduce additional interventions from them.

1. *Facilitate appropriate independence seeking.* Because becoming independent from the family is the primary developmental task of adolescence, and because ADHD individuals need extra guidance and learning trials to acquire new behaviors, parents need to look for opportunities to gradually give their adolescents more freedom in return for demonstrating responsibility. A parent might break the terminal independence response into small units and shape each behavior, moving on to the next step after the teenager has demonstrated responsibility on the last step. For example, one terminal behavior might be staying alone in the house for a weekend and taking proper care of the house (nothing left unlocked, nothing missing, lawn watered and pets fed, no wild parties, etc.). The parent might break this terminal behavior down into smaller units (staying in the house for an evening, a night, two nights, etc.). As the adolescent successfully accomplishes each step, the parent moves onto the next.

2. *Maintain adequate structure and supervision.* Parents often ask when they can relax the increased structure they have created to monitor their adolescent's academic performance and home behavior. The answer is that they need to *maintain structure and supervision for longer than they typically think they should.* ADHD individuals need to be more closely monitored for all their lives, but we expect them to learn to do some of their own monitoring and/or enlist the help of spouses and significant others in monitoring their actions by adulthood. Ideally, parents need to facilitate the transfer of monitoring to the adolescent throughout adolescence, but the reality is that most parents continue the extra structure until the adolescent graduates high school and, in some cases, beyond that.

Part of the structure involves *actively monitoring the adolescent's be-*

havior outside the home. Parents should always know the answer to these four basic questions: (1) Whom are your adolescents with? (2) Where are they? (3) What are they doing? (4) When will they be home. Research has shown that parents who cannot consistently answer these four questions have adolescents at risk for drifting into deviant peer groups, substance abuse, and delinquency (Patterson & Forgatch, 1987). Parents should also develop clear "street rules" or rules for how they expect their adolescents to conduct themselves in the community outside the home.

Another aspect of structure and monitoring is to *plan ahead for problem situations* before they occur. Because many conflicts between parents and adolescents are highly predictable, it behooves therapists to help parents learn to anticipate and plan in advance to handle these situations. In a family in which curfew violations have been a frequent problem, for example, the therapist might prepare the parents in advance for how they will respond at 2:00 A.M. when Sally comes home 2 hours late. Without such planning, parents and adolescents often react based on emotion and do a lot of damage to their relationships in the heat of the moment.

3. *Establish "the bottom line" rules for living in your home and enforce them consistently.* Regarding discipline, parents need to divide the world of issues into those that can be negotiated and those that cannot. There is an important distinction between issues that can be handled democratically and those that cannot. Each parent has a small set of bottom-line issues that relate to basic rules for living in civilized society, values, morality, and legality, which are not subject to negotiation. Such issues usually include drugs, alcohol, aspects of sexuality, religion, and perhaps several others. Each parent needs to clearly list and present to the teenager those issues that are nonnegotiable. Then, they need to enforce the rules around these issues consistently and fairly, through the wise use of consequences (see item 5).

4. *Negotiate all the other issues which are not bottom lines with your adolescent.* Parents need to involve their teenagers in decision making regarding the issues that can be negotiated. This is the single most important principle of parenting an adolescent, and one of the primary methods of shaping responsible independence behaviors. Teenagers are more likely to comply with rules and regulations they helped to create. Furthermore, they may have novel and creative perspectives on issues because of their youth and unique position in the family. Often, their perspectives lead them to suggest novel solutions. Problem-solving training, discussed in detail in Chapter 11, is the primary technique for involving adolescents in decision making. Parents need to remember, however, that involvement in decision making does not necessarily mean always being an equal partner with parents, and it certainly does not mean dictating to parents. In some cases, parents may retain the ultimate veto over decisions. In other cases, adolescents may be equal partners with parents. Parents need to gradually in-

crease the degree of involvement they give teenagers in decision making, through a shaping process.

5. *Use consequences wisely.* Parents need to become experts at behavior management in order to enforce their bottom-line rules, monitor and structure effectively, and discipline consistently. Barkley (1995c) outlined several aspects of the effective use of consequences with children who have ADHD:

a. *Give the adolescent more immediate feedback and consequences.* Adolescents with short attention spans and impaired delayed responding are more likely to stay on task when given immediate positive feedback contingent upon performance of boring and tedious tasks, coupled with mild negative consequences for shifting off task. Punishments given long after the misbehavior was committed are ineffective.

b. *Give the adolescent more frequent feedback.* ADHD adolescents benefit from frequently hearing nice things said about their actions and appearances, as well as from receiving frequent feedback and corrections for their errors. There are so many negatives in the life of the average ADHD adolescent which pull down his or her self-esteem, that he or she desperately needs to hear frequently what he or she did right. We may need to teach busy parents creative ways to remember to give their adolescents frequent feedback.

c. *Use incentives before punishments.* It is a knee-jerk reaction for parents to ground an adolescent until the end of the next marking period upon receiving a bad report card. Parents commonly load on immense punishments until they have used up all of their ammunition and the adolescent has little else to lose by misbehaving. When parents wish to modify a behavior such as poor study behavior, we need to train them to decide what positive behavior they wish to see the adolescent perform and then find a way to reinforce that positive behavior. Only after taking this step should they select a punishment for the negative behavior. However, in many cases, especially extreme oppositional behavior, incentives alone are not sufficient consequences; parents must also administer punishments.

d. *Strive for consistency.* ADHD parents often give up easily on behavior change interventions at the first sign of failure. ADHD adolescents incessantly bicker with their parents, sometimes wearing them down to the point where the parents back off. We need to help parents to stick with their interventions and demands, that is, to maintain consistency over time. "Divide and conquer" is also a motto of many ADHD adolescents, who have learned that if they can get Mom and Dad to disagree, they can avoid unpleasant effort and/or discipline. This principle is particularly common in stepfamilies and divorced families, where natural structural changes give the coercive adolescent a golden opportunity to manipulate the system. Therapists need to help mothers and fathers work as a team (i.e., to develop consistency across parents). I discuss how to build parental teamwork in more detail in Chapter 12.

e. *Act, do not yak.* Many parents repeat themselves incessantly when their adolescents fail to comply with their requests. Adolescents quickly learn that Mom or Dad are "all talk, no action." We need to teach parents that the time to talk is during family meetings and when negotiating solutions to disagreements, but after the rules have been stated and the consequences agreed on, it is the time to act, not yak. Parents need to state the consequences as if they mean them; this does not mean yelling but adequately projecting authority without meekness or hesitation.

6. *Maintain good communication.* Parents need to be available to listen when their adolescents wish to talk, but not to expect them to confide regularly in them. Parents and adolescents need to learn to listen to each other and express their ideas and feelings assertively but without putting down or hurting each other. Parents need to be clear and specific in making requests and giving feedback. Parents also need to learn when to "keep their mouths shut unless absolutely necessary" (Phelan, 1998). Parents of ADHD teenagers are tempted to comment continuously on their youngster's behavior, often slipping into nagging, lecturing, and arguing. Such frequent comments inevitably spur unnecessary conflict. Parents also believe that they should attempt to make pleasant conversation at the breakfast table, but sometimes, moody, irritable adolescents who are not "morning people" are better left alone at that time. Sometimes, the best guideline to communication is, "Silence is golden."

7. *Keep a disability perspective, and practice forgiveness.* This principle has to do with expectations and beliefs, which are considered in depth later. Therapists need to help parents remember that their adolescents with ADHD have a neurobiologically based disability, and that there is a "can't do" as well as a "won't do" component to their unthinking actions. Thus, parents can stop overreacting with anger when their adolescents inevitably make mistakes. Part of keeping a disability perspective involves refraining from *personalizing the adolescent's problems or disorder.* Parents need to refrain from blaming themselves or losing their personal sense of self-worth over their adolescent's problems. They also need to *practice forgiveness.* Parents need to forgive themselves for the mistakes they will inevitably make raising an ADHD adolescent, and to forgive their adolescent for his or her mistakes. Adolescents should, however, be held accountable for their actions, and consequences should be administered as planned, but afterward, parents should not "hold a grudge."

8. *Focus on the positive.* When in the throes of conflict dealing with very oppositional adolescents, it is difficult for parents to be positive. However, it is important to remind parents to *be their adolescent's cheerleading squad.* ADHD adolescents need unconditional positive regard from their parents and focused positive time with them. Follow-up studies (Weiss & Hechtman, 1993) have found that the single most important thing during successful ADHD adults' adolescence was having at least one parent, or, in some cases an adult outside the family, who truly believed in

their ability to succeed. ADHD adolescents need their parents to believe in them, to applaud their every positive achievement, and to be their cheerleading squad. They also need their parents to spend focused time with them; busy parents may not have a great deal of focused time to give, but it is the quality rather than the quantity of focused time that really matters. Parents need to find time to have fun with their teenager on a regular basis (Phelan, 1998).

A second important aspect of focusing on the positive is for parents to *encourage their adolescent to build on his or her strengths.* Many ADHD adolescents are so criticized that they actually begin to believe that they are lazy and unmotivated. They may be failing at school and in peer relationships but usually have at least one thing at which they excel. We need to teach parents to help the teenager identify those interests, hobbies, artistic pursuits, sports, and activities that are pockets of strength and help them pursue and succeed at these pursuits. Zeigler Dendy (1995) provides parents with detailed guidelines for encouraging ADHD adolescents to build on their strengths.

Introducing Principles of Parenting

To see how principle-centered parenting is introduced, let's rejoin Dr. Brown and the Santanas as she makes the transition in the discussion. Mr. and Mrs. Santana have now agreed that they should optimize their approach to childrearing, in accordance with Dr. Brown's recommendations.

DR. BROWN: You are probably thinking that this high-affection/moderate-structure philosophy is all well and good, but what do we do when we get home and Stephanie throws a fit when we ask her to clean up her room.

MR. SANTANA: You bet.

DR. BROWN: OK. Next, I'm going to introduce some principles which you can use as guidelines or a road map to chart your course through each decision you have to make as to how to deal with Stephanie, in times of crisis as well as normal times. We will go over the principles today, and in the next few meetings, with Stephanie present, we will put them into action. Here is a list of eight principles for parenting the adolescent with ADHD. (*Gives each parent a copy of Table 10.1.*) Let's review them one by one. I'll give you definitions and examples for each one, and I want you to tell me how you could apply them with Stephanie.

The therapist goes over the list of principles, elaborating on the material used earlier in this chapter along with Barkley's (1995c) discussion of principle-centered parenting, to help the parents understand each principle. After clarifying each principle and having the parents give illustrations of its applicability with their adolescent, the therapist explains the rationale for principle-centered parenting following Barkley (1995c), as follows:

DR. BROWN: Principle-centered parenting means that when a situation comes up with Stephanie that you need to deal with, before you act, you (1) pause for a moment; (2) use the delay to decide which principle is applicable to the situation; and (3) choose a response based upon that principle rather than your gut feeling, impulsive reaction.

MRS. SANTANA: What if we are in the middle of an argument and it is a crisis situation?

DR. BROWN: These are tough. You may call a timeout, a 5-minute recess for everyone to think things over, just like a timeout in a boxing match. We will come back to additional strategies for crisis situations later on.

The therapist closes the session by giving the parents a homework assignment related to principles of parenting. The parents are asked to track examples of situations in which they did or could apply these principles with their adolescent. Specifically, the therapist instructs the parents to take a short time each evening, together as a couple, and write down any examples of situations that arose that day in which one of the principles was applicable, to note which principle, and to record how they responded. Table 10.2 illustrates the type of monitoring form that might be used for this assignment, along with a model of the type of information to be recorded. The assignment is designed to increase parents' awareness and familiarity with the eight principles.

TABLE 10.2. Monitoring Form for Parenting Principles

Name _____

Date	Situation	Principle(s)	Response
9/29/98	Stephanie is upset about being dumped by her boyfriend and wants to talk, just as Mom is starting dinner.	Maintaining good communication. Make yourself available to listen when teens need to talk.	Mom postpones dinner 30 minutes and listens noncritically to Stephanie.
9/30/98	Mom finds Stephanie has lied when she said she had no math homework.	Act, don't yak. Give immediate consequences.	Without discussion, Mom tells Stephanie that she has lost telephone privileges for 2 nights.

Note. From *ADHD in Adolescents: Diagnosis and Treatment* by Arthur L. Robin. Copyright 1998 by The Guilford Press. Permission to photocopy this table is granted to purchasers of *ADHD in Adolescents* for personal use only (see copyright page for details).

EXPECTATIONS AND BELIEFS

After discussing the parents' overall approach to childrearing and presenting the 8 principles for parenting the adolescent with ADHD, the therapist moves to the next level of specificity in the inverted pyramid model of Figure 10.1. This next level involves the cognitions, beliefs, and attributions the parents and the adolescent have about growing up, family life, and how ADHD affects them. In session 11, the second session on home management, the therapist focuses primarily on the beliefs, expectations, and attitudes of the parents and the adolescent. This session is designed to further assess the family members' current cognitions and to help the family members develop reasonable expectations for performance at school and behavior at home. The therapist relies on cognitive restructuring techniques (Robin & Foster, 1989) to identify and change distorted thinking and encourage adherence to reasonable expectations. The session is divided into two portions. In the first half of the session, the therapist meets with the parents; in the second half, the therapist meets with the adolescent.

Parent Session

The portion of the session with the parents includes (1) a review of the homework assignment, (2) a "crash course" on adolescent development, (3) presentation of a rationale relating extreme thinking to extreme affect and behavioral overreactions, and (4) a review of common expectations and beliefs regarding ADHD and family life.

Reviewing Homework

The therapist asks the parents to pick several entries from the monitoring sheet and describe the situation, the principle that was applicable, and how they applied it in their response to their teenager. Correct applications are praised, and feedback is given about any incorrect applications.

Crash Course on Adolescent Development

Although most parents are vaguely aware that becoming independent from the family is the major developmental task of adolescence, they have not typically considered all the ramifications of this task, and they certainly have not pondered how the symptoms of ADHD interact with the adolescent's striving for independence. In addition, most parents are not familiar with the other major developmental tasks of adolescence. Lack of familiarity with the basics of adolescent development can lead to adherence to unreasonable expectations and incorrect attributions. Therefore, the therapist gives the parents a "crash course" in the basics of adolescent development.

From a cognitive restructuring point of view, the crash course also represents a normalizing or reframing with a positive intent of much of the negative behavior adolescents inevitably emit. By presenting this information within the context of adolescent development, the therapist makes it easier for the parents to accept it without activating any natural defensive reaction they might otherwise have. The therapist also helps them learn to apply the principle that they should not personalize the adolescent's problems—by distancing from the constant barrage of strange teenage behavior, having a developmental framework within which to understand it, and learning to prioritize what to respond to and what to ignore. The sensitive therapist is cognizant of this attitudinal portion of the agenda and monitors the parents' level of defensiveness and reactivity during the crash course, pacing his or her statements to shape their responses in productive directions. This is one of many examples of how the therapist operates simultaneously at multiple levels of analysis.

The therapist points out that there are five basic developmental tasks for the adolescent (Conger, 1977):

1. Becoming independent from the parents
2. Establishing an identity or finding out who they are and what they stand for
3. Learning how to make deep and close interpersonal bonds with members of the same and opposite sex
4. Understanding and coming to terms with their emerging sexuality
5. Completing their education and deciding on a career direction.

Becoming a productive, happy, and personally fulfilled adult depends on successful accomplishment of these tasks. The adolescent is supposed to accomplish these tasks while getting along with his or her family and doing his or her schoolwork. The therapist helps the parents to realize that the adolescent has a great deal of work to do.

The nature of independence seeking or individuation from parents is explored in more depth. I find it useful to present the metaphor of a nation establishing its independence:

> Imagine a nation establishing its independence, going from a dictatorship to a democracy. What often happens? This process does not typically go smoothly. There may be a bloody revolution with a great deal of fighting. Or if there isn't physical fighting, there is certainly a lot of verbal rhetoric and power plays. Why should you expect your family to make it through the independence seeking of your adolescence without a disturbance of the peace? A certain amount of conflict is inevitable and even healthy. I worry more about adolescents who never do anything rebellious than those who do rebel. This rebellion typically happens in early adolescence, between ages 12 and 14. In order to become independent, teenagers need to push against something, and

parents are the something that they push against. Usually, the teenagers typically rebel more strongly against their mothers than their fathers. Wise parents learn how to channel their conflicts into more innocuous areas that have no ultimate impact on life. It is much better, for example, to have conflicts with your adolescent over how clean the room is than over sexuality and drugs."

I go on to explain to parents that it is natural for adolescents to reject established parental and other adult societal values during this process of individuation, and to be embarrassed about being seen with their parents. To begin to establish their own identity, adolescents need to experiment with alternative ideas and values, usually those of their peers, and decide what they are comfortable with. At the same time this is happening, their bodies are changing rapidly and their minds are maturing to the point where they now can think more abstractly. The multiple influences of rapid physical maturation, cognitive development, and emotional change are unsettling to adolescents, leading them to have a fragile self-image. One response to this image is to project an air of omnipotence, that is, to shy away from anything or anyone who suggests they are less than perfect physically or mentally. Thus, it is natural for the developing adolescent to be less than enthusiastic about disabilities, psychiatric diagnoses, chronic physical illnesses, or any other condition which could be seen as a further insult to an already fragile self-image. Therapists should explain to parents that this is the basis for resistance to accepting the diagnosis of ADHD and its treatments.

The therapist then explains how ADHD interacts with these natural developmental tendencies during adolescence. Adolescents with ADHD undergo the same physical changes and face the same developmental challenges as do other teenagers. They may experience the same desires for independence and freedom as other teenagers. Yet their social and emotional maturity may lag behind that of other teenagers. They may be less ready to assume the responsibilities that accompany more independence.

Specifically, teenagers with ADHD may lag behind other teenagers in the overall development of self-control and organization. They may be less able to exercise hindsight, forethought, and planning and to engage in future-oriented, goal-oriented behavior. They may remain more likely to be victims of the moment, acting on impulse, being self-centered and insensitive to the needs of others. Poor attention and follow-through make it more difficult for them to stick to discussions or carry out agreements with their parents, and finish homework. Impulsivity translates into increased moodiness (severe PMS for many teenage girls), hypersensitivity to criticism, emotional overreactivity, poor judgment, and low resistance to temptations. Hyperactivity often continues more as minor motor restlessness and mental restlessness than as overt physical overactivity. Such restless behavior is easily misinterpreted as "disrespect" by parents. Repeatedly badgering parents to get their way is another manifestation of hyperactivity in some adolescents with ADHD.

The ADHD symptoms become inextricably intertwined with the developmental changes of adolescence. Many parents will ask a therapist whether a particular adolescent behavior is a result of ADHD or "just adolescence." They may be wondering whether to excuse or to punish the behavior. Did Stephanie really "forget" to put away the dishes, or was she just being "oppositional"? The answer is usually that the behavior is both an example of ADHD and the developmental changes of adolescence. I usually advise the parent to hold the adolescent accountable for his or her actions and apply whatever consequence is warranted, but that the parent might temper his or her affective response and avoid attributing the adolescent's behavior to malicious motives. I often use the example of a teenager getting stopped by a policeman for going through a red light shortly after getting his or her license. The adolescent may tell the policeman that he failed to notice the red light because he has a disability and is protected under the Americans with Disabilities Act, but the policeman does not care. The adolescent will be held accountable for adherence to the traffic laws, regardless of ADHD.

After covering these aspects of adolescent development and its interaction with ADHD, the therapist gives the parents an opportunity to ask questions and then moves on to address expectations and beliefs.

Cognitive Rationale and Coping Attitudes

The therapist might start off this discussion by reminding the parents of the seventh principle (Keep a disability perspective; don't personalize the adolescent's problems or disorder; practice forgiveness) and pointing out that they will now discuss the beliefs and attitudes underlying this principle in more depth. Then, the therapist might ask the parents to engage in the following mental imagery exercise, which vividly teaches people the connection between extreme thinking, negative affect, and behavioral overreactions:

> "Close your eyes, and imagine that you are opening the mail and you find a progress report from your son's school. The progress report indicates that he is failing English and Math, and has fifteen late assignments in History. Suddenly you can feel your blood begin to boil and the tension mount throughout your body. Your son lied to you again!!! He said he was up to date on homework and passing all of his courses. This is one more example of irresponsible behavior. He is always irresponsible. You told him to keep an assignment book. And get help from the teachers. He never does what he is told. He is so disobedient. If he keeps on going this way in school, he is going to fail out. He will never graduate, never go to college, and never get a good job. You will be supporting him until the day you die. And the thought of

confronting him is not appealing at all. He will deny it all at first, then blame it all on the teachers, showing you total disrespect. He is just doing all of this to get you mad and upset. He has no consideration for your feelings. Now open your eyes, and tell me how you feel and what you are thinking. And also, tell me how you would react if your son walked through the door at this very moment."

Through a Socratic discussion, the therapist helps the parents realize how the extreme thinking evokes extreme affect, and how difficult it would be to deal with the adolescent rationally, as a principle-centered parent is advised to do, in such a strong state of negative affect. Afterward, I suggest that the parents strive toward adherence to the following overall coping expectation: "We will encourage our adolescent with ADHD to go for the stars, to do his or her best, but we will accept that it is not a catastrophe when he or she fails to achieve perfection, and it does not mean that he or she is headed for certain ruination or is purposely trying to anger us."

Common Expectations and Beliefs

After discussing the cognitive rationale and the positive, coping attitude, I then distribute a copy of Table 10.3, Parents' Expectations and Beliefs, to each parent, and review the most common unreasonable beliefs. As we go through each belief, I ask the parents to rate their own adherence to this belief and to give examples of particular situations that activated the belief. I look at the reasonable alternative beliefs and expectations in the right-hand column and ask the parents whether they find them credible. If they do, we continue; otherwise, we review the evidence for the unreasonable versus the reasonable belief, and I suggest experiments the parents can do to test this evidence on their own after the session is over. The therapist does not usually have time to review every belief in Table 10.3; he or she may quickly survey the table and concentrate on the beliefs that seem most salient for a particular family.

Adolescent Session

Most teenagers with ADHD feel that their parents are unfair and restrictive of their freedom, and that those restrictions interfere with their life. In the portion of the session with the adolescent, the therapist's goals are (1) to assess the rigidity of these beliefs, (2) to determine how the amount of freedom given to the adolescent compares to the local norms for other adolescents of a similar age in the same schools and neighborhood, and (3) to correct any wildly unrealistic expectations the adolescent may have. The therapist should distribute Table 10.4 to the adolescent and use it as a springboard for discussion. The therapist should carry out the discussion in a lighthearted, tongue-in-cheek style, trying to remain animated and

TABLE 10.3. Parents' Expectations and Beliefs

Unreasonable beliefs	Reasonable beliefs
I. *Perfection/obedience*: Teens with ADHD should behave perfectly and obey their parents all the time without question	It is unrealistic to expect teens with ADHD to behave perfectly or obey all of the time; we strive for high standards, but accept imperfections.
A. School	
1. He should always complete homework on time.	1. I will encourage him to complete homework all the time but recognize this won't always happen.
2. She should study 2 hours every night, even when she has no homework.	2. If your attention span is short, you are lucky to get your basic homework done. Extra study is just unrealistic. These kids need a break after all the effort it takes to do basic homework.
3. He should always come to class prepared.	3. He will sometimes come to class unprepared, but I will help him learn good organizational techniques.
4. She should do papers for the love of learning.	4. Research shows teens with ADHD need salient, external reinforcers to motivate their behavior. *C'est la vie.*
B. Driving	
1. She should never get any speeding tickets.	1. All teens with ADHD get at least one speeding ticket. She should be responsible for paying it and take her medicine while driving.
2. She will never have an accident.	2. Research shows most teens with ADHD will get in at least one minor accident. She should take her medicine while driving and do her best. She should drive an old car.
3. Teens shouldn't adjust the radio tuner while driving down the highway.	3. She should avoid tuning the radio while driving as much as possible, but this may occasionally happen.
4. She will always stop completely for stop signs.	4. I should always stop completely at stop signs to model good behavior when my teen is in my car and only expect my teen to do as well as I do.
C. Conduct	
1. He should be a perfect angel in church.	1. This is unrealistic. As long as there are no major disturbances, I'm satisfied. Perhaps I should find a youth group service of more interest for him away.
2. She will impress all the relatives with her love for family gatherings.	2. Give her space. Teens just don't want to be with their families that much. This is normal. She should attend some family functions, but that is all I can reasonably expect.

(continued)

TABLE 10.3. *(continued)*

Unreasonable beliefs	Reasonable beliefs
3. He should never treat us disrespectfully.	3. You can't become your own person without some rebellion. Some backtalk is natural. He shouldn't curse or ridicule severely, and might be expected to apologize occasionally.
4. She should get out of a bad mood when we tell her to change her attitude.	4. People with ADHD are just moody and can't stop it. She should let us know when she is in a bad mood and keep to herself. We should not make a lot of demands on her at such times.
D. Chores	
1. She should put away the dishes the first time I ask.	1. It won't always happen the first time, but after several reminders, I should act, not yak (e.g., apply consequences).
2. He should always get the room spotless.	2. He should get it generally neat. Spotless isn't realistic.
3. She should not waste electricity by leaving the lights on.	3. She is just forgetful. We could work out a reminder system, but this is the least of my worries with a teen with ADHD.
4. He shouldn't be on the telephone when I've sent him to his room to clean it up.	4. Teens with ADHD will get off task; I will redirect him back to the task, and if it happens too much, assume it is opposition and ground him from the telephone.
II. *Ruination:* If I give my teen too much freedom, he/she will mess up, make bad judgments, get in big trouble, and ruin his/her life.	He or she will sometimes mess up with too much freedom, but this is how teenagers learn responsibility—a bit of freedom and a bit of responsibility. If they backslide, no big deal. I just pull back on the freedom for a while, and then give them another chance.
A. Room incompletely cleaned: he will grow up to be a slovenly, unemployed, aimless welfare case.	A. The state of his room has little to do with how he turns out when he grows up.
B. Home late: She will have unprotected sex, get pregnant, dump the baby on us, take drugs, and drink alcohol.	B. I have no evidence that she would do all these things. She is just self-centered and focused on having fun. So she will be punished as we agreed for coming home late.
C. Fighting with siblings: He will never learn to get along with others, have friends, have close relationships, or get married. He will end up a loser, and be severely depressed or commit suicide.	C. There is no scientific evidence that sibling fighting predicts later satisfaction in relationships. Siblings always fight. They will probably be closer when they grow up.

(continued)

TABLE 10.3. *(continued)*

Unreasonable beliefs	Reasonable beliefs
III. *Malicious intent*: My adolescent misbehaves on purpose to annoy me, hurt me, or get even with me for restricting him/her.	Most of the adolescents with ADHD just do things without thinking. They aren't planful enough to connive to upset parents on purpose.
A. Talking disrespectfully: She's mouthing off on purpose to get even with me for ———.	A. Impulsive teenagers just mouth off when frustrated. I'll try not to take it to heart.
B. Doesn't follow directions: He doesn't finish mowing the lawn just to bug me.	B. Teens with ADHD are allergic to effort. They don't take the time to plan to upset parents by not doing things.
C. Restless behavior: She shuffles her feet and plays with her hair to get on my nerves.	C. Teens with ADHD just can't contain themselves. I'll try not to attach meaning to her restlessness and ignore it.
D. Spending money impulsively: She bought $100 worth of CDs just to waste our money.	D. She probably just saw the CDs and had to have them. Poor delay of gratification is part of ADHD. She won't get any extra money for lunch or gas.
IV *Love/appreciation*: My teen should show love and appreciation for all the great sacrifices I make; If he or she really loved me, he or she would confide in me more.	Teens with ADHD are so self-centered that they don't easily show appreciation until they grow up and have their own children with ADHD. Only then will they realize what you did for them.
A. Money: What do you mean you want more allowance? You should be grateful for all the money I spend on you now. Some kids are not so lucky!	A. You will have to earn more allowance. I'd appreciate a thank you even though I understand you don't really think about what I do for you.
B. Communication: She never tells me anything anymore; she must not love me.	B. It's natural as teens individuate to keep more to themselves. As long as I am available when she wants to talk, that's all I can expect.
C. Spending time: If he really loved us, he wouldn't spend so much time alone in his room.	C. Spending time alone has nothing to do with love. It has to do with wanting privacy as he becomes more independent.

Note. From *ADHD in Adolescents: Diagnosis and Treatment* by Arthur L. Robin. Copyright 1998 by The Guilford Press. Permission to photocopy this table is granted to purchasers of *ADHD in Adolescents* for personal use only (see copyright page for details).

TABLE 10.4. Adolescents' Expectations and Beliefs

Unreasonable beliefs	Reasonable beliefs
I. *Unfairness/ruination*: My parents' rules are totally unfair. I'll never have a good time or any friends. My parents are ruining my life with their unfair rules. They just don't understand me.	Yes, I don't like my parents' rules and maybe they are sometimes unfair. But who said life is supposed to be fair? And how many other teenagers have gone through the same thing? They turned out OK. So will I. I'll just have to put up with it the best I can.
A. Curfew: Why should I have to come home earlier than my friends? They will think I'm a baby. I'll lose all my friends.	A. My friends are loyal. They will understand that my parents are creeps about curfew. I won't lose any friends.
B. Chores: Why do I get stuck doing all the work? Sam [brother] doesn't have to do anything. That's unfair!	B. Sam has some chores too. I'll count them up and if I have more, I'll talk nicely to my parents about it.
C. School: My teacher is unfair. She picks on me all the time. I always get stuck doing extra homework. I'll never have time for fun. Life is one big homework assignment.	C. Maybe she does pick on me. There could be a reason. I never am with the class or know the answer when she calls on me. Maybe if I kept up with the work she wouldn't call on me so much.
II. *Autonomy*: I ought to have complete and total freedom. My parents shouldn't boss me around or tell me what to do. I'm old enough for freedom now.	No teen has complete freedom. No adult really does either. Sometimes I need my parents, like for money or God forbid, even to talk to in times of trouble. I want a lot of freedom, but not total freedom.
A. Chores: I don't need any reminders. I can do it totally on my own.	A. I have not been getting them done on my own. I need to stop being a jerk and accept a little help.
B. Medicine: I don't need Ritalin anymore. I'm grown up now and can handle everything on my own.	B. Maybe I need to see whether I do better or worse on or off medicine. I'll keep an open mind about it.
C. Smoking: It's my body. I can do whatever I want with it. You have no right to tell me not to smoke.	C. It is my body. But do I really want to mess it up? My friends have gotten hooked on smoking. It costs a lot. And it tastes terrible when you kiss someone.
III. *Love/appreciation*: Getting material things is a sign that your parents love you. Getting your way is a sign that your parents really love you.	Material things don't tell you whether someone really cares about you. It's how you are inside that makes the difference.

(continued)

TABLE 10.4. *(continued)*

Unreasonable beliefs	Reasonable beliefs
A. Clothes: If my parents really cared about me, they would buy me those designer clothes.	A. I would like designer clothes, but that's not how I tell whether my parents love me. I can tell from how they act towards me and the affection they show.
B. Concert: If my parents really loved me, they would let me go to the rock concert with my friends.	B. If they really love me and think it is dangerous to go to the concert, they would try to stop me. I won't use this to judge how they feel.
C. Sexuality: If I have sex with my boyfriend, then he will really love me forever.	C. Love does not equal sex. I need to judge from how my boyfriend acts and expresses his feelings to me. All boys want sex. So this tells me nothing about love.

Note. From *ADHD in Adolescents: Diagnosis and Treatment* by Arthur L. Robin. Copyright 1998 by The Guilford Press. Permission to photocopy this table is granted to purchasers of *ADHD in Adolescents* for personal use only (see copyright page for details).

keep the adolescent's attention. He or she should make liberal use of exaggerations for effect. The therapist should abbreviate the session or shift gears if he or she senses that the adolescent is drifting. The therapist should not conduct a monologue and should not worry if the subtleties of his or her points are missed. The extent to which the therapist will be able to accomplish these goals vary greatly from adolescent to adolescent, depending on the adolescent's attention span, level of resistance, and general maturity (or immaturity).

Let's look in on Dr. Sam as he conducts the beliefs session with Abe, a 15-year-old recently diagnosed as having ADHD.

DR. SAM: Look at the first thing on the list, the idea that your parents' rules are totally unfair and will mess up your life. Have you ever felt that way?

ABE: Yep. Just like the curfew one. They made me come home early from the homecoming dance. My friends probably thought I was a real nerd.

DR. SAM: If you keep thinking "my parents are unfair, my parents are unfair, they're going to mess me up, and so on," how are you going to feel?

ABE: Pissed off at them. I do feel that way.

DR. SAM: So if you are pissed at them and go to try to get a later curfew, are you going to have a nice, calm discussion?

ABE: We always have a yelling match. And I get grounded.

DR. SAM: So maybe you can do something to keep from getting so pissed off at them that you lose your cool and then your privileges. If I were you, I'd try thinking to myself something like, "Yes, I don't like coming home early from the dance, but parents always worry too much about what could happen. Yes, it's unfair, but it's not the end of the world. My friends are loyal and will understand. There will be more dances, and maybe I can get a later curfew. I'm going to tell myself to stay cool and calm when I approach them to discuss this. I'm not going to blow it and get grounded again."

ABE: Do you really think I can convince them to change my curfew for the Halloween dance?

DR. SAM: I don't know, but if you stay calm and don't think the worst, you might. I'll help you and your parents to try to work it out to everyone's liking. What about the idea that you should have as much freedom as you want all the time. Do you ever feel that way?

ABE: Yes, it's like they are always bossing me around. Especially about homework. My mother keeps bugging me to start my homework.

DR. SAM: So your mom is the big bad slave driver on homework. Now I want you to be totally honest, and I will never tell, but do you really think you would get your homework done without your mother bugging you?

ABE: Well, I don't know. . . . Doc, probably you're right. Nope.

DR. SAM: ADD people need structure to get things done. So how can we get you the structure around homework without you feeling like she is taking away your freedom? Any ideas?

ABE: I could set an alarm clock to go off when it's time to do homework.

DR. SAM: Great idea. We can talk that over with your parents.

ABE: Can we talk that over next week? How much longer till we stop?

DR. SAM: You've done a great job with this discussion. Let's stop right now.

Dr. Sam discussed unfairness/ruination and autonomy with Abe. He used practical motivations (e.g., the possibility of a later curfew and getting Abe's parents to stop nagging him about homework) to help reinforce the utility of considering more reasonable beliefs. Teenagers respond better to such tangible contingencies than to an abstract discussion such as why the world is intrinsically unfair or why unlimited autonomy is bad for adolescents. After a reasonable effort, when Abe indicated he was losing interest in the discussion, the therapist stopped the session. Covering one or two of the expectations and beliefs may be as much as it is reasonable to expect in a session with an inattentive adolescent.

CONCLUSION

For most families, the therapist can cover the materials presented in this chapter in two sessions. In some cases, the therapist may need to devote more time to selected portions of the material. In addition, even though the discussion of expectations is presented before the therapist moves into specific conflict and behavior management techniques, many families benefit from incorporating further discussion of expectations into later sessions. Unreasonable expectations and malicious attributions are likely to crop up repeatedly as the therapist is working on problem solving and communication. With the foundation laid before beginning skill training, the therapist is in an excellent position to refresh the family's memories and reintroduce cognitive restructuring.

CHAPTER ELEVEN

○

Family and Home Management Techniques

After covering childrearing philosophy, principles of parenting, and beliefs/expectations, the therapist introduces specific techniques for resolving parent–adolescent conflict and managing the problems of daily life at home with an adolescent diagnosed as having ADHD. These techniques include problem-solving training, communication training, behavior management, and structural family therapy interventions. During problem-solving training, I teach the family a four-step heuristic for negotiating compromise agreements to specific disputes and guide the family to integrate a problem-solving framework into their daily interactions. This is the primary technique for translating into action the basic parenting principles of shaping independence-related behavior and involving adolescents in decision making. During communication training, we identify and correct specific negative habits in how the parents and adolescents send and receive messages and help them generalize these corrections to their life at home. Behavior management training guides the parents in utilizing Barkley's principles of immediate, frequent, and highly salient consequences, involving the use of reward before punishments. Behavior management techniques are useful in place of problem-solving communication training for the families of young adolescents not mature enough to participate meaningfully in a truly interactive family therapy and when integrated into a behavioral family therapy context.

In many families, after the therapist teaches them to resolve their conflicts, improve their communication, and develop a creative grab-bag of behavior management tricks to deploy flexibly as the situation warrants, life at home with an ADHD adolescent improves, and the therapist can shift gears into the follow-up mode. However, a certain proportion of families do not benefit sufficiently from these techniques unless the therapist also attends to their unique structural problems. Families that have experienced a recent divorce, stepfamilies, single-parent families, and families with major parental disagreements and/or marital conflict need help with issues of taking sides, putting people in the middle, disengagement, and enmeshment. I draw on the wealth of strategic/structural family therapy techniques to help these families. Problem-solving training, communication training, and behavior management are strategically implemented within the context of structural family therapy interventions. Strategic/structural interventions can be seen as addressing Barkley's principle of parental consistency, helping parents work as a team.

Other things being equal, I typically prefer to teach families problem-solving skills first, communication skills second, and behavior management integrated with the other two on an ongoing basis. I prefer this sequence because the families can rapidly resolve many of their specific conflicts through problem solving, providing relatively immediate relief. It takes longer to see tangible results from communication training. However, in those cases in which communication is so negative that it is difficult to conduct a problem-solving discussion, I prefer to introduce communication training first, then move to problem-solving training.

The interventions aimed at family structure are discussed in Chapter 12 (this volume). There is no set time to introduce these interventions; it depends on clinical need. The therapist assesses the structural problems and the functions of problem behavior in the family on an ongoing basis and targets structure and function throughout all the family conflict and home management sessions. For example, in stepfamilies where the adolescent is dividing the mother and stepfather and the stepmother is stuck in the middle, the therapist might need to address this issue early, and possibly repeatedly, in the therapy.

PROBLEM-SOLVING TRAINING

Problem-solving training is a central component of the home-based family intervention for adolescents with ADHD. It is a direct application of the principle of involving the adolescent in the decision making that affects his or her life, as a means of recognizing the natural developmental push toward adolescent independence and teaching responsible independence-related skills to the adolescent. The therapist teaches parents and adolescents a set of heuristic steps for negotiating mutually acceptable solutions to disagreements or conflicts and helps the family integrate these steps into their everyday life through the use of family meetings and informal application of individual problem-solving components in daily interchanges. The cognitive-behavioral conceptualization of problem solving as a framework for individuals to follow when faced with interpersonal conflicts guided the development of these procedures (D'Zurilla & Goldfried, 1971; Spivack, Platt, & Shure, 1976). The problem-solving model, adapted for use with families, consists of four steps: (1) problem definition, (2) generation of alternative solutions, (3) decision making, and (4) planning solution implementation. A fifth step, renegotiation, is invoked when the family is unsuccessful in resolving the dispute through implementation of the initial solution. In the following discussion, I guide readers, in a manualized form, through each step of problem-solving training.

Training Procedures

Families are taught problem solving through instruction, modeling, behavior rehearsal, and feedback over the course of several sessions. The therapist introduces problem solving in a session in which the family is guided through an initial problem-solving discussion with an issue of moderate anger/intensity. First, the therapist gives a brief rationale with instructions for each step of problem solving. Second, he or she models appropriate verbalizations at each step. Third, he or she asks each family member to rehearse the appropriate problem-solving response. Finally, the therapist praises appropriate statements and suggests corrective feedback for inappropriate behaviors. It is expected that family members' initial responses will not meet criteria but that the therapist will be prepared to shape terminal responses through successive approximations.

Introducing Rationale for Problem Solving

The therapist should say something like this:

> "We are entering a stage of treatment where you will learn new problem-solving skills for negotiating solutions to disagreements that you can all live with. In problem solving, each of you will take turns defining a specific problem. You will then list some solutions, decide which ones you would like to try, and plan to carry them out. If you do not at first succeed, you will try again or renegotiate. We will learn to use these steps of problem solving to resolve disputes around specific issues such as curfew, chores, dating, and so on."

Selecting an Issue for an Initial Problem-Solving Discussion

The therapist should select an issue with an anger-intensity level of two or three on the Issues Checklist, if the family has completed this measure. Such an issue would be meaningful but of moderate intensity. Moderate-intensity issues are ideal for skill acquisition; high-intensity issues arouse too much affect. Alternatively, the therapist should ask the family to pick a significant but not tremendously conflictual issue. He or she should distribute the Family Outline of Problem Solving and Problem-Solving Worksheet (see Tables 11.1 and 11.2) to each family member and/or post a large-print copy of the outline on the wall.

TABLE 11.1. Family Outline of Problem Solving

I. Define the problem

   A. You each tell the others what they are doing that bothers you and why.
     1. Be brief.
     2. Be positive, not accusing.

   B. You each repeat the others' statements of the problem to check out your understanding of what they said.

II. Generate alternative solutions

   A. You take turns listing possible solutions.

   B. You follow three rules for listing solutions:
     1. List as many ideas as possible.
     2. Don't evaluate the ideas.
     3. Be creative; suggest crazy ideas.

   C. You won't have to do it just because you say it.

III. Evaluate/decide on the best idea

   A. You take turns evaluating each idea.
     1. Would this idea solve the problem for you?
     2. Would this idea solve the problem for the others?
     3. Rate the idea "plus" or "minus" on the worksheet.

   B. You select the best idea.
     1. Look for ideas rated "plus" by all.
       a. Select one such idea.
       b. Combine several such ideas.
     2. If none rated "plus" by all, see where you came closest to agreement and negotiate a compromise. If two parents are participating, look for ideas rated "plus" by one parent and the teenager.

IV. Plan to implement the selected solution.

   A. You decide who will do what, when, where, and how.

   B. Plan reminders for task completion.

   C. Plan consequences for compliance or noncompliance.

Note. From *ADHD in Adolescents: Diagnosis and Treatment* by Arthur L. Robin. Copyright 1998 by The Guilford Press. Permission to photocopy this table is granted to purchasers of *ADHD in Adolescents* for personal use only (see copyright page for details).

Teaching Problem Definition and Paraphrasing

The therapist should give the rationale for problem definition:

> "We have selected chores [substitute your issue] for discussion. First, we each must define the problem. We define the problem by starting with an 'I,' and making a short, clear statement of how we feel and what is happening that is a problem. Try not to be blaming. Take responsibility for your own feelings and actions."

TABLE 11.2. Problem-Solving Worksheet

Name_____ Date_____

Problem or topic_____

SOLUTIONS	EVALUATIONS		
	Teen	Mom	Dad
_____			
_____			
_____			
_____			
_____			
_____			
_____			

Agreement _____

_____

_____

Implementation plan

A. Teen will do_____ by the
following time_____.

B. Mom will do_____ by the
following time _____ .

C. Dad will do_____by the
following time_____.

D. Plan for monitoring whether this happens_____

_____

E. Any reminders that will be given. By whom? When? How many?

_____

_____

F. Consequences for compliance and noncompliance

   1. Teen_____

   2. Mom_____

   3. Dad_____

Note. From *ADHD in Adolescents: Diagnosis and Treatment* by Arthur L. Robin. Copyright 1998 by The Guilford Press. Permission to photocopy this table is granted to purchasers of *ADHD in Adolescents* for personal use only (see copyright page for details).

He or she should model a plausible problem definition:

"For example, Mr. Jones, if I were you, I might say, 'I am angry at you, Andrew, because I asked you to mow the lawn and take out the trash by sunset, but it's bedtime and you haven't done either.' "

The therapist should ask Mr. Jones to rehearse the problem definition:

THERAPIST: Mr. Jones, please define the chores problem in your own words, following these guidelines.

MR. JONES: Andrew, you are so irresponsible and you never take the garbage out or mow the lawn when I ask you.

He or she should give Mr. Jones feedback. Because he did not adequately define the problem, the therapist would give Mr. Jones the following corrective feedback, asking him to try again:

THERAPIST: That's a start. But, starting with a "You" makes it sound blaming. Try again, starting with an "I" and just saying what Andrew does that bothers you.

MR. JONES: I get mad at you for being irresponsible about not taking out the trash or mowing the lawn.

Even though Mr. Jones's definition was not perfect, the therapist might accept it as a reasonable first approximation and move on. He or she might say:

"That's much better. You started with an 'I' and got specific about what he does. Next time, though, you might want to try a less put-downish word than 'irresponsible.' "

If Mr. Jones's initial definition had been adequate, the therapist would have praised him and moved on.

As each person defines the problem, the therapist asks at least one listener to paraphrase the speaker to check for understanding. For example:

THERAPIST: Andrew, to make sure you understood your dad, please tell me exactly what he said.

ANDREW: He said I don't do the dumb chores when he tries to make me.

Because Andrew embellished his father's statement in a put-downish, accusatory manner, the therapist gives him corrective feedback.

THERAPIST: You added some negative stuff. Just repeat what your dad said; you get to give your opinion next.

ANDREW: He said I don't do the grass and trash on time.

THERAPIST: Much better. Mr. Jones, is that what you said?

MR. JONES: Yes.

The therapist asked the father to verify the son's paraphrase. Next, he would ask Mrs. Jones to define the problem, followed by her husband paraphrasing her definition. We usually ask the adolescent last, because teenagers need several examples of problem definition statements. When it is Andrew's turn, the therapist should proceed as follows:

THERAPIST: Now, Andrew, it is your turn to define the problem. If I were you, I might say, "Mom and Dad, I get mad when you ask me to do the lawn or the garbage at a bad time, like when my favorite show is on TV." Andrew, start with an "I," keep it short. Go ahead.

ANDREW: Uh. What? (*Stares at the ceiling and is lost in thought.*)

THERAPIST: Your turn to define to problem.

ANDREW: My dad's the one with the problem. I'm not having any problem.

MR. JONES: See, Doc, that's what always happens. . . .

THERAPIST: Sorry to interrupt, Mr. Jones. I totally understand. Andrew, this isn't put-down Dad hour. Listen again while I show you what I have in mind by defining the problem. You might say, "I get mad when you ask me to do the lawn at bad times, while I'm busy."

ANDREW: Dad, you bug me too much about the stupid lawn.

THERAPIST: Getting better. But one more time, listen to me. I start with an "I" and tell him what bugs me without accusing or blaming: "Dad, I get mad when you ask me to do the lawn and I am busy doing other things." Now, Andrew, your turn.

ANDREW: I get pissed when I'm watching TV and you ask me to do the lawn right away.

THERAPIST: Great!

Persistence paid off; it often takes several attempts before ADHD teens get on the same wave length with the therapist and even come close to a decent problem definition. The therapist should persevere in an objective, noncritical manner; by doing so, the therapist not only helps the adolescent learn to express him- or herself but also models patience and appropriate structuring skills for the parents, who have been dealing with this for years.

After everyone has had an opportunity to define the problem, the therapist should reiterate that it is natural for family members to have different opinions about an issue, but it is not necessary for one person to persuade another to accept his or her opinion in order to discuss the issue.

Teaching Solution-Listing Skills

The therapist should begin by providing a rationale and instructions:

> "Now that you have defined the problem, you need to think of some solutions. You will take turns listing as many ideas as possible. Suggest anything that comes to mind, even if it seems silly. Don't judge the ideas yet; that comes later. You don't have to do it just because you said it. That is called brainstorming."

The therapist should ask the adolescent to record the ideas in writing on the worksheet. If the adolescent refuses, he or she should ask another family member rather than creating a confrontation now. Over time, the therapist should rotate the recording chore. If the therapist has reasons to expect the adolescent not to cooperate with the request to record the ideas, he or she should ask another family member.

It is wise for the therapist to prompt the family to take turns suggesting ideas, keep the floor open to all ideas, and block any attempt to evaluate the ideas, critically or positively. He or she should keep the mood light and the pace of the session moving, keep an eye on the adolescent, and ask him or her a question or solicit a comment if his or her attention is wandering. The therapist should not permit anyone to monopolize the conversation or use solution listing as a forum to criticize other family members. Although it is not the therapist's responsibility to suggest ideas, he or she may make several suggestions to keep things moving or lighten the atmosphere. The ideas can be outlandish, to spur creativity and interject humor. The therapist may also prompt family members to suggest compromises that address each other's perspectives on the problem, if they are sticking to one-sided solutions:

> "Andrew, can you think of any ideas that would solve the problem for your dad?"

The therapist should continue solution listing until the family has listed six to eight ideas and/or he or she judges their ideas to be going beyond their initial positions. Typically, family members first list their initial positions as ideas and, as time goes on, begin to list ideas that are possible compromise solutions. If too many solutions are listed, it will not be feasible to evaluate them all within one meeting.

Teaching Evaluation/Decision-Making Skills

The therapist should introduce evaluation/decision making by asking the family to review the ideas on the worksheet. He or she should ask each family member to evaluate each idea, indicating whether it will solve the problem, whether it is practical, and whether he or she likes it. Then, the

therapist should ask the family members to rate the idea "plus" or "minus," recording the ratings in the appropriate columns on the worksheet.
It is important to model a correct evaluation:

> "The first idea to address the chores problem is, 'Andrew finishes the lawn before he watches television.' As a teenager, I might say, 'That's OK as long as I don't miss my favorite shows; I guess it solves the problem. I'll give it a plus.' "

Then, the therapist can guide the family members in evaluating and rating each idea, carefully controlling the interaction. He or she should not let it deteriorate into an argument. The therapist must help family members clarify ideas, as needed. Sometimes, additional solutions are mentioned. It is helpful to add them to the list and ask the family to evaluate them.
After all the ideas have been evaluated, the therapist can lead the family in the decision-making phase:

1. Explain to the family that the goal is to reach a decision everyone can live with, and that everyone will have to give up something to get something; this is the essence of negotiation.
2. Ask the secretary to read aloud the ideas rated "plus" by everyone. If one or more ideas were rated positively by all, congratulate the family on reaching an agreement and ask them to combine these ideas into an overall solution.
3. Proceed to implementation planning. If no ideas were rated positively by all, the therapist will have to help them negotiate a compromise.

If the therapist has carefully selected an issue of moderate intensity for the first problem-solving discussion, the chances are good that an agreement will be reached. Later, as the family negotiates more intensely anger-producing issues, consensus may be less likely to occur. If there was no agreement reached, it is important to try the following approach to negotiation:

1. Find an idea on which the family came close to an agreement (e.g., an idea endorsed positively by one parent and an adolescent).
2. Clearly state the gap between the various positions.
3. Ask the family to bridge the gap between their various positions by suggesting additional ideas in between their positions.
4. Ask the family to evaluate these additional ideas and try to reach a compromise.

Consider the chores problem. Andrew and his parents agreed that he should mow the lawn and take out the garbage, but they failed to agree on the timing and reminders. As is common with ADHD teens who procrastinate, Andrew insisted that he should not have to do these chores until late Sunday afternoon or evening. But, based on past experience, when Andrew left things for the last minute, he failed to do them. Thus Mr. Jones insisted that the lawn be mowed early Saturday morning and that the trash cans be at the curb by 4:00 P.M. Sunday afternoon. Andrew wanted several reminders, but Mr. Jones felt Andrew would be shirking his responsibilities if he received any reminders; he insisted that his son remember on his own. Mrs. Jones backed her husband up in the session but did not seem as rigid about the time and the reminders as her husband.

The therapist understood where Mr. Jones was coming from and suspected that Andrew was not really taking the discussion too seriously, probably figuring nothing would happen if he did not do the chores. The therapist also believed that Mr. Jones was forgetting the nature of ADHD when he refused to permit reminders. However, it was not appropriate to voice these concerns in the context of a problem-solving discussion because the therapist wished to take a neutral stance and facilitate a compromise so that the family could learn from its implementation efforts what worked and what did not work.

The therapist fractionated or divided the issue into its elements and asked the family to negotiate each element separately: (1) the time for completing the chores and (2) the reminders. The father and son were asked to negotiate with each other a time for completing the chores in between Saturday morning and Sunday evening. With the therapist blocking put-downs and criticisms, they eventually compromised on Sunday morning at 10:00 A.M. for the lawn and dinnertime on Sunday for the garbage. Then, the therapist asked Andrew to wait outside while he briefly reviewed the need for performance reminders on the basis of ADHD as a neurobiological disorder with the parents. Mr. Jones adhered to the belief that any reminder was a somehow a sign of weakness but after a brief discussion was able to see the need for one strategically timed reminder. Andrew was called back into the room, and it was agreed that his father would leave him a single written reminder on Sunday morning about the lawn and on Sunday afternoon about the garbage.

This example illustrates how to foster negotiation as well as how the therapist occasionally needs to deal with beliefs that make negotiation more difficult. Talking to Mr. Jones without his son in the room also permitted the therapist to be frank and the father to save face. Fractionating the conflict into its elements also is often a helpful approach. Robin and Foster (1989) discuss fractionating the conflict, as well as several additional approaches to resolving impasses, in more detail.

Implementation Planning

The goal of implementation planning is for the family to specify the details that are necessary to put the agreed-on solution into operation.

These details include (1) who will do what, when, and where; (2) who will monitor compliance with the agreement, and how monitoring will be carried out (with charts or graphs, or verbally); (3) the consequences for compliance or noncompliance with the agreement; (4) what, if any, performance reminders will be given, if these have not already been built into the solution; (5) exactly what constitutes compliance (e.g., how clean must a room be?); and (6) what difficulties are anticipated in carrying out the agreement.

Effective implementation planning is central to the success of problem-solving training with ADHD teens, as they need the structure of performance prompts and immediate consequences to maintain their behavior and they may take advantage of any ambiguity in the agreed-on solution to manipulate their parents and avoid effort. Some parents may also use ambiguities as opportunities for lectures and/or extra punishments. The "Implementation Plan" section of the Problem-Solving Worksheet guides the therapist in fleshing out the details of the agreed-on solution and recording these details in writing.

Let's examine the implementation planning process for Andrew and the Jones family. Table 11.3 depicts their completed Problem-Solving Worksheet. First, each person's actions for implementing the solution are clearly specified, along with the time for completing them. Andrew is to cut the grass, bag the cuttings, and clean and return the lawn mower to the garage by 10:00 A.M. He is also to take the trash cans to the curb by dinnertime or 7:00 P.M. Sunday, whichever comes first. The therapist prompted the family to specify the details about bagging the cuttings and cleaning and putting away the lawn mower by asking Dad to define what "doing the lawn" included. The therapist suspected Andrew might cut the lawn and simply stop there. Also, the time for the trash includes two alternatives because the family mentioned that they often ate out late on Sunday and Mr. Jones thought this might be an excuse for Andrew to avoid the trash chore. The therapist must decide in each case how much detail to go into. Even though Mrs. Jones does not have a major task to do, she was given a role in reminding her husband, to help prompt and reinforce his behavior, and to include her in the solution implementation. The therapist should always create a role for each family member in implementing the solution. Mr. Jones's responsibility also built in some safeguards for Andrew against lecturing, which frequently occurred in the past when Andrew failed to complete the chores.

A plan for the parents to share the monitoring and write the results down was included. In addition, the therapist prompted the family to work out consequences for compliance and noncompliance with the solution. Such consequences include incentives and punishments. The therapist typically asks the adolescent to suggest the incentives and the parents to suggest the punishments. The standard types of consequences discussed in the section of the chapter on behavior management can be attached to agree-

TABLE 11.3. Problem-Solving Worksheet for Andrew Jones

Name <u>Andrew Jones & Parents</u>   Date <u>9/19/98</u>

Problem or topic <u>Chores problem, e.g., Dad says Andrew does not mow the lawn or take out the garbage reliably and on time. Mom agrees. Andrew says his parents ask him to do the chores during his favorite TV shows or at other inconvenient times.</u>

EVALUATIONS

SOLUTIONS	Teen	Mom	Dad
1. No television until the lawn is done	−	+	+
2. Andrew does the lawn and garbage any time he wants	+	−	−
3. Andrew does the lawn right after school on Friday	−	−	+
4. Mom takes out trash; Dad does lawn	+		−
5. Hire a lawn service	+	+	−
6. Pay Andrew $30 for doing lawn and trash	+	−	−
7. Replace lawn with rocks	−	−	−

Agreement <u>Andrew does the lawn by 10:00 A.M. Sunday and takes the trash to the curb by dinnertime Sunday.</u>

Implementation plan

A. Teen will do <u>Cut the grass, bag the cuttings, clean & return mower to garage by 10:00 A.M. Sunday from May to November. Andrew will take the big trash cans from the garage to the curb by dinnertime or 7:00 P.M. Sunday, whichever comes first.</u>

B. Mom will do <u>Remind Dad not to lecture Andrew about chores and to give Andrew only one reminder as planned below. Mom will do this on Friday and Saturday evenings.</u>

C. Dad will do <u>Remind Andrew one time Sunday morning by 9:00 A.M. of need to do the lawn and remind him one time by 4:00 P.M. Sunday afternoon of need to take out garbage. Dad will not lecture on these topics.</u>

D. Plan for monitoring whether this happens <u>Dad will check on Sunday morning for the lawn. Mom will check on Sunday evening for the garbage. Will write on calendar on refrigerator whether Andrew did each of these chores.</u>

E. Any reminders that will be given. By whom? When? How many? <u>See above.</u>

F. Consequences for compliance and noncompliance

1. Teen <u>Andrew will earn $10 per week of his $20 allowance for doing the lawn. Praise is the positive consequence for doing the garbage. Andrew will lose all television privileges on Sunday night if he fails to do either chore on time, and will still have to do the chores.</u>

2. Mom <u>Dad and Andrew will both thank Mom for doing her part and helping them deal well with each other.</u>

3. Dad <u>Mom will do something nice for Dad if he keeps from lecturing Andrew about these chores. Andrew will say something nice to his dad for not lecturing.</u>

ments negotiated through problem solving. It is important to specify consequences for each member of the family, even if these may primarily consist of verbal feedback for the parents. The implementation plan is essentially a form of a behavioral contract. I return to behavioral contracts later in this chapter.

Summarizing and Assigning Homework

The therapist should bring the initial problem-solving training session to a close by congratulating the family on successfully reaching an agreement to the problem, giving them brief feedback about the strengths and weaknesses of their interaction, and assigning as homework implementation of the solution:

> "You worked hard and reached a solution to this problem. Congratulations! Mr. Jones, I was impressed by your willingness to be flexible about things you belief in strongly. Mrs. Jones, you backed your husband up well. And Andrew, you stuck in there with me on defining the problem. I'd like you to go home and put this solution into effect, and come back next week and tell me how it went. After I make myself a photocopy, I will give you the Problem Worksheet to take home. Use this as your written instructions for carrying out the solution. We will continue working on problem solving then, and I'll be asking you in the future to start to have family meetings to use these skills at home. Any questions?"

If the family did not use a Problem Worksheet, the therapist might consider writing down the homework assignment so that they will have a written record of their homework assignment.

Building Problem-Solving Skills: Two Follow-Up Sessions

Most families with ADHD adolescents need at least two more opportunities to practice problem-solving skills with the therapist's coaching to learn to apply these skills at home. In addition, they need graduated assignments in implementing problem solving at home, through family meetings, impromptu problem-solving sessions, and informal application of problem-solving components. After completing each assignment, the family will benefit from the opportunity to report back to the therapist and receive feedback and suggestions for fine-tuning their future efforts.

I prefer to conduct the two additional sessions over the next 2 weeks after introducing problem solving, to maintain momentum, although it also works well to intersperse these sessions with communication training, described later in this chapter. Each of these sessions is typically divided into three portions: (1) review of the previous week's homework; (2) a new problem-solving discussion; and (3) summarization/assignment of new homework. I describe this agenda to the family at the beginning of each session.

Homework Review

After greeting the family, the therapist should ask for a report of the previous week's homework. Did they successfully implement the solution negotiated during the previous week's session? If assigned, did they conduct a family meeting or otherwise practice problem-solving skills? I ask each family member to give an independent report. If the homework was successfully completed, I praise the family and move on to a new problem-solving discussion. If the homework was not completed, I investigate what went wrong, objectively but persistently. In the case of the assignment to implement the agreement reached last week, I ask the following questions:

1. Did the family try to implement the solution? If yes, where did it break down? If they didn't try to implement the solution, why not?
2. Was there resistance to the solution from one or more members? Who, and what type of resistance?
3. Did negative communication sidetrack them?
4. Was there general mistrust and hostility?
5. Did they "forget" to implement the solution?
6. Did a new crisis with the adolescent arise and eclipse the solution implementation (a run-in with the law, a failing report card, drugs or alcohol, etc.)?
7. Did real-life circumstances (out-of-town business trips, a busy adolescent sports schedule, visits from relatives, holidays, etc.) interfere?
8. Did "the family ADHD" do them in (one or both parents with ADHD got overwhelmed, distracted, off-task; show generally poor follow-through, family chaos, etc.)?

Parents and adolescents with ADHD often try to minimize the impact of failure to carry through on solutions they committed to implement; this is especially likely in families with multiple ADHD members, where chaos reigns supreme and little ever gets accomplished in an orderly fashion. Homework assignments are, after all, examples of a request for delayed responding, and impaired delayed responding is central to ADHD (Barkley, 1997b). Because coping with impaired delayed responding involves programming behavior change at the point of performance and the therapist usually is not present when the solution needs to be implemented, a great deal of effort may need to be devoted to developing family reminder systems to facilitating solution implementation. Such systems may range from setting timers or personal organizers to give off audible reminders throughout the week, using Post-its and other written reminders, people reminding each other, or writing the assignment on a calendar. The therapist should not simply ignore the failure to do the homework; this sets up a precedent for the family to fail to cooperate with future assignments and reinforces what may be their natural but unfortunate style of operating.

Sometimes, the solution was partially implemented but did not work. Impulsive families may get easily frustrated and give up, or further arguments may erupt. The therapist must help the family reframe the problem as insufficient problem solving rather than malicious intent or sabotage. Perhaps they failed to evaluate adequately the solutions, and picked an unrealistic one. Perhaps they did not define the problem along its most salient dimension. The therapist should be appropriately empathetic and definitely not critical. In such cases, he or she should coach the family to cycle through the steps of problem solving again, figuring out where they went wrong and helping them renegotiate a more viable solution. Renegotiation then becomes the major agenda item for this session, instead of a new problem-solving discussion.

New Problem-Solving Discussion

It is helpful to select another issue of moderate intensity to problem-solve. If the first issue was one of greater concern to the parents than the adolescent, the therapist should try to balance it out by giving the adolescent an opportunity to pick the next issue. He or she should coach the family to follow the outline of problem-solving steps and focus efforts on intensive skills building. It is important to tighten up criteria for adequate problem definitions, thorough evaluations, and so on. The therapist should give as much feedback as necessary to shape improved responses. These two sessions provide the opportunity to refine the family members' ability to apply the components of problem solving.

It is wise to tailor elements of the model to increase the involvement of inattentive, restless adolescents who may not be able to sit through an entire problem-solving discussion. The therapist must recognize when the adolescent's yawning, fidgety, whining behavior represents the mental fatigue and burnout common with ADHD adolescents instead of truly oppositional behavior and not let the parents overreact inappropriately. The therapist should keep his or her comments and the parents' comments brief and to the point, talk in an animated and humorous style, and bring the adolescent into the discussion often. It is wise to gauge the amount of time the adolescent can "last" and consider having more frequent, shorter sessions or sending the adolescent to the waiting room and working on parent management issues in the second half of each session. The therapist can simplify the steps of problem solving to accommodate the adolescent by having the parents brainstorm and evaluate the solutions, then presenting the adolescent with two or three choices to consider. Finally, whenever possible, the therapist should time the therapy appointment so that stimulant medication is in effect during the session.

New Homework Assignments

Following the second and third problem-solving sessions, I assign homework designed to increase the chances that the family will generalize the use of problem solving to the home environment. In addition to implementing agreed-on solutions, I ask the family to establish a regular family meeting time. I extract a specific commitment from them as to when they will hold the first meeting. During these meetings, the family should attempt to problem-solve gripes that have accumulated since the last meeting. I ask them to tape-record the first few meetings, and then I review the tapes and give them feedback. Ideally, families with ADHD adolescents ought to have at least one such meeting per week. Realistically, most ADHD families are either so busy or chaotic that it is difficult to schedule any meetings. The therapist should help them creatively plan how to find time to practice problem solving—in the car on the way to the session or shopping, early morning or late evening, at mealtime, by conference call, through a private chat room of an online service at three terminals in separate cities, or by E-mail from around the world. The therapist should help them see the possibilities for using technology to facilitate problem-solving interactions.

Another invaluable type of assignment involves daily application of component problem-solving skills. The goal is to have the family start to act "principle centered," as Barkley would say. For example, whenever the parents approach their adolescent, they should be thinking, "How do I actively involve my teenager in this issue, and how do I apply problem solving to it?" The therapist should suggest that they try to use problem definition statements whenever something is bothering them about another family member's behavior. He or she can ask them to consider suggesting at least two alternatives when approaching each other about issues, or to prompt each other, saying, "What are our choices?" For example, if a mother needs to approach her daughter about doing the dishes, she could say, "Sally, I need for you to help me with the dishes. We can do it now, or we could find another choice." Having family members develop private cues for engaging in problem-solving behavior may also be helpful. To help William evaluate ideas before he acted on an impulse, Mrs. Smith, for instance, reached an agreement with William that she would say "What would happen if . . . " whenever she felt he needed to think before he acted.

The therapist has to carefully tailor such tasks to the styles of particular families to increase their chances of success. Without such attempts at generalization programming, many families with ADHD adolescents will not integrate problem-solving skills into their natural repertoires.

COMMUNICATION TRAINING

"Maintain good communication" is one of the most basic principles parents and ADHD adolescents need to become aware of and act on in their daily relationships. Communication is the glue that binds relationships together, the vehicle through which parents and adolescents make their needs known to each other and meet those needs. It is easy for the impulsive, restless person to do a great deal of damage to a relationship in moments by flying off the handle in a monumental burst of negative communication; such damage could take months, if not years, to repair. By the same token, it is all too easy for an inattentive person to give the impression of aloofness, indifference, or not caring when he or she is spaced out, distracted, or daydreaming instead of listening effectively. After school and in the evening, when adolescents are mentally and physically fatigued from school and parents are burned out from a hard day at the office, it is likely that impulsive outbursts and spaced-out listening will occur. Thus, ADHD symptoms can very easily impair interpersonal communication in family relationships, even under the best of circumstances. When the associated information processing, learning problems, and psychiatric comorbidities that many ADHD adolescents and their families display are added to ADHD symptoms, family communication becomes even more fragile. It is amazing that any meaningful communication takes place under such conditions.

It is also important for families to understand the carefully researched principle of reciprocity in interpersonal communication (Patterson, 1982), which basically boils down to "You get what you give." Parents who are negative to their adolescents will have adolescents who are negative back to their parents; parents who are positive to their adolescents will have adolescents who are more positive back to their parents. Researchers have found that there is a matching of intensity and rate of negative communication in marriages and parent–child interactions (Patterson, 1982). Such reciprocity takes place both in moment-to-moment interactions and over longer time spans. The impaired response inhibition of ADHD individuals, coupled with the natural adolescent striving for autonomy, fuels rapid escalation of chains of negative interactions, resulting in some of the most florid shouting matches one can imagine. Naive listeners might easily think an ADHD adolescent and her ADHD parent in one of these bursts of reciprocal negative communication were raving lunatics.

Practically, to change reciprocally negative interactions, it is helpful to break down the principle of "maintain good communication" into a short list of general guidelines which are first introduced to the family, followed by a more lengthy, formal retraining of negative communication habits. A minimum of two therapy sessions is necessary to teach communication skills, with associated homework assignments and follow-up in later sessions. The therapist should present the following general principles to the family.

General Guidelines for Maintaining Good Communication

1. *Listen when the other person is in the mood to talk, but don't try to force the other person to open up to you.* Adolescents may go for days or even weeks without having the urge to open up and confide in their parents, even if they have a generally positive relationship with them. They may be confiding in their friends or keeping things to themselves. Then, for seemingly no reason a parent can discern, suddenly, often at the most inconvenient times for parents (or therapists), the teenager wants to talk. Therapists need to normalize this adolescent reaction and teach parents to put a high priority on listening at those times the teenager wants to talk, even if the parent has other plans. Many parents of ADHD adolescents get upset because their youngsters won't confide in them or even talk in more than monosyllables to them most of the time; their concerns are usually unfounded and their expectations are unrealistic. But when one assesses the situation further, the adolescents' complaints that their parents have not been willing to listen on the few occasions when they wanted to talk are sometimes justified. For ADHD adolescents, this principle usually translates into exerting the mental effort necessary to inhibit the impulse to interrupt their parents when they vehemently disagree with what their parents' are saying and to try to hear and process their parents' ideas even though they disagree.

2. *Use active listening to encourage the other person to express his or her opinion and help the other person feel understood.* Active listening is the cornerstone of most communication training programs (Gordon, 1970; Robin & Foster, 1989). Active listening involves paraphrasing back the content and emotional tone of the speaker without adding any of one's own ideas or feelings. ADHD adolescents and their parents both need to incorporate this skill into their daily interchanges.

3. *Honestly express how you feel, good or bad, in language that gets the point across without hurting the other person.* Expression, not suppression, of affect is the goal of the communication training. Most of the time, nonhurtful expression of negative, critical affect involves making clear-cut "I statements" that are essentially similar to problem definition statements.

4. *Distinguish between truly negative and truly ADHD communication. Deal with the truly negative communication, and ignore or work around the truly ADHD communication.* Most ADHD adolescents, especially when medication is not in effect, continually do so many things that could conceivably be considered examples of negative communication that if a therapist or a parent attempted to correct all these behaviors, it would be a full-time job taxing the patience of even the most reflective adult with a high tolerance for frustration. These behaviors just happen, often with-

out planning or awareness of the part of the adolescent; that is the biological legacy of ADHD. If the adult managed to give feedback on each inappropriate communication behavior, it would be difficult to keep from damaging the adolescent's self-esteem, because the high frequency of corrections would inevitably leave a negative global impression. Instead, the therapist must teach parents how to prioritize which communication targets to correct and which to ignore (i.e., pick battles wisely). I find it useful to distinguish between *truly negative* communication and *truly ADHD* communication. Truly negative communication is intentional, premeditated, proactive, critical, and demeaning, aimed at weaknesses of the other person, designed to manipulate the other person into doing what the speaker wants, and often part of long-standing negative attitudes toward the other person. Truly ADHD communication is also negative and hurtful, but it is reactive, spontaneous, impulsive, nonsensical, poorly timed, not part of a long-standing pattern of negative attitudes toward the other person, and stupidly executed in a manner which is unlikely to get the other person to do what the speaker wants. It occurs under conditions of fatigue, external stress, or threat, when external circumstances further erode the ADHD individual's already impaired inhibitory control. Family members need to give a high priority to targeting the truly negative communication and only deal with the truly ADHD communication when all the truly negative communication rarely occurs (this never happens with most ADHD adolescents).

Consider the following example to help clarify this distinction. Fourteen-year-old Alice, the identified ADHD adolescent patient, and her parents, Mr. and Mrs. Wardsworth, were attending a family therapy session at 5:00 P.M. on a school day after Alice had two final exams and soccer practice; she was fatigued and her noon dose of Ritalin had worn off long ago. She participated reasonably well for the first 25 minutes of the therapy session but then became increasingly restless and started making sarcastic remarks after everything her parents said. Her parents became enraged by her sarcastic remarks and demanded an apology. The therapist helped them to see that the fatigue, the confining situation of the therapy session, the hard day at school, and the medication being worn off were all factors contributing to her sarcasm. Those conditions did not excuse her sarcasm, but they did help explain it. It was better to make light of her sarcasm, end the discussion, and finish the session without Alice in the room because her negative communication was truly ADHD induced.

By contrast, at the next therapy session, at 10:00 A.M. on a Saturday morning, when Alice had taken her Ritalin, she began to attack her parents when they brought up the need to discuss her poor choice of friends. She cursed them out and threatened to run away if they did not back off. The therapist considered her behavior to be truly negative communication and intervened immediately to modify it.

Systematic Communication Training

After presenting these four principles to the family and thoroughly discussing them, the therapist then begins systematic communication training. The goals of this training are (1) to increase family members' awareness of their specific negative communication habits and the deleterious impact of negative communication on parent–adolescent relations; (2) to pinpoint the most salient negative communication habits for this family; (3) to teach positive communication habits, using instructions, modeling, behavior rehearsal, and feedback; and (4) to assign home practice of positive communication skills.

The therapist should distribute the Family Negative Communication Handout in Table 11.4. Family members are asked to recall recent examples of the specific negative communication habits on the handout, to describe the impact of these examples on their relationship, and to suggest more constructive ways to express the same feelings and thoughts.

TABLE 11.4. Family Negative Communication Handout

Check if your family does this:	Try to do this instead:
1. ___Call each other names.	Express anger without hurt.
2. ___Put each other down.	"I am angry that you did ____."
3. ___Interrupt each other.	Take turns; keep it short.
4. ___Criticize too much.	Point out the good and bad.
5. ___Get defensive.	Listen, then calmly disagree.
6. ___Lecture.	Tell it straight and short.
7. ___Look away from speaker.	Make eye contact.
8. ___Slouch.	Sit up, look attentive.
9. ___Talk in sarcastic tone.	Talk in normal tone.
10. ___Get off the topic.	Finish one topic, then go on.
11. ___Think the worst.	Don't jump to conclusions.
12. ___Dredge up the past.	Stick to the present.
13. ___Read others' minds.	Ask others' opinions.
14. ___Command, order.	Request nicely.
15. ___Give the silent treatment.	Say what's bothering you.
16. ___Make light of something.	Take it seriously.
17. ___Deny you did it.	Admit you did it, or nicely explain you didn't.
18. ___Nag about small mistakes.	Admit no one is perfect; overlook small things.

Note. From *ADHD in Adolescents: Diagnosis and Treatment* by Arthur L. Robin. Copyright 1998 by The Guilford Press. Permission to photocopy this table is granted to purchasers of *ADHD in Adolescents* for personal use only (see copyright page for details).

The following example illustrates these steps:

THERAPIST: Today we will work on how you communicate with each other. I've noticed that you sometimes get really upset about the way you talk to each other. This leads to a build up of anger, yelling, and screaming, and sometimes ends up in a big fight or family crisis. Having ADHD family members makes it even worse as they lose it more easily than non-ADHD folks. Look at this handout. On the left side are negative communication habits; on the right side are positive alternatives. Give me some recent examples of the negative habits which occurred in your family.

ALICE: That's easy. My mom yells at me all the time, don't you, Mom (*sarcastic*)?

MRS. WARDSWORTH: There you have it, Doc. She's doing everything on the list right this minute.

ALICE: Am not. You always exaggerate. I only counted yelling.

THERAPIST: You are so helpful in quickly identifying negative communication habits (*dead serious, no sarcasm*). So, Alice, how do you feel and what do you do when your mom yells at you?

ALICE: I give it right back to her, and then some.

THERAPIST: Sounds like you give what you get; this is they way it goes in families.

MR. WARDSWORTH: They make all the noise. I get a headache.

THERAPIST: So their yelling matches affect you by giving you a headache. Sounds like yelling affects everyone. Now let's consider what Alice and her mom can do instead of yelling. Any ideas?

MRS. WARDSWORTH: It says on this list that we could make a nonblaming "I" statement. Isn't that like when we defined problems?

THERAPIST: Very good. You start with an "I" and express your feeling, but it doesn't have to be a description of a problem, just whatever you need to. . . .

ALICE: (*interrupting*) Mom, I feel you are a creep (*sarcastic*)!

THERAPIST: Stop! Alice, I don't think you're taking this seriously. I'm disappointed.

ALICE: So can we go home now?

THERAPIST: Not until the hour is up. Acting sarcastic won't get you out of here early. If you are bored and annoyed, start with an "I" and tell us without sarcasm.

ALICE: I'm bored and annoyed.

THERAPIST: Much better.

MRS. WARDSWORTH: Doc, I don't know how you put up with it.

THERAPIST: It's a challenge, but I am used to it. Now, Mrs. Wardsworth, start with an "I" and tell Alice how you feel about her behavior in this session. And Alice, don't say anything until your mom is done.

MRS. WARDSWORTH: Alice, I am annoyed and frustrated because you are not taking this discussion seriously.

MR. WARDSWORTH: I am upset by the way you treat your mother.

THERAPIST: Now you folks are starting to get the hang of "I" statements. And Alice, you are being a lot more cooperative.

The action moved rapidly, as is usually the case, in this vignette. Alice identified yelling, and everyone else immediately identified Alice's mocking, sarcastic tone as negative communication habits. The impact on the family was made apparent, including Mr. Wardsworth's somatic complaints. The therapist quickly corrected Alice and pointed out that she could not end the session through sarcasm; instead, he required her to emit a more appropriate "I" statement. By the end of the interaction, family members were beginning to practice "I" statements and Alice had calmed down somewhat.

After the negative communication habits and positive replacement behaviors have been pinpointed, the therapist guides the family through an intense practice of correcting the negative behaviors, picking a few at a time. The family may be asked to problem-solve an issue or discuss recent events in family life. The therapist stops the discussion as soon as a family member emits a targeted negative communication behavior, reminds them of the positive alternative response, and asks them to replay the scene utilizing the positive instead of the negative behavior.

The success of communication training depends on the persistence of the therapist. It is important to correct every instance of a targeted negative communication pattern assertively but respectfully. It is also important to balance targets across family members. The therapist should not repeatedly single out one family member if it can be avoided. He or she should liberally praise positive communication behaviors.

At the end of each communication training session, the therapist assigns homework to practice correcting the targeted negative behaviors throughout the week.

BEHAVIORAL PARENT MANAGEMENT

Behavioral parent management techniques have been extensively researched and repeatedly found to be effective in helping parents increase compliance and other prosocial behaviors and decrease aggression and other negative behaviors in preschoolers and school-age children with ADHD (Anastopoulous, Barkley, & Sheldon, 1996). A number of manualized, highly teachable and replicable behavioral parent management protocols have been tailored for the parents of children with ADHD, such as Barkley's (1997) defiant child approach. Barkley has evaluated the effectiveness of a modified version of the defiant child approach with adolescents in a study reviewed in Chapter 12 (this volume).

Dr. Gerald Patterson, a preeminent social learning researcher, and his colleague Marion Forgatch, have written the most articulate account of how parents can apply behavior management with adolescents in their two-volume series, Parents and Adolescents Living Together (Forgatch & Patterson, 1989; Patterson & Forgatch, 1987). Although the series was ostensibly written for parents, it is written at a level of great value to professionals. They integrate the use of behavior management with problem-solving and communication skills, an integration I also strongly advocate. Many of the ideas in this section are based on Patterson and Forgatch's suggestions. A *Defiant Teen* training manual which also integrates behavior management with problem-solving communication training is forthcoming (Barkley, Edwards, & Robin, in press).

Behavioral parent management training with adolescents typically includes the following techniques: (1) monitoring and tracking behavior, (2) building positive parent–adolescent interaction, (3) positive incentive systems, (4) shaping behavior, and (5) punishment systems. Positive incentive systems include the contingent use of praise, point systems or token economies, and behavioral contracts. Shaping a terminal response through reinforcement of successive approximations of the terminal response is often a variation on the positive incentive systems. For adolescents, punishment techniques include ignoring minor negative behaviors, taking away privileges, grounding, work chores, and making restitution. Time out, in the form of isolation in a chair or room, is not usually developmentally appropriate. In addition to the techniques just mentioned, a number of family management techniques (message centers, reminder systems, design and allocation of physical space in the home, etc.) may be particularly helpful to the families with a parent and an adolescent with ADHD (Dixon, 1995; Nadeau, 1995).

I integrate these techniques into the parenting and home management phase of my comprehensive intervention. With the 11- to 13-year-old youngsters, I decide before I begin working on issues at home whether the case is appropriate for mutual problem solving or whether this is primarily a parent management case. Is the adolescent mature enough, and are his or her ADHD symptoms in sufficient control that he or she can participate meaningfully in family therapy sessions? Minimal participation during family sessions; highly impoverished verbalizations due to cognitive or emotional limitations; resistance to accepting or even discussing how to deal with ADHD; delay in the onset of formal, abstract thought processes; lack of interest in becoming independent; and predominant interests in the kinds of toys and play activities characteristic of 8–10-year-old children would be the clinical indicators for taking a management approach rather than a problem-solving approach. If these indicators are present, I find it more effective to implement the modified Barkley defiant child approach than to intervene with problem-solving communication training. I help the parents manage the adolescent as they would manage a young child. I have learned through difficult experience that problem-solving communication does not work with such immature, highly resistant 11- and 12-year-olds.

In the majority of cases, I do intervene with problem-solving communication training. When there is a high rate of reciprocal negative communication and coercion between parent and adolescent, it is often helpful to precede problem-solving communication training with a session using one of the techniques for building positive parent–adolescent interaction. After learning problem-solving skills, many families benefit from learning behavioral contracting, punishment, and monitoring/tracking skills, which they can then apply to implementing the solutions negotiated through problem solving and to managing their interactions on a day-to-day basis. During the review of the principles of parenting early in the parenting/home management phase of intervention, the therapist may spend some time guiding parents in the appropriate use of rewards and punishments. A brief summary is given here of each of the major behavior management techniques as it might be implemented with adolescents.

Monitoring and Tracking Behavior

Monitoring refers to keeping track of an adolescent's whereabouts—what they are doing, with whom, when and where. Tracking refers to counting or recording a particular adolescent behavior. Taken alone, monitoring and tracking are not behavioral interventions that will necessarily change adolescent problem behavior, but they are essential in parenting adolescents. Too often today busy parents do not know their adolescent's whereabouts; impulsive adolescents can easy get into trouble (Moffit & Silva, 1988). Too often, parents and adolescents negotiate a solution to a problem but do not monitor its implementation effectively. The therapist should call the parents' attention to the need to monitor the adolescent's general whereabouts, as well as specific agreements reached with the adolescent. Creative routines may be worked out to facilitate monitoring. If Sally and her parents reached an agreement that Sally will come home by 1:00 A.M. on Saturday, a parent needs to be awake and waiting at 1:00 A.M. to determine whether Sally complied. If Aaron is supposed to take his Ritalin at 6:30 A.M., a parent should be around to check on whether he took the medication. The therapist should caution parents not to undertake agreements they cannot see through to the end with adequate monitoring and tracking.

Building Positive Parent–Adolescent Interaction

Many researchers and clinicians who work with adolescents have noted how important it is for parents to spend focused positive time with the teenagers (Alexander-Roberts, 1995; Patterson & Forgatch, 1987; Zeigler Dendy, 1995). Not only does spending focused positive time build a positive parent–adolescent relationship, it also communicates caring and love to the adolescent, who may be accustomed to hearing primarily critical comments from adults, and contributes to the development of positive self-esteem and a sense of security. As discussed in Chapter 10, a disengaged parenting style promotes insecurity among adolescents.

The therapist might assign a Barkley-style parent attending task (Barkley, 1997c). The therapist may introduce the attending task by asking the parent to think about the characteristics of positive and negative supervisors with whom they have worked and honestly evaluate which characteristics they display in interactions with their adolescent. Then, the therapist indicates that the objective of the attending task is to help them learn to give positive attention to their problem adolescent and improve general relations. The parents are then asked to schedule 15 to 20 minutes at least three times in the next week when they will observe and/or participate with their adolescent engaging in a pleasant activity and give their adolescent positive feedback. The adolescent should be permitted to choose the activity, within reason. It is essential for the parents to understand that they are not to direct the activity, take charge of it, or respond critically but just to observe or participate, depending on the activity. Possible activities might include sports, working on a hobby, computers, video games, and going for a walk or a bike ride. Passive endeavors such as watching television or a movie at home would be the only ones not appropriate for this assignment, although for the parent to take the adolescent on an outing that included going to movies could work well.

Braswell and Bloomquist (1991) described a Positive Activity and Interaction Schedule, which is an alternative format for helping parents and adolescents with ADHD spend positive, focused time together. Table 11.5 summarizes the five steps of their schedule. The therapist goes through these five steps with the parent and adolescent together.

The Positive Activity and Interaction Schedule and the Barkley attending tasks essentially accomplish the same thing—building positive interaction—and might be employed flexibly by the therapist. Given the hectic pace of life for many families with ADHD adolescents, the therapist may need to help the family creatively brainstorm how to fit such activities into their lives. For some families, a single, longer outing on a weekend or weekday evening might work better than several shorter interactions. The

TABLE 11.5. Positive Activity and Interaction Schedule

Directions: The parent and adolescent should complete each step together. Both should give equal input and effort to make sure each step is accomplished.

Step 1: List as many activities as possible that the parent and adolescent enjoy doing together that can be accomplished in 30 minutes or less.

_____   _____   _____

_____   _____   _____

Step 2: Schedule two or more 30-minute periods per week when the parent and adolescent will engage in one or more of the above activities together (indicate day, date, and time).

_____   _____   _____

_____   _____   _____

Step 3: Parent lists specific positive behaviors he or she will try to do more of during the activity period (listening, praising, giving feedback, hugs, etc.). Get input from the adolescent.

_____   _____   _____

_____   _____   _____

Step 4: Adolescent lists specific positive behaviors he or she will try to do more of during the activity period (talking, eye contact, expressing feelings, discussing events at school, etc.). Get input from the parent.

_____   _____   _____

_____   _____   _____

Step 5: Parent and adolescent write down comments about their perceptions of each activity period. Both should write down observations and feelings about themselves and the other. (Use the back of this form if necessary.)

Activity time 1:_____

_____

Activity time 2:_____

_____

Note. From Braswell & Bloomquist (1991). Copyright 1991 by The Guilford Press. Reprinted in *ADHD in Adolescents: Diagnosis and Treatment* by Arthur L. Robin. Permission to photocopy this table is granted to purchasers of *ADHD in Adolescents* for personal use only (see copyright page for details).

Positive Parent Adolescent Interaction Schedule also lends itself nicely to being integrated into communication training. During a session when the therapist has targeted one or two specific negative communication habits, he or she might introduce the task of going through the interaction schedule, stopping, and correctly identifying the negative communication targets. Then, as part of the schedule and activity, the parent–adolescent dyad might practice the specific positive communication skills targeted during the session.

Positive Incentive Systems

Praise

Praising an adolescent contingent upon the emission of a desired behavior is clearly the most straightforward and, in many cases, powerful positive incentive. Patterson and Forgatch (1987) point out that although parents may use encouragement, they do not necessarily use it in a consistently contingent manner. To their comments, I would add that for an adolescent to praise a parent is truly a powerful consequence, and most adolescents with ADHD do not consistently use praise when their parents do something they like or appreciate. The therapist needs to encourage parents and adolescents to create a contingent positive environment where each regularly praises the other for actions and behaviors they like. Parents may need to control their bad moods and track their own behavior and their adolescent's behavior to create a contingent positive environment.

It is useful to point out to the family the four types of noncontingent family environments cited by Patterson and Forgatch (1987): (1) the misers—family members rarely or never encourage each other; (2) warm fuzzies—family members receive praise, hugs, smiles, and encouragement no matter what they do, good or bad; (3) nasties—no matter what family members do, they are greeted with sarcasm and criticism; and (4) you are a failure—parents send mixed messages that although high achievement and cooperation are good, the children could have done even better. This discussion can be conducted in a humorous manner, which helps maintain the inattentive youngster's interest, by asking each family member to speculate about the extent to which each type of environment applies to the family.

The therapist might ask the parent and adolescent to tell each other what forms of positive verbal and nonverbal feedback they are comfortable with. Sometimes, effusive parents may overwhelm adolescents who are more comfortable with more indirect positive feedback. Adolescents with poor self-esteem may not feel deserving of praise and sometimes say they prefer other types of feedback. Similarly, parents may be hungry for even a single appreciative comment from their adolescent. Most adolescents with ADHD are self-centered and would not normally think of praising their parents; Barkley (1997a) argues that self-centeredness is one of the traits that follows from poor self-regulation affect/arousal motivation.

Point Systems

Point systems or token economies may be appropriate for 11- to 13-year-old adolescents but typically are perceived as trivial and childlike for older adolescents, for whom other positive incentives may be more effective. Designing a point system begins with the following steps: (1) the parent decides what chores, tasks, and social behaviors the adolescent will earn points for; (2) the parent determines how many points can be earned; (3)

the adolescent lists potential rewards; (4) the parent, with some input from the adolescent, decides how many points must be earned to receive a specific privilege, and how often the privilege can be earned; (5) the parent monitors the adolescent's behavior and awards the points as decided; and (6) the parent and adolescent review the point chart or book and the adolescent either receives or does not receive the decided-on privileges. Based on 20 years of clinical experience with such systems, Barkley (1996d) has made a number of suggestions for how to enhance the effectiveness of point systems:

1. Introduce the program on a positive, upbeat note that emphasizes privileges to be gained rather than lost.
2. Keep the list of behaviors at a reasonable length, rather than overloading it with trivial items.
3. Have at least 15 items on the list of rewards and emphasize those that can be earned on a daily rather than weekly basis because ADHD adolescents satiate easily on any particular reward and do not delay gratification easily. Don't include basic necessities such as regular meals, snack after school, reasonable clothing, etc., on the list, but do include the adolescent's weekly allowance. If the youth loses interest in some rewards after several weeks, replace them with new items on the list.
4. Be sure at least one-third of the privileges are available every day if the adolescent earns sufficient points to purchase them.
5. Use points tracked with a checkbook register or notebook that does not look too childish. The chart on the refrigerator may be demeaning to adolescents.
6. With adolescents, use a large number of points, such as 25 points for a chore and 100–200 per day. Large numbers look better to youngsters than do smaller numbers.
7. Do the math for the system such that the youngster spends twothirds of his or her daily income on his or her daily privileges; thus although they can accrue some points toward long-term rewards, they don't save so many points that motivation dwindles.
8. Build in bonuses for a positive attitude.
9. Schedule frequent opportunities for the exchange of points.
10. Pay only for compliance to the first request.
11. Dispense the points liberally but contingently. Don't be a miser. The therapist might need to provide a minimum quota of points for the parents to dispense if they might otherwise be miserly about it.
12. Don't implement point fines in the first week, and if you do later implement fines for problem behavior, keep the system in approximately a 2:1 rewards to fines balance (i.e., give out twice as many points as you take back in fines).

13. Don't fall into a punishment spiral where all the points are taken away in one bad episode.
14. Make sure that the parents do not give out the points unless the work has been done.

The therapist should become familiar with these guidelines and build them into the development of a point system with a family. The actual point system needs to be reasonably simple to have any chance of being effectively implemented, even though it reflects a sophisticated understanding of reinforcement principles applied to ADHD. When using point systems even with immature, young adolescents, the therapist needs to set it up in such a way that the adolescent does not perceive it as silly or childish. When one or both parents also have ADHD, point systems often require too much coordination for the parent to follow consistently, and the therapist might accomplish the same goal by using behavioral contracting.

Behavioral Contracts

A behavioral contract is simply a written agreement between a parent and an adolescent specifying an exchange of behavior for privileges. Spelling out a verbal agreement in writing underscores each party's commitment to change and prevents later misunderstanding of the terms of the agreement. The contract can be short or long, simple or complex; it can cover one specific exchange or many different exchanges (similar to a point system), depending on the therapist's judgment of the family's interaction style and ability to carry it out effectively. The therapist can quickly and spontaneously guide a family to write a simple contract with no advance preparation or planning, making it a useful technique when dealing with impulsive families that frequently change topics in midstream and bring up major crises in the last 20 seconds of a therapy session. Similarly, the parents can be taught to "think contract" as they deal with the vicissitudes of adolescent behavior at home and, whenever a spontaneously developing problem seems amenable to a contract, to write one on the spur of the moment. Even if the contract does not solve all the family's problems, it may avert an immediate showdown and carry the family until the next therapy session, when problem-solving and/or other techniques can be used to deal more extensively with the issue. As indicated earlier in the chapter, behavioral contracts also dovetail nicely with problem solving in that agreements reached through problem solving may be formalized in behavioral contracts, which then govern their implementation.

The therapist should first prompt the parents and the adolescent together to write a draft of the agreement. Then, they review the first draft and discuss the details of the wording, making sure to get everyone's perspective. Afterward, a final draft of the contract should be written, signed, and dated by everyone involved. The contract should clearly specify the behaviors to be performed by the adolescent, the date and time the behaviors are to be performed, and the consequences for complying with and not complying with the terms of the contract. The therapist needs to decide based on clinical experience with each family the degree of detail necessary for a given family. The spontaneously negotiated variety of contracts are likely to begin with less detail, and if implementation problems arise, add more details. The family should keep the contract handy. Patterson and Forgatch (1987) suggest that families might start a binder in which they keep all of their contracts and monitoring forms.

Following are several examples of contracts that families negotiated:

I, Bill Peterson, agree to come home on Saturday nights by 12:00 A.M. If I am more than 5 minutes late, I understand that I will be grounded from the telephone Sunday through Tuesday.

Signed, *Bill Peterson Randy Peterson Molly Peterson* Date: 11/3/98

I, Sally Jones [teenager], agree to clear the dishes from the table, rinse them off, put them in the dishwasher with soap, and turn the dishwasher on by 8:00 P.M. on Sundays through Fridays. In return, I, Patricia Jones [mother] agree to drive Sally to and from a maximum of three school sports events or dances per week; Sally needs to give me two days notice of when she wants to be driven to a game.

Signed, *Sally Jones Patricia Jones* Date: October 1, 1998

Amanda Arnold agrees to clean up her room every Saturday by noon. We consider the room to be clean if:

a. The bed is made with four hospital corners.
b. The trash basket has nothing in it.
c. All books, papers, CDs, makeup, etc., is off the floor and in a drawer or neatly placed on a bookshelf.
d. The carpet has been vacuumed (i.e., we heard the vacuum cleaner running for at least 5 minutes and there is no visible dirt on the carpet).

Mrs. Sandy Arnold will inspect the room at noon on Saturday. If the room meets all the criteria in this agreement, Amanda earns anyone of the following privileges:

a. Go to the movies with a girlfriend that evening. Parents pay for her ticket.
b. Rent two videos that evening.
c. Five dollars allowance.

This contract will be in effect for 2 weeks from the date it is signed, and then it will be reviewed for modifications in a family meeting.

Signed, *Amanda Arnold Sandy Arnold* Date: March 5, 1998

The first contract is very brief and was spontaneously negotiated by the family on Saturday evening at 7:00 P.M., when Bill got a last-minute date with the pretty blond who was in his math class. It specified a loss of a privilege if what was a later-than-normal curfew is not adhered to. The second contract provides a little more detail about the behaviors to be performed and the privilege to be earned, including the safeguard for the mother of the 48-hour notification. This contract specifies an exchange of activities between parent and adolescent. The third contract more obsessively covers all the details and even specifies a trial period after which it will be reviewed and revised; such a trial period is often a good idea for parents who feel they are taking a risk in permitting more freedom and adolescents who feel they are being asked to do too many chores. Many things could go wrong because of missing details in the first two contracts. The therapist should teach the family to deal with these problems as they arise. In my experience, it is better to teach families with ADHD adolescents to quickly reach some contractual agreement, get it going, and then refine it over time than to deal with a bored, restless adolescent during a long therapy session working out all the possible problems and planning to work around them.

Allowance

Monetary allowances are a powerful positive incentive which serve dual purposes: (1) encouraging compliance and positive behavior and (2) teaching the adolescent the value of money. An ADHD adolescent should always earn his or her allowance by completing household responsibilities. Because of the impaired delayed responding associated with ADHD, it is also desirable that the allowance be paid, at least in part, daily, rather than weekly. The total weekly allowance could be divided, with a small portion paid for daily chores and another portion paid for weekly responsibilities. The therapist needs to help the parents decide how much allowance will be earned per week, to select the chores or responsibilities the adolescent will be required to complete, and to assign a monetary value to each task. Then, a system for tracking completion of the daily and/or weekly chores needs to be established, and the system needs to implemented and evaluated over several weeks.

Several factors need to be carefully considered with regard to the goal of teaching the adolescent the value of money. The amount of money to be paid per week should depend on what the family can afford, what the allowance is meant to cover, how much money the teen earns independent of the allowance, and how hard the adolescent is willing work around the house. The amount should increase as the adolescent gets older. The parent and adolescent need to discuss whether the allowance is meant to cover gas money, lunch money, clothing, cosmetics, or just miscellaneous spending money. If the adolescent earns money outside the home through a part-time job, the parents should take this into account. The therapist needs to develop local norms for what common allowances are in his or her community, taking income into account, so that he or she can help parents make such determinations. No family, however, should pay more than they can afford because of pressure from the adolescent.

Adolescents with ADHD initially may spend all their allowance as soon as they receive it. One of the advantages of a daily allowance compared to a weekly allowance is that the adolescent cannot spend it all at once. The therapist may wish to work with parents to have the family require that the adolescent save part of the allowance and have the remainder available for spending. If the adolescent who is receiving a weekly allowance spends it all at the beginning of the week and asks for more money, the answer must be "no." Otherwise, the adolescent will not be forced to learn how to handle money.

Sometimes pitfalls arise as a result of relying too much on money as a reinforcer. Some adolescents may belittle the value of money received from their parents, reducing its effectiveness. Others may become too materialistic, demanding large sums of money to perform even trivial behaviors. Giving money also may become an easy out for parents who wish to avoid doing more time-consuming but relationship-building activities with their adolescents. The therapist needs to judge each family individually with regard to the extent to which money becomes a recommended reinforcer.

Shaping

The principle of shaping involves reinforcing successive approximations to a desired goal response and shaping the behavior in the direction of that goal. Shaping is applicable to all the positive incentives discussed in this chapter. The therapist needs to teach the family to shape each other's behaviors gradually in desired directions rather than waiting until a big change occurs, which may take forever. For example, Mrs. Jones was writing a contract with Jennifer for practicing the violin. Currently, Jennifer practices for 5 to 10 minutes once or twice a week; her violin teacher asked her to practice for half an hour five times a week. Mrs. Jones recognizes that this will be a large change for her daughter, and she decides to apply the principle of shaping. They write a contract to require 10 minutes of practice a day for the first week, 20 minutes a day for the second week, and 30 minutes a day afterward. The contract worked well because it eased Jennifer into more frequent practice and permitted her to earn privileges immediately, motivating her to keep working harder over time.

Punishment Systems

The therapist needs to remind the family of Barkley's principle, "Incentives before punishments." Adolescents with ADHD need a combination of the carrot and the stick, but the stick without the carrot is less effective than the combination of positive incentives and punishments. Effective punishments need to be small and enforceable and to fit the crime and the family environment. Such punishments include grounding, taking away privileges, work chores, and making restitution/overcorrection. Parents also need to learn to focus on the need for action when issuing a punishment—many adolescents impulsively say "no way" but then comply within a few minutes; issuing backup punishments without waiting a few minutes to see if compliance is forthcoming is counterproductive in such situations.

Grounding

Grounding the adolescent to the house for a period of time is a common and often effective punishing consequence. Parents unfortunately have a tendency to issue long groundings (e.g., the adolescent is grounded until the next report card arrives or for 2 weeks or a month). Such an extended grounding loses its meaning, ends up being unenforceable and more punishing for the parents than the adolescent, and demonstrates no evidence to support its greater effectiveness than a shorter grounding. I recommend that parents ground an adolescent 1 day at a time.

Parents may also want to create a hierarchy of levels of grounding to have a variety of consequences available for repeated offenses. For example, level one might be grounding from the telephone, level two might be grounding from the television, level three might be grounding to the house, and level four might be grounding to the adolescent's room.

Taking Away Privileges

Grounding represents one example of taking away privileges. Parents can creatively remove an infinite variety of privileges contingent upon problem behavior or failure to carry out responsibilities. Examples include telephone usage (1 day at a time), television time, CD player, computer use, video games, having a friend over, borrowing things, special foods, bicycle or skateboard, use of the car, and parental rides to special events. As with grounding, taking away privileges for extended periods is counterproductive and not more effective than removing them for shorter periods of time. The therapist should discuss with the parents and the adolescent which privileges are most meaningful. Parents should only remove those privileges they can control and see through to the end, and they should remove the privilege the same day the negative behavior took place.

For example, it is not effective for a single parent who works until 6:00 P.M. to tell her 15-year-old son that he cannot watch television after school, unless she has some mechanism to monitor his compliance with the punishment. In this case, either another adult would have to be present until the mother came home, or she would have to purchase one of the devices that prevents the television from being turned on unless she enters the appropriate code.

Work Chores

Effortful work around the house is another form of punishment often effective with adolescents. Such work might include dusting, vacuuming, cleaning the toilets, mopping, laundry, and so on. Adolescents with ADHD often seem "allergic" to effort, rendering work chores very effective. The therapist needs to gauge the degree of oppositionality of a particular adolescent and the parents' ability to get the adolescent to do the work chores. In some cases, the parental effort involved in getting the adolescent to start and stick with the work chore may outweigh its value as a punishment. This will be an individual clinical decision in each case. Patterson and Forgatch (1987) recommend a work chore of 5 minutes' duration; whether the chore takes 5, 10, or 15 minutes, similar to grounding, the chore should not be of long duration and should be imposed on the same day as the infraction. These authors outline eight steps for parents when imposing a work chore:

1. Set the stage so you may not have to impose the work chore.
2. Warn the adolescent that you will impose a work chore as soon as your request is not met with compliance.
3. Don't argue or lecture. (Act, don't yak.)
4. Each time you are about to make a request, have two work chores in mind to impose, if needed.
5. Impose no more than two work chores before going to a backup punishment such as withdrawing a privilege.
6. Make sure the chore is brief.
7. Stay out of the way while the adolescent is doing the chore.
8. Stay calm and neutral.

These work chore guidelines might easily be generalized to administering any punishing consequence. Parents often are so upset and angry by the adolescent's problem behavior that they issue punishments in sarcastic, demeaning, baiting ways which invite aggressive counterattacks from their adolescents. The therapist might ask the parents and adolescent to role-play issuing each of the punishments in this chapter in a calm, neutral, yet assertive manner. Such practice will not only prepare the family for the real thing but make salient to the adolescent the parents' commitment to consistent follow-through with consequences for their behavior. Such practice could even be integrated into communication training.

The guideline about staying out of the way after issuing a work chore cannot be overemphasized. Many parents are so angry at their adolescents that after issuing a punishment, they hound them and try to spur more interaction. Such a tactic often backfires, with an escalation of coercive, negative interactions. The therapist should advise parents to give adolescents plenty of space while they are doing the work chore. Afterward, parents need to check on the quality of the work, and if it was not adequately completed, require that it be redone.

Overcorrection

Overcorrection is a behavioral technique that involves making restitution for a problem behavior by repeatedly practicing a prosocial alternative response. This is the official behavior modification version of the timeless teacher punishment of writing "I will not talk out of turn" 100 times. In situations in which adolescents have destroyed property or stolen property that did not belong to them, restitution is an essential part of the punishment package. Sometimes, restitution is a sufficient consequence by itself; other times, the therapist might advise parents to also take away privileges or ground the adolescent. Because restitution typically involves unpleasant work, it can also be seen as a variation on work chores. An angry adolescent who kicks a hole in the wall should be expected to clean up the mess and help repair the damage; they may also be asked to make further restitution by washing all the walls in the house or doing another onerous clean-up chore. A parent might ask an adolescent to do community service for the poor as a form of restitution for stealing money.

CONCLUSION

This chapter extensively discussed intervention to reduce parent–adolescent conflict when the problems are negotiable. That is, parents and adolescents can work them out best through mutual discussion and agreement. Chapter 10, in discussing principles of parenting the ADHD adolescent, made the important distinction between those issues subject to negotiation and those that are not. Basic house rules and street rules are not subject to negotiation (e.g., parents are still basically in charge of adolescents, and it is not subject to negotiation). The next chapter discusses how the clinician can intervene to bolster parental authority and help parents deal with non-negotiable issues, as well as how to deal with common structural problems which some families encounter.

CHAPTER TWELVE

———— O ————

Restoring Parental Control and Other Structural Interventions

In the Introduction to Section III the first two questions about prioritizing therapeutic goals were whether the adolescent was out of control and whether he or she was abusing substances. If the answer to either question was "yes," I recommended that the therapist address these issues before proceeding with any other component of the intervention. In essence, I am referring here to adolescents with comorbid severe ODD, CD, and/or Substance Use Disorders. If substance use is more than occasional and recreational, practitioners should refer the adolescent to a substance abuse treatment program. If his or her use is recreational and some motivation to change is apparent, the therapist should arrange for careful monitoring of possible substance use while continuing therapy. When the parents have very little control over the adolescent, I recommend an intensive family-oriented intervention.

This chapter addresses techniques for restoring parental control as a prime example of structural/functional interventions within the family. In addition, I address structural problems such as those that commonly arise in stepfamilies. In Chapter 2, I introduced the concepts of hierarchy, alignment, coalitions, triangulation, and cohesion within the family systems model of parent–adolescent relations. Before we can discuss specific interventions for restoring parental control or other problems of ADHD adolescents related to family structure, we need to expand on these concepts.

STRUCTURAL/FUNCTIONAL PROBLEMS

Structural/functional problems are fundamentally problems of hierarchy, alignment, and sequence within families. The biology of ADHD predisposes families to problems of hierarchy, alignment, and sequencing; therefore, it is important for the practitioner to understand these constructs and how they interact with the core symptoms of ADHD in order to develop effective interventions.

All families have a hierarchy or pecking order which either explicitly or implicitly defines the distribution of power within the family. In Western civilization, parents are generally supposed to be in charge of children, even adolescent children, and are thus supposed to be elevated in the power hierarchy to the top position. Adolescents are not supposed to be dictating to their parents. In two-parent families, mothers and fathers are supposed to work as a team in childrearing; parental consistency makes life easier for everyone. Parent–adolescent arguments, rebellious adolescent behavior, family fights, bursts of negative communication, inadequate problem solving, and distorted thinking take place within the context and stream of ongoing interactions between family members.

Within a behavioral family systems model of parent–adolescent relations, the concepts of hierarchy, alignment, coalition, triangulation, cohesion, disengagement, and enmeshment have proven most clinically useful (Robin & Foster, 1989). As mentioned previously, hierarchy refers to the pecking order or distribution of power in a family. If the parents are in charge of the children, we say that the hierarchy is correct; in the most common problematic situation in families with adolescents who have ADHD, the teenagers are in charge of the parents or have too much power. We call this "hierarchy reversal." Hierarchy reversal is clearly a problem because impulsive adolescents may make dangerous, unwise decisions in the absence of effective parental controls. Clearly, the out-of-control adolescent with ADHD and comorbid CD and his or her parents represent a severe example of hierarchy reversal.

Alignment refers to a family member joining or opposing another family member who is carrying out some function in the family. In a coalition, two family members consistently take sides against the third on some issue or action. Therapists encourage parents to take sides against the adolescent in childrearing; this represents a within-generational coalition and is synonymous with parental consistency. However, when a parent and adolescent consistently take sides against the other parent, this type of cross-generational coalition may become problematic because the adolescent may avoid important responsibilities or misbehave unchecked. Triangulation is essentially a sequence of unstable coalitions—two family members place the third in the middle, and the third vacillates, first siding with one and then with the other. Similarly to cross-generational coalitions, the adolescent in a triangulated family interaction may effectively manipulate the situation to avoid important responsibilities or get away with serious misbehaviors.

Cohesion refers to the degree of closeness or distance in relationships between family members. Cohesion is best thought of as a bipolar continuum, with disengagement or great distance between family members at the one extreme and enmeshment or a high degree of closeness and overin-volvement between family members at the other extreme. A father–son dyad would be disengaged when the father never knows his son's where-abouts and the son rarely interacts with his dad. A mother–daughter dyad would be enmeshed if the mother or daughter could not go for more than 5 or 10 minutes without touching base with each other about something, good or bad. Family interaction researchers have generally found that a moderate degree of cohesion promotes positive interaction in most West-ern families (Robin & Foster, 1989).

There is one more very important aspect to structure—the sequencing of structures in time, which creates function. We can best understand se-quencing through the use of a videotape or motion picture analogy. A videotape is made up of many individual frames; the image on each frame consists of thousands of pixels or binary points. When the videotape is played, the frames go by in very rapid succession, creating the sensation of continuous motion or the stream of action in real time. The structure of the family at any one point in time is similar to a single frame of the videotape. The skills and cognitions of the family members are equivalent to the pix-els or binary points on a single frame. As family members behave in real time, each frame of structure goes through the videocassette recorder, cre-ating the stream of family interaction. When the clinician constructs a pic-ture of family structure involving hierarchy, alignment, and cohesion, he or she looks at a cross-section of the video. If the clinician repeatedly samples cross-sections by stopping the video of family life on numerous occasions, he or she will start to see regularities or cycles of structure over time. Through observation and analysis of these cycles, the clinician draws infer-ences about the functions of each person's behavior within the family sys-tem.

I find the social learning framework (Patterson, 1982) useful to de-scribe the functions of family members' responses within such repetitive, interlocking sequences. The most common functions are positive reinforce-ment, negative reinforcement, punishment, escape, avoidance, coercion, and reciprocity (Robin & Foster, 1989). Following is a clinical example of each function:

1. *Positive reinforcement.* When Mr. and Mrs. McMillan took a unit-ed stand with Sally, telling her together she had to work harder at getting her homework done on time, she began to spend 2 hours a night on home-work and within 2 weeks was getting it all done on time. Mr. and Mrs. McMillan's behavior of taking a strong, united stand was positively rein-forced by Sally's compliance, and the couple went on to do the same thing with other issues. In positive reinforcement, the contingent administration of a consequence increases the future probability of the behavior that pro-duced the consequence. Mr. and Mrs. McMillan's behavior also illustrates, structurally speaking, a strong parental coalition.

2. *Negative reinforcement/escape.* Damon constantly badgers his mother to let him get his license. She gets so sick and tired of his badgering that she finally gives in and permits him to get his license. Damon's badgering was an aversive stimulus to his mother; when she gave in, he stopped badgering or removed the aversive stimulus. His mother's behavior of giving in and taking him to get his license was negatively reinforced because it removed an aversive stimulus. The contingent removal of an aversive stimulus, increasing the future probability of the behavior that removed it, constitutes negative reinforcement. Damon's mother also *escaped* the aversive stimulus of his badgering by giving in.

3. *Punishment.* Mary argues with her father when he asks her to do her chores. He grounds her from the telephone for the evening. Mary stops arguing with him afterward. The grounding punished his daughter's arguing behavior. A contingent stimulus which decreases the future probability of emission of a behavior constitutes punishment.

4. *Avoidance.* Avoidance behavior is a response which prevents the occurrence of an anticipated aversive stimulus or event. Many children with ADHD act out in public places, embarrassing their parents. Many parents stop taking those children to malls and stores. Not taking the child would be an example of avoidance behavior because it is designed to avoid the anticipated negative consequence of the child's misbehaving in the public building.

5. *Coercion.* Coercion (Patterson, 1982) represents a combination of negative and positive reinforcement, and escape. As mentioned in Chapter 2, coercion is one of the major processes through which repertoires of aggressive behavior are shaped in children with ADHD, as a function of many family interactions over a number of years. Thus, coercion is a central function in families with ADHD members. Rodney is belligerent, demanding, and argumentative toward his parents. Whenever he wants something, he throws a major tantrum, yelling, screaming, cursing, and constantly nagging his mother. At first, she tries to ignore him, but he persists. Next, she yells at him, but he persists. Eventually, she gets to the end of her rope and caves in to appease him, permitting him to have whatever he wants just to get him off her back. Rodney's demanding behavior is positively reinforced by his mother getting him whatever he wants; his mother's appeasing behavior is negatively reinforced by removing the aversive stimulus of his tantrums and nagging, permitting her to escape from his aversive behavior. The combination of positive reinforcement of demanding behavior and negative reinforcement of the response to the demanding behavior constitutes coercion. Over time, substantial repertoires of negative interactions may be built up and maintained through coercion. As Barkley (1990) has eloquently pointed out, family members quickly learn to skip the early, less intense responses in the chain of coercive behavior, over time more rapidly escalating to the most severe responses.

6. *Reciprocity.* Reciprocity basically refers to an equity in the exchange of positive or negative behavior over time between two family members (e.g., "you get what you give in family relations"). Sara and her mother, Mrs. Antonio, for example, pick at each other frequently. Sara loses it and calls her mother "stupid" and "mean." Her mother yells at Sara a lot for not doing her chores adequately. They frequently exchange or reciprocate negative behaviors and eventually build up grudges and negative perceptions of each other. By contrast, Mr. Antonio is more laid back and overlooks Sara's incomplete chores and slovenly appearance. He rarely says anything to his daughter about these issues, and he hardly ever yells at her. Sara rarely talks back to him. Their conversations are marked by more neutral or positive exchanges. They reciprocate positive behaviors. The difference in style between Mr. and Mrs. Antonio may also inadvertently lead Sara to seek out a cross-generational coalition with her father against her mother. Even if Mr. Antonio does nothing to encourage this coalition, his wife may view his intransigence as tacit side taking against her, fueling marital conflict.

Case Example of Multiple Structural/Functional Problems

The Morass family consists of 15-year-old Mitchell, his natural mother, Belinda, and his stepfather, Adam. Adam and Belinda married 6 months ago. Belinda was divorced from Mitchell's natural father, Bill, 2 years ago, after a bitter fight. Belinda always suspected that Bill had ADHD, but he would never agree to be evaluated or to deal with any of his problems. His hot temper, verbal abusiveness, infidelity, and inability to hold down a job and consistently provide for his family contributed to her decision to divorce him. Bill is very angry that Belinda divorced him, and he frequently bad-mouths Belinda to Mitchell during visits and gets angry if Mitchell says positive things about Adam.

Adam was married before but did not have any children. He is not at all familiar with ADHD and generally believes that wayward teenagers need strict discipline to get straightened out. During their courtship, Belinda did not go into any detail about her son's problems, and the couple did not talk extensively about what Adam's role would be in parenting Mitchell or how they would deal with Bill's potential interference.

Mitchell now lives with his mother and stepfather but visits his natural father, Bill, every other weekend. Mitchell was diagnosed as having ADHD at age 8 and has been treated intermittently with Ritalin and individual and family therapy since that time. Mitchell's current presenting problems include family conflict, especially with Adam, poor school performance, and angry outbursts involving destruction of property in the home. Through careful interviewing, the therapist discerned the following repetitive sequence:

1. Mitchell returns from a weekend visit with Bill. It is always a difficult transition.
2. His homework is not completed and he is "wired." He does a lot of physical activities with his dad. The rules are also very different in the two household. He can do whatever he wants at his dad's, but he must watch his language and behavior at his mom's house.
3. Belinda discovers that Bill did not give Mitchell his Ritalin over the weekend and made no attempt to get Mitchell to do his homework. She manages to avoid badmouthing her ex-husband but gruffly asks Mitchell to complete his homework.
4. Mitchell refuses, saying he is too tired now and will do it during first-period Learning Resource Center (LRC) class Monday.
5. Adam steps in and tells Mitchell to do what his mother asked.
6. Mitchell blows up and tells Adam he does not have to listen to him because Adam is not his real father. Adam yells at Mitchell to get to work on his homework and stop the nasty language or else. . . . An argument ensues.
7. Belinda tries to stay out of it, but after a few minutes she begins to worry that her son and husband might hurt each other, or that perhaps Adam does not really appreciate how to deal with a teenager with ADHD. She has been trying to get Adam to go a CH.A.D.D. meeting or read about ADHD, but he has not yet done either. Her vision of the happy stepfamily vanishes before her eyes as she listens to her son and husband going at each other. She tries to calm the two of them down.
8. Adam accuses Belinda of interfering in his attempts to discipline Mitchell. He storms out of the room with Belinda trailing him. They have an argument upstairs. Adam blames it all on Bill's interference in their parenting of Mitchell. Belinda agrees but gently asks her husband to consider learning more about ADHD. He agrees. They calm down. The couple makes up and have some very tender moments afterward. They totally forget about Mitchell's undone homework for now.
9. Mitchell goes to his room and plays video games. He is on total overload, between his dad badmouthing his mom and Adam, Adam telling him to do his homework, the differences between the two households, and his loyalty conflicts to his mom and dad. His mind is racing and he really does not fully understand why or what to do to calm down. He blots everything out by playing Mortal Combat on his Sega. It feels good to get his aggressions out this way. By the next morning, he has totally forgotten about the incomplete homework and receives a failing grade on it.
10. Bill calls Mitchell the next day to see how things are going and Mitchell tells his dad everything that happened that night before. Bill lets Mitchell know that he is pleased about the argument be-

tween Belinda and Adam and Adam's poor treatment of Mitchell. It confirms his view of his ex-wife as an incompetent parent. He promises to protect Mitchell from Adam. Mitchell gets frustrated with his dad because his dad has made and failed to keep many promises in the past, but he is afraid to tell his dad about his anger and frustration. Instead, when he gets off the phone, he kicks the cat and pulls its tail. He feels like kicking a hole in the wall, but he knows that would get him in big trouble and he does remember that his therapist, Dr. Jones, told him to try to get his anger out in a safe way.

What structural patterns are present? The within-generational coalition between Belinda and Adam is fragile, and it falls apart when Mitchell manipulates the situation by picking an argument with his stepfather. Adam is attempting to discipline Mitchell too soon in his relationship with his stepson. He does not understand that he cannot discipline Mitchell until he has a stronger relationship with him, and until Bill's interference has been more effectively neutralized. He also does not understand or know how to cope with Mitchell's ADHD. Belinda is triangulated between her husband and son, sometimes siding with one and sometimes with another. When Belinda worries that her husband is not responding to her son appropriately, she interferes protectively. This spurs marital conflict. She and her husband are also in a coalition against her ex-husband; they find it easy to blame Bill for Mitchell's behavior. At another level of analysis, Bill is in a cross-generational coalition with his son against his ex-wife and her new husband. He badmouths his ex-wife and her new husband to his son and instigates his son to misbehave at home, increasing the chances of this happening by failing to give Mitchell his Ritalin and responsibly supervising him on homework. It is no coincidence that the conflict occurred shortly after Mitchell's return from a visitation weekend. Impulsive youngsters have a difficult time with transitions between households and are likely to act out just before or after such transitions.

What functions might these interactions serve for the participants? Homework is an aversive stimulus which Mitchell avoids by starting an argument with his mother and stepfather. Bill also positively reinforces Mitchell's behavior of fostering conflict between his mother and stepfather. At another level, Bill and Belinda reciprocate negative interactions through their son. Mitchell and Adam reciprocate negative behavior directly, and Mitchell's defiance also is coercive to his mother and stepfather. When they back off and argue with each other, Mitchell stops arguing with them, negatively reinforcing them for backing off. Bill also reaffirms his control over Mitchell and creates problems for his ex-wife; furthermore, he can avoid dealing with his son's handicapping condition of ADHD and blame his son's problems on his ex-wife. Belinda and Adam also externalize blame on Bill for Mitchell's failure to do his homework and avoid the difficult responsibility of effectively structuring the study environment for an adolescent with ADHD. In addition, as with many couples, making up after an argument puts Belinda and Adam in a very amorous mood. Leaving Mitchell to his own devices and forgetting about his homework is therefore strongly negatively reinforced for the couple because it indirectly sets the stage for intimacy.

Of course, these functions must be regarded as hypotheses, which are subject to further clinical examination as the therapist gets to know the family. Nonetheless, they illustrate how each person's behavior interlocks with the others', and how Mitchell's ADHD, not to mention his father's possible ADHD, becomes an organizing factor in a sequence of structural difficulties encountered by this stepfamily.

Throughout this chapter, I highlight the interplay between structure and function in analysis and intervention of recurring, circular interaction patterns in family systems with members diagnosed as having ADHD. Specifically, I consider five types of structural/functional patterns the practitioner often encounters in families with adolescents diagnosed as having ADHD: (1) weak parental coalitions/parental inconsistency; (2) the out-of-control adolescent with severe hierarchy reversal; (3) children acting better for their fathers than for their mothers; (4) a mother feels like she has two children (teen and husband); and (5) stepfamily issues. Table 12.1 summarizes these five, common underlying structural dimensions and the pre-

TABLE 12.1. Common Structural Problems

Problem	Structural pattern	Intervention
1. Parental inconsistency	Weak parental coalition Cross-generational coalition	1. Prompt, reinforce teamwork 2. Block teen's interference
2. Out-of-control teen	Hierarchy reversal Weak parental coalition Cross-generational coalition	1. Reinforce parental authority 2. Build parental coalition 3. Behavioral contracting 4. Extrafamilial controls
3. Kids act better for Dad than for Mom	Cross-generational coalition	1. Educate Dad 2. Get Dad to back Mom
4. "I have two kids— my son and my husband"	Inverted hierarchy	1. Get Dad evaluated for ADHD 2. Reallocate spousal roles 3. Damage control
5. Stepfamily problems	Triangulation Cross-generational coalitions	1. Deal with both families 2. Address loyalty issues 3. Address environmental issues

ferred interventions. During the discussion of stepfamilies, we return to Mitchell, Belinda, Adam, and Bill, and develop approaches to intervene to change aspects of their situation.

INCONSISTENCY/WEAK PARENTAL COALITION

A weak parental coalition refers to a situation in which two parents disagree about how to discipline an adolescent, and the adolescent takes advantage of this disagreement to disobey parental rules and commands or to avoid parent-imposed responsibilities. The following pattern typifies this situation: (1) the adolescent misbehaves or disobeys the parents' rules; (2) one parent attempts to impose a consequence; (3) either the adolescent complains about the first parent's actions to the second parent or the second parent spontaneously notices the situation; (4) the second parent reacts to the adolescent differently than does the first parent; (5) the two parents either overtly or covertly disagree about how to handle the situation, resulting in either no action or ineffective action actually being taken; and (6) the adolescent ignores both parents' interventions and continues to do as he or she pleases. Sometimes one of the parents sides with the adolescent against the other parent. Then, we are also dealing with a cross-generational coalition.

The therapist's goals are to educate the parents about the harmful impact of such inconsistency and/or side taking and to build a strong parental coalition, blocking any interference from the adolescent. The therapist might ask the parents to reach an agreement concerning rules or regulations pertaining to the issue under consideration, while instructing the adolescent to listen quietly. If the adolescent interrupts the parents, tries to sidetrack the conversation or, through nonverbal behavior, to distract from the agreement being reached, the therapist bluntly prevents the interruption from being successful and redirects the parents back to the task of reaching an agreement. The parents are asked how the adolescent interferes with their acting as a team at home, and they are prepared to resist such interruptions when they need to work together at home in the future. The therapist might use problem solving, communication training, and behavior management techniques strategically to accomplish these goals. For example, the couple could be asked to problem-solve the issue of how to respond consistently when an adolescent throws a tantrum or kicks a hole in the wall. Making statements indicative of cross-generational side taking might be defined as a negative communication target, and each parent might be asked to correct the other when side-taking statements are made. A clearly specified behavioral contract with an accompanying behavior chart system for monitoring might be written to help two parents work as a team in enforcing the rules concerning curfew or chores.

Often, parental inconsistencies and disagreements about how to deal with adolescent problem behaviors stem from factors that may not be immediately apparent to the therapist, such as the parents' belief systems and family of origin experiences. Parents may have been grappling with their inconsistencies for many years, and may even realize that they ought to be more consistent, but may be unaware of why they automatically fall into the same pattern over and over again and are just unable to change. Impulsive, hyperactive, challenging youngsters bring out and magnify even the most minute parental inconsistencies, as if the parents were under a microscope. Ideally, some of these distorted beliefs and family-of-origin issues would have been identified during the sessions devoted to childrearing approaches, parenting principles, and beliefs/expectations. Nonetheless, the therapist may need to investigate what underlies such differences to help the parents resolve them. A case I recently treated illustrates my approach to the weak parental coalition, with additional factors underlying parental inconsistencies.

Case Example of Weak Parental Coalition

Mr. and Mrs. Cheyne and 13-year-old Valerie, the identified ADHD patient, showed up for a family therapy session very distraught. As soon as they sat down, Valerie blurted out that she hated her mother, who had been very mean to her last night. When her mother had asked her to put the dishes away, Valerie had responded "in a few minutes," in her best 13-year-old intense and gruff voice tone. As always, Mrs. Cheyne thought her daughter was purposely being sarcastic, and she told Valerie to watch her tongue. When Valerie returned her mother's fire in an escalating, critical manner, a yelling match ensued, culminating in the mother and daughter vowing that they hated each other. Mr. Cheyne heard the argument and called a family meeting. He wanted Valerie to apologize to her mother, and then he wanted to drop the whole incident. Mrs. Cheyne wanted Valerie grounded for 2 weeks, during which time Valerie alone would do the dishes. Valerie accused her mother of being unfair to her and bossing her father around, and she told her father that he was the parent she really cared about. Mr. Cheyne did not know what to do or say, but before he could act, Mrs. Cheyne stormed out of the family meeting because she felt that her husband's intransigence reflected his siding with their daughter. Meanwhile, Valerie avoided any punishment. The dishes were still waiting to be put away 24 hours later. This type of situation recurred regularly with the Cheyne family—Valerie and her mother getting into it; Mrs. Cheyne wanting to punish Valerie more severely than her husband did; and the parents disagreeing, with Valerie avoiding any consequences for her rude behavior.

I strongly suspected that there was more than meets the eye to the parental differences, in part because this couple seemed to genuinely care about each other and their daughter, but they nonetheless repeatedly got stuck in such traps. I also suspected that Mrs. Cheyne had many of the same impulsive tendencies as Valerie, even though she might not meet clinical criteria for ADHD. After sending Valerie to the waiting room for a few minutes so that Mr. and Mrs. Cheyne would not have to lose face in front of their daughter, I pointed out to the parents that their inconsistencies were setting them up for failure; Valerie was dividing and conquering, setting herself up in a coalition with her father against her mother when it suited her fancy. I noted that Valerie did generally come across "like gangbusters," using a disrespectful, accusing tone of voice, but that this was not unusual for an ADHD 13-year-old, and perhaps Mrs. Cheyne could learn to "roll with the punches" a little more. Conceptually, she agreed, but Mrs. Cheyne felt that Valerie just pushed all her buttons and she had to respond. I asked Mrs. Cheyne whether this situation reminded her of anything in her family of origin. She seemed puzzled, but after pondering my question for a few moments, she slowly and painfully recalled that she used to get very upset when her older sister Rosa talked disrespectfully to their mother. It turned out that Rosa had treated her mother rudely for many years. Rosa was now an alcoholic, had two children out of wedlock, did not have a job, could not maintain any long-term relationships, and also had many other emotional problems. Mrs. Cheyne tearfully verbalized that she had vowed never to let anyone treat her the way her Rosa treated their mother. Valerie's disrespectful mannerisms reminded her of her sister. She feared that if Valerie did not change, she too would turn out to be a failure. Mr. Cheyne was totally surprised by this revelation; he knew nothing about Rosa's treatment of Mrs. Cheyne's mother. Thus, Mrs. Cheyne's ruinous beliefs were based on her family-of-origin experiences and were mediating her difficulty in responding more rationally to her daughter's rather typical 13-year-old negative communication style. I was able to help her put these beliefs in the perspective of present-day reality, to point out the differences between Valerie and Rosa, and to prepare Mrs. Cheyne to cognitively restructure her thoughts so she could react more reasonably to her daughter's provocative mannerisms in the future.

Next, I asked Mr. Cheyne if he could think of any factors in his family of origin that would have caused him to tolerate disrespectful adolescent behavior. He indicated that there was so much yelling in his family of origin that he just learned to tune it all out. He had just let it go by without any reaction then, as he did now. Mr. and Mrs. Cheyne agreed to work on moderating their opposite but nonetheless extreme reactions so they could be on the same wave length with Valerie. Afterward, I brought Valerie back into the session and asked her to listen quietly while her parents reached an agreement on a consistent reaction when they believed her voice tone was out of line. She interrupted their discussion 10 times in 15 minutes, but I blocked her interruptions, telling her that it was her parents' turn to talk. The couple agreed to give Valerie one opportunity to tone down her disrespect, and if she did not, to fine her 25 cents for every subsequent negative comment. Despite her bitter protestations of the inequity of this plan, she has not lost more than 75 cents a week since her parents adopted this plan.

This case illustrates the importance of investigating underlying cognitive distortions and family-of-origin issues when dealing with structural problems in ADHD families. It also illustrates the manner in which the therapist must operate simultaneously at multiple levels of analysis.

Another variation on the weak parental coalition arises when the mother and the father are both unassertive, even though they agree on what to do. At times there seems to be a bad fit between a hyperactive, controlling, type A teenager and two laid-back, passive parents. Similarly to parental inconsistency, the therapist's task is to prompt and reinforce a strong parental coalition and to block any interference by the adolescent. The techniques used in this situation are identical to those used in the earlier example of parental inconsistency.

RESTORING PARENTAL CONTROL

All the strategies discussed for weak or inconsistent parental coalitions are also applicable to restoring parental control, except that the parents are opposing a much stronger force in their belligerent, aggressive teenager. What exactly do we mean by "out of control" in an ADHD adolescent? We are referring to adolescents who are extremely noncompliant toward their parents, overtly and covertly, and who regularly engage in one or more of the following target behaviors: (1) running away from home overnight, (2) staying out all night, (3) sneaking out of the house in the middle of the night without permission, (4) engaging in physically assaultive or aggressive acts toward parents and/or siblings, (5) destroying property in the house, (6) stealing money or other things from their parents or siblings, (7) relentlessly cursing out parents in foul language directly in their presence, (8) going joy riding in the family car without a license, (9) using drugs or alcohol in the house, or (10) repeatedly and purposely lying to parents about their whereabouts or other important issues. The phrase "out of control" really refers to an inversion of the parental hierarchy, as discussed earlier in this chapter; the teenager does whatever he or she wants, and parental comments, rewards, or punishments have little impact on his or her behavior. These adolescents may often be diagnosed with CD or bipolar disorder in addition to ADHD.

There is a paucity of empirically proven, tried-and-true interventions that reliably restore parental control in the out-of-control adolescent with ADHD. In a recent volume highlighting advances in empirically based, psychosocial treatment strategies for children and adolescents (Hibbs & Jensen, 1996), clinical researchers working with conduct disorders reported limited success with preadolescents using such techniques as cognitive interpersonal problem solving and parent management training (Kazdin, 1996) and family problem-solving/structural interventions (Vuchinich, Wood, & Angelelli, 1996). Henggler, Schoenwald, Borduin, Rowland, and Cunningham's (1998) multisystemic treatment also represents a promising start at addressing these issues.

I present the strategies most commonly used clinically. These strategies include (1) building a strong parental coalition and reinforcing parental authority through structural/strategic family interventions; (2) behavioral contracting for basic house rules and street rules; (3) problem-solving training at the individual adolescent and family level; and (4) judicious use of extrafamilial controls (e.g., inpatient hospitalization, the police, and the juvenile justice system).

In two-parent families, such adolescents have typically "divided and conquered" their parents, spurring parental inconsistency and causing escalation of marital discord. The therapist's first goal is to get the parents working on the same team in setting and enforcing consequences for basic house rules and street rules. The therapist draws up a hierarchy of the out-of-control adolescent behaviors, from least to most difficult to deal with, based on the parents' and the therapist's judgment of the situation. Then, the therapist helps the parents select one of the easier behaviors from the hierarchy and guides the parents in developing a behavioral contract specifying consequences for complying with and not complying with the demand to stop the antisocial and start the prosocial behavior. These steps are taken in a session with the parents without the adolescent present. Next, the adolescent is brought in and the therapist coaches the parents in presenting the rules and the contract, blocking acting out by the adolescent. The therapist backs the parents up and exhorts them to carry out the contract at home. Usually, it is wise to arrange for telephone contact or a short interval between sessions during this week. Typically, the adolescent finds a loophole or way around the parental contingency. The therapist then helps the parents plug all the loopholes, until the adolescent has no choice but to comply. When the parents have successfully enforced one house rule or street rule, the therapist guides them to move on to a more difficult behavior. If the therapist–parent team is unable to close off the loopholes, the therapist helps the parents creatively employ extrafamilial controls, which may include a short-term placement of the adolescent in an institutional setting. This process continues until all the out-of-control behaviors have been dealt with.

Case Example of Restoring Parental Control

Dr. and Mrs. Donovan sought help with their 14-year-old ADHD son, Barry, who was sneaking out his bedroom window two times a week in the middle of the night and hanging out with his friends, entertaining girls in his bedroom during his school lunch hour and the afternoon classes he skipped, while the Donovans were at work, and cursing his parents out when they confronted him. Despite Barry's superior intellectual ability and the absence of any learning disability, he was also receiving failing grades in school and, in addition to his truancy, getting in trouble for disrespectful behavior toward teachers at least once a week. He was diagnosed as having ADHD at age 6 and had been treated with Ritalin until he refused to take it at age 12. Four previous attempts at therapy had been unsuccessful; Barry refused to talk to the therapist, and his parents eventually stopped the therapy.

Dr. Donovan was a highly intellectualized man who would endlessly lecture to his son and threaten extreme punishments which later turned out to be impossible to carry out consistently. Mrs. Donovan disagreed strongly with her husband's approach to discipline. She preferred to provide reinforcements for good behavior and short-term groundings or other similar punishments for bad behavior; she felt her husband was all talk and no real action. Barry knew exactly how to get his parents into an argument and avoid any real consequences for his out-of-control behaviors. Mrs. Donovan was becoming increasingly depressed, while Dr. Donovan was starting to avoid his family, spending long hours at the hospital seeing patients.

The situation reached crisis proportions when Barry sneaked out one night and took the family car joy riding without a license. He was stopped by the local police for speeding and going through a red light and charged as a juvenile for driving without a license. Barry wanted his parents to get him a lawyer who would get him off the hook. He threatened to destroy his father's favorite lounge chair and run away if his father did not do what he wanted. Dr. Donovan wanted his son to face whatever punishment the court would give. Mrs. Donovan wanted her husband to get her son a good lawyer and then deal with the behavior at the family level. The Donovans consulted me at this point, shortly before the juvenile hearing was scheduled.

When initially consulted by a family under these type of circumstances, I do not conduct my normal comprehensive evaluation, described in Chapters 3 through 6 (this volume), first, due to the crisis. Nonetheless, I mail out the rating scales, get releases to talk to previous therapists and obtain previous reports, and pick up as many elements of the rest of the evaluation as I need after the immediate crisis is stabilized. I instructed the parents to come to the first session without Barry. After getting a brief history of the situation, we moved to drawing up a hierarchy of the out-of-control behaviors and prioritizing our interventions. We drew up the following hierarchy:

1. Help the parents reach a decision about how to proceed regarding the current juvenile court heaving on Barry's joy-riding episode.
2. Increase school attendance and stop truancy, which would simultaneously solve the problem of Barry entertaining his girlfriend at home during the schoolday.

3. Stop Barry from sneaking out of the house in the middle of the night.
4. Replace Barry's cursing at parents with respectful communication.

In addition to correcting these antisocial behaviors, we also agreed that increasing completion of schoolwork, general compliance with parental requests, and encouraging Barry to take stimulant medication again would be later targets for change.

We started with the business of dealing with the mother and father's disagreement about how to deal with the juvenile court situation. I asked what would happen when they had such a disagreement in the past. They both agreed that Dr. Donovan would say he was going to follow through on his position but never get around to it. Mrs. Donovan would follow through on her position, but before she could administer any consequences, her husband and she would get into an argument, and Barry would disappear. Let's join the session as I am trying to get the parents working on the same team regarding this issue.

DR. ROBIN: So what outcome do you each want to see happen as a result of the joy-riding episode?

DR. DOVOVAN: I want Barry to face the medicine for what he has done and never go joy riding again.

MRS. DOVOVAN: I also want him to stop taking the car out, but I don't want him to have a police record.

DR. ROBIN: Let's get the two of you on the same team. You both want Barry to face the consequences for his actions, but you disagree about how to do this. Have you had much success getting consequences to work at home lately?

BOTH PARENTS: No!

DR. ROBIN: Then I think it is very important for the judge, as an authority outside the home, to have a chance to impose consequences. This is an opportunity to reinforce your authority with the authority of the court, and I think you should take it. But I think we ought to work to link those consequences back to the family situation, and build in a safety net so it won't ruin Barry's future.

MRS. DOVOVAN: How do we prevent a police record?

DR. ROBIN: We don't have to, because the juvenile record will be destroyed when he turns 18 if there are no additional charges. We will have your lawyer talk to the judge beforehand, and ask the judge to consider incorporating some of your house rules into his ruling. For example, in addition to whatever consequence the judge is going to impose, we could ask that he order Barry to attend school regularly, not sneak out of the house in the middle of the night, and participate in family counseling, or face more serious consequences in the future. Most judges like these kinds of contingencies.

The Donovans agreed to go along with my suggestion. The judge ordered that (1) Barry not be permitted to get his license until his 18th birthday instead of his 16th birthday; (2) he serve 30 hours of community service; and (3) he be placed on probation for 6 months with the terms being that he must attend school every day all day, must not sneak out at night, and must attend family counseling sessions. If Barry broke any terms of this probation, he would be sent to the county youth home.

Barry was very angry at his parents for not "getting him off," but he had heard how bad it was in the youth home and knew that he would not be able to see his friends if he was placed there, so he decided to comply with the terms of probation. I told his parents to bring him in for a family session. He said that he would attend but would not talk because the judge had only ordered attendance, not talking. I told his parents to ignore his manipulations and to bring him in anyway. In the session his parents decided that they wished to target Barry's extremely rude, disrespectful communication style toward his mother next. They indicated that their primary target for change was his obscene verbal outbursts and threats of violent behavior.

DR. ROBIN: Tell Barry what kind of language you expect him to use when he wishes to talk to you, Mrs. Donovan.

MRS. DOVOVAN: I expect you to talk to me with respect—no four-letter words, no threats of violence, and no demeaning comments about women.

BARRY: You worthless piece of crap. You stink!

DR. DOVOVAN: Don't talk to your mother that way!

DR. ROBIN: Good, Dr. Donovan. You need to make it clear to Barry how you feel about his behavior. Now, please talk to your wife about the consequences for such behavior.

BARRY: They can't make me stop anything. They never. . . .

DR. ROBIN: This is between your mom and dad. Sit quietly until your turn!

DR. DOVOVAN: I think we should ground Barry for 4 months every time he curses you out.

BARRY: You can't keep me in the house for 4 minutes, you old fart.

DR. ROBIN: Butt out, now! Mrs. Donovan, talk to your husband about his suggestion.

MRS. DOVOVAN: Dear, don't you think that is a little stiff. He curses all day. We would soon have him grounded for life, and how would we enforce it?

DR. DOVOVAN: I guess you're right. . . .

BARRY: No, I'm the one who is right. The two of you are. . . .

DR. ROBIN: . . . Please continue, Dr. Donovan.

DR. DOVOVAN: Barry makes me so angry that I want to ground him forever or kick his butt, but I know that isn't going to work. Why don't we fine him 50 cents off his allowance for each curse word?

MRS. DOVOVAN: OK, why don't we also make him earn his rides to his job at the pizza place by talking respectfully?

BARRY: I'll walk before I talk nicely.

DR. ROBIN: Ignore him and keep up the good discussion. You don't need a another fruitless power struggle.

DR. DOVOVAN: Sounds good to me. He will earn his rides and pay 50 cents per curse.

MRS. DOVOVAN: Then we are agreed.

BARRY: Just you try, you shitheads. . . .

DR. DOVOVAN: Enjoy your walk to work today. That will be 50 cents.

MRS. DOVOVAN: I can't believe you actually followed through.

DR. ROBIN: He really wants to see your son treat you properly.

BARRY: This is bull! I'm out of here. (*Gets up and angrily storms out of the session, slamming the door behind him.*)

MRS. DOVOVAN: Now what do we do?

DR. DOVOVAN: Nothing. He walks home if he isn't at the car when we leave.

MRS. DOVOVAN: But he will catch a cold.

DR. ROBIN: You have to be consistent. He may catch a cold, but you will keep catching hell if you don't follow through. You are doing very well working as a team. If he doesn't want to freeze his butt off, he will be at the car waiting. Teenagers often need to blow off steam and make a point by storming out of sessions like this. Let him go.

MRS. DOVOVAN: You're right, Dr. Robin. But it is sometimes hard not to give in to the urge to help him out. He is such a good boy underneath.

DR. ROBIN: Mrs. Donovan, he is a man, and you need to see his behavior for exactly what it is—rude and demeaning to you and women. The two of you have a good plan for now. Carry it out best you can, and I will help you modify it as needed.

DR. DOVOVAN: I really feel like we are working as a team now.

DR. ROBIN: You are. I congratulate you both.

It always feels as if we are walking in deep mud when conducting such a session. Every step takes such effort. Each time I made a statement designed to get the parents working as a team on establishing consequences for cursing and demeaning behavior, Barry tried to sidetrack the discussion or manipulate the situation. I did my best to interrupt his antics and keep his parents on task, without unnecessarily antagonizing Barry. When he saw he was not going to get anywhere, he stormed out of the session, as many such adolescents do, figuring his parents would come after him and then cave in. I prevented them from doing so and praised the parents for their teamwork.

Over the next week, Barry walked to work every day and lost $10 of his $12 allowance for cursing. He did not come home from school on time on the day of the next session, and therefore his parents had to attend without him. I reported his failure to attend the counseling session to his probation officer, who read him the riot act. He attended the next session after that, and slowly began to earn a few of his rides (the wind chill was −50 on the days he refrained from cursing; it takes a lot of motivation for such youth to make changes). We continued to work on parental agreements to enforce consequences for basic house rules and street rules, with mixed outcomes.

This case example illustrates how the therapist helps to restore parental control in such cases. It takes a great deal of effort, stamina, and stick-to-itiveness. Extrafamilial authority is often necessary to back up the parents (e.g., the juvenile court in this case). In past years, it used to be possible to hospitalize such youth in inpatient psychiatric or residential placements when they became extremely violent or abusive to their parents, but nowadays such hospitalization is typically no longer possible. It is still possible to work with the juvenile justice system or other community agencies at times in a productive manner, when brief out-of-home placements are needed.

It is instructive to note the similarities and differences between the approaches in the Cheyne and Donovan cases. The parents in both families had weak parental coalitions, inconsistent approaches to discipline, and power struggles with their adolescent, although Barry was actively antisocial and Valerie was not. Both teenagers "divided and conquered" their parents, although the stakes were much higher with Barry than Valerie. In both cases, I prompted and reinforced the parents for working as a team, blocked any interference by the adolescent, and helped the parents establish a behavioral contract for the target behaviors. I spent more time on attempting to give the Cheynes insight into the underlying distorted cognitions and family-of-origin factors that may have precipitated parental inconsistency. With the Donovans, I focused primarily on direct action in the session. I was much more forceful in blocking Barry than Valerie when they attempted to sidetrack their parents' discussions. The practitioner takes the same general approach with these two kinds of cases but must crank up the intensity and immediacy of the structure and be much more action oriented with the more flagrant antisocial behavior.

MOM CATCHES MORE FLAK THAN DAD

Research suggests that children with ADHD comply less and misbehave more in interactions with their mothers than with their fathers (Barkley, 1998). If the father is away at work most of the day and the mother has more contact with the child, the father will not witness as much of the defiant behavior as the mother, although he will hear his wife's frequent complaints. Under these circumstances, some fathers who are not that familiar with ADHD may doubt their wife's reports because the child acts fine for them. They do not take action to back up their wives in handling a difficult child, and the child learns to appeal to his or her father to avoid or mitigate any consequences imposed by the mother. As a result, it is easy for a cross-generational coalition to inadvertently arise between the father and child against the mother. At best, the father may fail to follow through with consequences imposed by his wife, perhaps because he wants to have some enjoyable time with his child. At worst, he may actively undermine his wife's disciplinary efforts and deny his child's disability. When a father undoes or softens the mother's discipline, he negatively reinforces the child's misbehavior and certainly fuels marital conflict. Such cross-generational coalitions are usually well entrenched by the adolescent years and usually put a great strain on the parents' marriages. The fathers often withdraw into their work worlds and spend little time with their wives or children. The mother gradually becomes overinvolved with the adolescent and the father becomes disengaged. Triangulation may also abound. Upon the father's arrival home in the evening, he is faced with the latest tales of horror from his wife about the adolescent's behavior and the latest stories of maternal inequities and unfair rules presented by the adolescent. He lands squarely in the middle between his teenager and his wife.

The therapist's goal is to break up the cross-generational coalition and build a strong within-generational, mother–father coalition. First, in a couple session, the therapist needs to explore the reasons why the father does not completely believe his wife's report of the behavioral problems that occurred earlier during the day in his absence. Does the father deny the existence of ADHD in the adolescent? Is the adolescent a convincing liar? Has the mother failed to be truthful in the past? Is there a long history of marital problems such that the parents do not believe each other? Does the father mistakenly believe that children will act the same in all situations? In answering these question, the therapist should ask the father what type of evidence of the adolescent's negative interactions with his wife would be convincing? Perhaps an audiotape or videotape would be helpful, or a phone call to the office with the adolescent screaming in the background. Sometimes, simply facilitating open communication between the spouses helps the father see that his wife needs his support.

Second, the therapist needs to help the couple develop a plan for the father to back up the mother in handling difficult behavioral problems during his absence. The adolescent needs to believe that his parents are working as a team, and that failure to behave appropriately with either parent will result in identical consequences. Central to this plan is clear and timely communication between the spouses concerning developing problem situations. At a minimum, the husband and wife need to review the day's events with each other in the evening, before the father acts on any partial information supplied by the teenager. In some cases, the mother may need to call, page, or E-mail her husband during the day, or while he is out of town on business. The couple also needs to define a range of discipline each is comfortable with the other unilaterally implementing, as well as certain consequences they wish to discuss before implementing; this definition helps them avoid a situation in which they absolutely cannot live with the other's unilateral action and undermine it later on.

Third, the therapist needs to help the couple decide in what situations the mother will say to the adolescent, "Your father will handle this when he comes home." Too frequent use of deferring to the spouse undermines the mother's parenting effectiveness. But failure to have this option available may also undermine her effectiveness given the research finding on differential reactions of ADHD children to fathers versus mothers. I typically help the parents define a short list of severe misbehaviors (aggression, destruction of property, antisocial behavior such as stealing or alcohol use, etc.) for which the mother may decide to defer action until her husband returns home, reminding parents about the ineffectiveness of delayed consequences with ADHD individuals. The therapist needs to guide the couple in implementing the strategies they have developed, blocking the adolescent's inevitable attempts to sabotage the strong parental coalition. Such guidance typically involves repeated discussion of the loopholes that have arisen between sessions, monitoring of parental communication, and aggressively preempting any backsliding toward cross-generational coalitions.

Fourth, the couple might be asked to carefully examine the distribution of fun versus instrumental task activities that each parent is doing with the adolescent. In many contemporary families, fathers spend more time doing fun/recreational activities, such as taking adolescents to sporting events, and mothers spend more time supervising chores and homework. This makes Mom "the heavy" too much. It may help improve mother–adolescent relations to have Dad take over some of the supervision of chores and homework and have Mom do more of the fun/recreational activities with the adolescent.

Fathers might also be asked to read *Voices from Fatherhood: Fathers,*

Sons, and ADHD (Kilcarr & Quinn, 1997) to deepen their understanding of ADHD.

"I HAVE TWO CHILDREN: MY SON AND MY HUSBAND"

In families that have both a parent and an adolescent diagnosed as having ADHD (or the parent is suspected but not yet formally diagnosed) the non-ADHD spouse often feels as if he or she has two children: the adolescent and the spouse with ADHD. Let's take the case of a family in which the father and son are diagnosed as having ADHD, and the mother is the non-ADHD spouse (although the dynamics are similar when the mother is the ADHD parent). The father often has difficulty with organization, follow-through, forgetfulness, temper control, mood control, emotional intensity, and consistency in parenting and managing a household. He often has to work twice as hard at his job to accomplish half as much, and he may have to bring home work from the job which he was not able to complete during work hours. As a result, he has less time for attending to his marriage and parenting responsibilities. His wife ends up doing more than her fair share of the household management and parenting, not to mention picking up the slack whenever he fails to carry out the chores he committed to complete. He often seems immature and childlike to his wife. Before long, she feels burned out and dumped on. She begins to feel as if she has two children: her adolescent and her childlike, immature husband.

Structurally, this is problem of hierarchy. Normally, the husband and wife are supposed to be at an equal level of shared executive power in the hierarchy, elevated above the children. Because ADHD impedes the husband's efficient completion of adult responsibilities, he functions at a similarly dependent level in the hierarchy as his son. This may be further reinforced by some ADHD fathers' tendencies to bicker with their adolescents more like two siblings than like a parent and a child. The hierarchy is inappropriately structured here, with the adolescent and the father at an equal, sibling level, below the mother. The therapist's goal are (1) to elevate the ADHD father to the appropriate coexecutive position with his wife in the family hierarchy, as much as possible; (2) to help the ADHD father face and cope with his own disability; and (3) to help the parents share more equitably and effectively in the executive management of the family.

If the father is suspected of having ADHD but not yet formally diagnosed and treated, the therapist should tactfully assess his openness to evaluation. Therapists trained to work with ADHD across the life span can do such adult evaluations themselves, increasing efficiency and combating rapport difficulties. Approaching the father in an individual meeting works best to avoid putting him on the defensive. The therapist should gently point out the similarities between father and son and relate these similarities to the symptoms of ADHD. The therapist might suggest that the father read a book such as *Driven to Distraction* (Hallowell, 1994b) or *Adventures in Fast Forward* (Nadeau, 1996), or if he cannot easily get through a book without distraction (a common situation for ADHD adults), suggest that he attend an adult support group meeting and talk to other adults in similar situations. The therapist must help him overcome the sometimes natural masculine tendency not to admit weakness or not to want to be dependent on others for assistance. He or she should point out that the son feels the same way, and that by exploring and coping effectively with his own possible ADHD, the father will not only improve his own life and his marriage but will also serve as a stellar model for his son. In my experience, after such a father has been correctly diagnosed and treated medically for ADHD, the situation improves dramatically. The steps the father makes set in motion a positive chain of events, culminating in an increase in reciprocity of positive behaviors. In my experience, mothers suspected of having ADHD are more amenable to undergoing evaluations than are fathers, although I follow the same procedures outlined previously. The mothers benefit most from reading *Women with Attention Deficit Disorder* (Solden, 1995).

In addition to diagnosis and medical treatment of the father's ADHD, the therapist might implement the following interventions: (1) psychoeducational explanation of the role of hierarchy in the family and how the father's ADHD is impeding coexecutive leadership functions in the family, (2) role reallocation of selected parenting tasks, and (3) instruction in ADHD compensatory techniques. I use Barkley's concept of executive parenting to explain the importance of parents' functioning at an equal level of the power hierarchy. It is helpful to illustrate how an ADHD father might slip to a lower level of the hierarchy and how this negatively affects the marriage. The therapist should ask the couple to become aware of and strive to compensate for specific instances in which the ADHD parent is slipping into the sibling level of the hierarchy. This framework provides a natural opening to discuss role reallocation and compensatory techniques.

Reallocation of roles involves a review of all the parenting responsibilities and who currently carries them out, followed by a reallocation of roles based on which responsibilities are best suited to an ADHD parent versus a non-ADHD parent. For example, a father with ADHD might thrive on such activities as driving the adolescent to weekday evening and weekend sporting activities, getting the adolescent up and going in the morning, and chaperoning the adolescent at dances. The non-ADHD parent might do better at checking up on whether homework was done, taking the adolescent clothing shopping, and monitoring school performance.

Compensatory techniques which the ADHD father can apply to work around ADHD symptoms include but certainly are not limited to the use of lists, electronic personal organizers, timers, breaking down tasks into their components and scheduling each component. Many of the books written for adults with ADHD contain a multitude of useful advice (Gordon, 1995b; Kelly & Ramundo, 1993; Nadeau, 1995, 1996).

By placing the issue of the ADHD parent within the framework of structural problems, we can more easily understand its tremendous impact on the family with an adolescent with ADHD. Because ADHD is biologically and genetically based, the practitioner should become adept at dealing with families with more than one ADHD member. They are much more common than practitioners may realize.

STEPFAMILIES

Under even the best of circumstances, stepfamilies and second marriages are replete with multiple complexities of instrumental coordination problems, emotional loyalty issues, side taking, triangulation, unclear hierarchies, and role confusion. Add ADHD to these already muddied waters and we have a veritable tidal wave of potential conflict, as demonstrated by the description of the Morass family earlier in this chapter. In addition, adolescence is a difficult developmental period for children to adjust to second marriages and stepfamily life.

Given the high divorce and remarriage rates in today's society, the practitioner is likely to encounter a fair number of adolescents with ADHD residing in stepfamilies, and he or she needs to know how to adapt the approaches described in this book to the unique problems of these families. In addressing the issues of ADHD stepfamilies, we need to consider the factors that make stepfamily life difficult for all families and the unique ways in which the symptoms of ADHD further complicate stepfamily life. Many of the suggestions given here are based in part on the excellent discussion of ADHD adolescents residing in stepfamilies by Zeigler Dendy (1995). I organize this discussion in terms of four broad and certainly not mutually exclusive domains: (1) approach to therapy, (2) structural problems/role confusion, (3) loyalty issues, and (4) living arrangements/environmental problems.

Approach to Therapy

The therapist needs to conduct family therapy sessions with the adolescent and each of two families in which he or she resides and/or visits. The therapist needs to determine firsthand, not based on rumor and hearsay, how the adolescent interacts with each family, and what issues the adults in each family have with the adults in the other family. He or she also needs to assess firsthand the impact of ADHD symptoms in each family, and the knowledge and skills of each family for coping with an adolescent diagnosed as having ADHD. Either I see the adolescent with each family on alternate weeks or apportion the sessions to the noncustodial family in proportion to the frequency of visitation. The therapist also needs some time alone with the parents and stepparents. Whether the therapist brings the two natural parents and their new spouses together in a session with the adolescent depends on the level of acrimony that exists. Usually, such a session is too threatening and counterproductive. However, I have worked with a small number of families in which it was possible, usually a number of years after the divorce and remarriages, to have all the relevant adults in the room productively at one time. One important detail concerns payment arrangements in stepfamilies. Typically, the custodial parent, most commonly a natural mother, brings the adolescent for treatment, but the natural father is often the responsible financial party with regard to health insurance and payment. Experience suggests that unless unambiguous arrangements are made at the start of therapy to collect copays and/or fees from the noncustodial parent, the therapist will end up giving away some or all of his services without reimbursement. Such families are usually financially strained, and paying the therapist is not their highest priority.

Consider the common situation in which the adolescent resides with the natural mother and the stepfather during the week and visits with the natural father for two weekends per month. This is the situation in the Morass family. Ideally, in such a situation, the therapist should go through all the phases of the comprehensive burst of intervention outlined in this book for a newly diagnosed adolescent with ADHD, with the adolescent and each family participating in each phase of treatment. Then, each family will have participated meaningfully in ADHD education, school intervention, and home intervention and will have the knowledge, attitudes, and skills to help parent the adolescent effectively. Under such circumstances, the therapist also has a considerable number of opportunities to bridge the gaps where there are major inconsistencies across households, or to figure out how to help the adolescent adjust to these inconsistencies. The special problems inherent in stepfamilies can then be addressed as needed on an ongoing basis throughout the therapy, rather than on a crisis basis when an explosion occurs. Realistically, the therapist may not always have this opportunity available, either because of geographical distance of one of the two families or resistance from, most often, the noncustodial natural parent and/or stepparent. We approximate this ideal as closely as we can. In the following discussion, we will assume that the therapist is integrating work on the stepfamily-specific factors into the general 15- to 20-session intervention for adolescents diagnosed as having ADHD.

Structural Problems/Role Confusion

Early in the therapy, during the sessions when the therapeutic contract is being formulated and family ADHD education is being undertaken, the therapist should make some comments about the stepparent's role in disciplining the adolescent with ADHD. In recently remarried families, the therapist needs to point out the importance of the biological parent retaining most disciplinary responsibility for a period of time, sometimes over a year or two, to permit the relationship between the stepparent and the adolescent to develop gradually. The therapist should also point out the importance of the biological parent backing up the stepparent in the presence of the adolescent and deal with any concerns about the stepparent's approach to the adolescent privately at a later time. If ex-spouses are interfering with the development of new relationships between an adolescent and a stepparent, the therapist needs to do whatever is possible to neutralize this interference. In families in which the remarriage took place many years ago, this is not usually an issue. Irrational beliefs couples may have about "instant togetherness" and "teenagers should accept stepparents quickly" also need to be challenged.

During the sessions that focus on problem solving, communication training, and behavior management, the therapist should identify and target directly structural difficulties with coalitions and triangulation. Triangulated interactions, for example, could be targeted for change in a manner similar to negative communication habits (e.g., through the use of modeling, instructions, behavior rehearsal, and feedback). Let's reconsider the Morass family, for instance. Recall that Adam interfered with Belinda's attempt to get Mitchell to do his homework. Adam was taking on a disciplinary role too early in his relationship as a stepfather with Mitchell, and without any effective steps having been taken to neutralize Bill's covert attempts to sabotage the stepfather–stepson relationship. Anyway, Belinda repeatedly found herself triangulated between her husband and son, when Mitchell refused to do what Adam said and Adam turned to Belinda for support. The therapist might decide to conduct a problem-solving discussion of how to handle incomplete homework on Sunday evening after Mitchell returns from a visit with his father. He might proceed as follows to target triangulated interactions during this discussion:

DR. JONES: I've noticed that Belinda often ends up stuck in the middle when Mitchell refuses to do what she says and Adam gets into the act to try to help Belinda out. This happens a lot in stepfamilies. The stepfather tries to help the natural mother out, but the teenager says he doesn't have to listen to the stepfather because he isn't his real father.

MITCHELL: But Adam isn't my real father. . . .

DR. JONES: I know. Neither is your math teacher your father, but you do what he says. I understand that you have a thing about Adam taking over your father's role, but I don't think he really wants to do that. Adam, are you trying to be Mitchell's father?

ADAM: Absolutely not. Mitchell has one father, Bill. I'm trying to help his mother.

DR. JONES: Belinda, what help do you want from Adam when Mitchell disobeys you?

BELINDA: I need him to back me up but not to try to issue the consequences.

DR. JONES: Well, Adam?

ADAM: All right, I'll do my best.

DR. JONES: Explain to Mitchell that you don't want to be his father.

ADAM: Mitchell, I'm not your dad. I'm just concerned about your homework.

MITCHELL: OK.

DR. JONES: We are going to have a problem-solving discussion to help you, Mitchell, and your mother solve the problem of homework that is not yet done when you get home from a visit at your dad's. Adam has agreed to help your mom out, but basically this is between you and your mom. If anyone puts anyone else in the middle, I'll stop the action, point it out, and ask that person to try to handle his feelings directly.

The therapist should handle other structural problems in a similar manner, using skills training interventions strategically.

Loyalty Issues

During the first few home management sessions, when the therapist is discussing belief systems and expectations, he or she should bring up loyalty and displacement issues in stepfamilies. The therapist should normalize the adolescent's inevitable wish to get his or her natural parents back together again, should explain to the parents how the adolescent will feel torn between them and may feel that forming a relationship with a stepmother represents disloyalty to a natural mother. Parents should be advised not to require that the adolescent address the stepparent "Mom" or "Dad" unless the adolescent chooses to do so; this seemingly simple point can easily aggravate loyalty conflicts and trigger negative reactions from ex-spouses. The therapist should strongly advise each natural parent not to put the adolescent in loyalty conflicts by asking him or her to do things such as spy on the ex-spouse, tell lies, pump the ex-spouse for information, or withhold information. The negative impact of such behaviors should be clearly depicted.

Displacement refers to the feelings some adolescents, particularly boys, may have when their custodial mother, who may have been a single parent for a number of years since the divorce, remarries. These young men often viewed themselves as the "man of the house" while their mother was single. In fact, the mothers may have needed their help with many household management and babysitting chores and may have elevated them in the power hierarchy. When a stepfather comes on the scene and the adolescent's assistance is no longer needed, the adolescent naturally feels displaced. A moody, impulsive adolescent is likely to act out such feelings of displacement, perhaps through conflict with his stepfather, or through angry rebellion against his natural mother. The parents should be helped to understand what the adolescent is going through, and to give the adolescent opportunities to discuss his or her feelings. Stepparents especially need to learn not to be threatened when adolescents feel displaced.

The therapist should spend some time individually with the adolescent discussing loyalty issues and feelings of displacement. Some adolescents may be willing to talk about such feelings, but others may refuse. Immature, impulsive adolescents may not really understand what they are feeling or why. The therapist should take an empathetic stance and bring up possible scenarios and normalize what the adolescent experiences.

Environmental Factors

Living arrangements, visitations arrangements, family routines, and transitions between households are practical environmental factors to which he therapist must attend in stepfamilies. Forgetful, inattentive adolescents are likely to leave stimulant medication, schoolbooks, assignments, homework, materials, library books, backpacks, clothes, tapes, CDs, video games, and other things at one household when they need them at the other household. Sometimes, such "forgetfulness" is planned avoidance, as in the case of the adolescent who conveniently comes to visit his father for the weekend without any of the materials he needs for an unpleasant homework assignment. If parents have rules restricting the adolescent from removing certain possessions from one household to the other, these are likely to be broken, either inadvertently or on purpose. The therapist should establish an exit and entrance checking routine in each household to help prevent such difficulties. Shortly before it is time to depart for the other household, the parent should ask the adolescent to review what needs to be taken, pack it, and leave it near the door. Keeping a running packing list throughout the week may work for some families. Each family should also establish clear guidelines about the circumstances under which a parent will or won't make an extra trip to bring something to the other household that was left behind; otherwise, teenagers (and ex-spouses) will attempt to manipulate one parent to bring the things that were left behind.

Regarding schoolwork, upon picking up an adolescent for visitation, before pulling out of the driveway, the noncustodial parent should ask what homework there is and what books are needed and, if the adolescent has lied about having the materials in the past, should demand to see the books and papers in question. When communication between ex-spouses permits and the adolescent cannot be trusted, the custodial parent might need to send a note summarizing the current status of homework and what needs to accomplished over the visitation period. In our modern era of computer technology, the therapist might suggest that families that have the appropriate equipment available make full use of E-mail and faxing to communicate information during visitations. For example, if an adolescent left a report that was on her hard disk at her mother's house during a visitation to her father, her mother could send it to her as a file attached to an E-mail.

It may be difficult for adolescents with ADHD to remember and to accept the different rules and routines at two households, resulting in unnecessary conflicts when the adults interpret forgetfulness and confusion as malicious intent and oppositional behavior. The therapist should review major areas of family life where routines are common—getting up in the morning, mealtimes, bedtimes, religious service attendance, chores, curfew, self-care activities, such as showers and baths, etc.—and clarify the routines at each household. The therapist might guide the adolescent to make charts, tables, and lists with two columns—one for their mother's house and one for the father's house—highlighting what they are expected to do in each home. Computerwise adolescents might make this tedious experience more interesting by using computer graphics to accomplish it. The therapist should guide the parents and stepparents to make the routines as similar as possible, recognizing that this is not always feasible.

Families also need help realizing that transitions from one household to another are times of high risk for conflict and problem behaviors. For one thing, ADHD individuals do not make transitions easily; they either shift tasks too quickly and frequently or often get overfocused on one task and refuse to shift gears. In addition, adolescents quickly learn that parents may not be able to discipline effectively just before a transition, because the other parent "rescues" the adolescent. Everyone is likely to be feeling loyalty conflicts at such times too. The therapist should help the family anticipate such difficulties and prepare to prevent unnecessary conflicts. For example, agreements concerning chores should specify that they be completed far in advance of a transition time. Parents should remind teenagers to gather their belongings in advance, and the time before transitions should be a low-demand time.

In some cases, the adolescent has no problem remembering the different rules in the two households but believes that the differences are unfair and refuses to comply with the more effortful rules. The therapist should clearly emphasize that there will be differences between households on rules, that everyone will have to accept this, and that it is counterproductive for one parent to try to interfere with the routines at the other parent's home, or for the adolescent to expect things to be the same across the two households. The therapist can use problem-solving techniques to help the adolescent negotiate mutually acceptable routines in each household.

OUTCOME RESEARCH

Behavioral family systems therapy interventions such as those discussed in Chapters 10, 11, and this chapter have been extensively evaluated and found to be effective in reducing parent–adolescent conflict in families selected on the basis of family conflict rather than formal DSM-IV diagnoses (Robin & Foster, 1989; Stern, in press). However, only a single published study specifically evaluated this form of treatment with adolescents specifically diagnosed as having ADHD. Barkley, Guevremont, Anastopoulos, and Fletcher (1992) conducted a comparison of three family therapy programs for treating family conflicts in adolescents with ADHD. Sixty-one 12- to 18-year-olds were randomly assigned to 8–10 sessions of behavior management training (BMT), problem-solving communication training (PSCT), or structural family therapy. To be eligible, the adolescents had to (1) be referred to the investigators' ADHD clinic; (2) meet DSM-III-R criteria for ADHD and have parent or teacher complaints of inattention, impulsivity, and restlessness; (3) be willing to be off psychoactive medication for the duration of the study; and (4) have T-scores greater than 65 on the hyperactivity scale of the Child Behavior Checklist. The treatments were conducted by two licensed clinical psychologists trained and supervised by senior clinicians expert in each treatment (I supervised the PSCT therapy and Barkley supervised the BMT). The adolescent and at least one parent (usually the mother) participated in each BMT and PSCT session; the parent(s) participated in the BMT sessions without the adolescent.

The BMT approach followed Barkley's (1987) *Defiant Children* manual with several modifications: (1) when learning positive attending skills, parents were asked to observe the adolescent participating in an activity and provide positive feedback to the adolescent rather than playing with their child; and (2) grounding at home for brief periods replaced time out as a punishment technique. Successive sessions focused on the use of positive parent attention, point systems or token reinforcement, daily home–school report cards linked with the home token system, groundings for unacceptable behavior, and instructions for parents on how to anticipate impending problem situations and establish plans in advance to deal with them. Regular homework was assigned following Barkley's (1987) protocol.

The PSCT approach followed the guidelines outlined throughout this book and included three main activities: (1) problem-solving training, (2) communication training, and (3) cognitive restructuring of extreme beliefs and unreasonable expectations. Homework assignments were given in later sessions; these involved applications and practice of problem-solving and communication skills. There was no systematic inclusion of ADHD family education, childrearing frameworks, or principles of parenting.

The structural family therapy (SFT) approach helped families identify and alter maladaptive family systems or interaction patterns, such as trans-generational coalitions, scapegoating, and triangulation. The therapists focused on creating transactions, joining with the family's transactions, and helping to restructure maladaptive transactions, relying on analysis and targeting of family boundaries, alignments, and power. Homework assignments typically involved instructions to replace ineffective transactions with novel strategies. Some of the structural interventions described in this chapter were included in Barkley's treatment condition, but it should not be construed to include all these elements and is not therefore a definitive test of the role of family structure interventions in behavioral family systems therapy.

Each family was assessed before and after treatment and at a 3-month follow-up on the following dependent measures: (1) the Child Behavior Checklist parent and youth self-report version social competence scales and broad-band internalizing and externalizing psychopathology scales; (2) the Conflict Behavior Questionnaire (CBQ); (3) the Issues Checklist (IC); (4) the Locke–Wallace Marital Adjustment Test; (5) the Beck Depression Inventory; and (6) videotaped interactions during a neutral and a conflict topic discussion coded with the Parent–Adolescent Interaction Coding System—Revised (PAICS-R). The PAICS yielded summary scores for the frequency of two negative communication categories (put-downs/commands, defends/complains), and four positive communication categories (problem-solves, defines/evaluates, facilitates, and talks). The Family Beliefs Inventory (FBI) was given at pre- and postassessment, and a five-item consumer satisfaction survey was given at the end of treatment. The therapists rated family cooperation on a five-item scale at the end of each session.

In general, analyses revealed that all three treatments resulted in significant improvements on most measures from before to after treatment, with further gains in many cases from postassessment to follow-up. There were few differences between treatments. Specifically, parents and adolescents reported improvement on the Internalizing and Externalizing scales of the Child Behavior Checklist, with further improvement during the follow-up interval on the Internalizing scale. Parents also reported significant improvement on school adjustment from before to after treatment. On the parent adjustment measures, there were improvements before to after treatment on the Beck Depression Inventory but not on the Locke–Wallace Marital Adjustment Test.

On self-reported family conflict, mothers and adolescents consistently reported significant gains in their interactions and levels of specific disputes on the CBQ and the IC, and teens reported some improvements in their relationships with their fathers during the follow-up interval. These results were clear-cut and indicative of amelioration of parent–adolescent conflict as seen by both the teenager and the mother and by follow-up generalizing to the teenager's perception of the father–adolescent relationship, even though the fathers were not typically involved in the treatments.

The results were more variable and difficult to interpret on the observed family interactions. One would have predicted that the negative categories should decrease and the positive categories should increase following treatment, but this did not consistently occur. During the neutral topic discussion, mothers displayed decreases in problem solves and increases in talks from pre- to postassessment, along with increases in facilitates and decreases in define/evaluates from postassessment to follow-up. Teenagers displayed increases in defends/commands and define/evaluates and decreases in problem-solves and facilitates from pre- to postassessment; Talk increased from postassessment to follow up. During the conflict discussion, there was no change for the teenagers but a treatment by assessment period interaction for the mothers on facilitates and talks. Only SFT mothers decreased on facilitates, but they had differed from the other two groups at preassessment. For talks, the BMT and PSCT groups decreased between postassessment and follow-up. At follow-up, the PSCT group showed more talks than the BMT or the SFT groups. The decreases in categories such as defines/evaluates, facilitates, and problem-solves and the increases in defends/commands are contrary to predictions and suggestive of a deterioration of interactions; however, Barkley, Guevremont, et al. (1992) did not comment on this finding.

Surprising results counter to predictions were obtained on the FBI. There were no significant decreases in adherence to rigid, unrealistic ideas for either parents or adolescents after treatment. However, there was a significant interaction of treatment and assessment period. Parental adherence to beliefs about perfection and obedience increased from pre- to postassessment for the PSCT group but stayed the same for the BMT and SFT groups. There were, however, no significant differences between the three groups either before or after treatment. PSCT was the only treatment to target unreasonable beliefs; we would have predicted an improvement rather than a deterioration on the FBI for this group. Several interpretations are plausible: (1) An initial emphasis upon negative attributions without more time to deal with them may have exacerbated rather than improved these beliefs, or (2) the parents may have been unaware of such beliefs until the therapist brought them up in the PSCT group, leading to increased reports on the postassessment FBI. At least one other investigation with PSCT treating volunteer families with parent–adolescent conflict found reductions in extreme beliefs on the FBI (Nayar, 1985). Further research is needed to determine the robustness of this finding and if it replicates, what it means.

Barkley determined the clinical significance of the results following Jacobson and Truax's (1991) recommendations, by computing the index of Reliable Change (magnitude of the improvement) and the Recovery Index (is client within the normal range?), using the IC quantity and weighted anger-intensity scores. For the number of conflicts, the percentages of subjects showing a reliable change were 10% for BMT, 24% for PSCT, and 10% for SFT; none showed deterioration. For the Recovery Index, the percentages of subjects who moved into the normal range were 5% for BMT, 19% for PSCT, and 10% for SFT. Comparable percentages were obtained for the weighted anger-intensity score. There were no significant differences between treatments on these indices.

Consumer satisfaction ratings were high and did not vary significantly across the three treatments. However, therapist ratings of family cooperation did differ significantly. The therapists rated the PSCT families as significantly less cooperative than either the BMT or the SFT families. Perhaps the greater amount of effort required of the PSCT group influenced these ratings.

The lack of either a no-treatment or an attention-placebo control leaves ambiguous the question whether the positive gains were due to the treatments or other factors such as the passing of time, therapist attention, or measurement artifact, and the relatively small sample sizes limits the power to obtain significant subtle differences between treatments.

The results of this study were promising in that they did indicate that all three treatment approaches resulted in statistically significant amelioration of self-reported parent–adolescent conflicts and negative communication, decreases in externalizing and internalizing behavior problems and maternal depression, and a high degree of consumer satisfaction with the treatments. At the same time, the results are very sobering when the stringent criteria of reliable change and movement into the normal range were applied, in that 80–95% of the families with ADHD adolescents did not make any clinically significant improvements through any of these family-based interventions. Nonetheless, the high degree of parental satisfaction suggests that even if clinically significant results were not obtained for the majority of families on the dependent measures, the families felt they benefited. Barkley, Guevremont, et al. (1992) speculated that perhaps the parents felt better prepared to cope with the problems inherent in raising adolescents with ADHD, even if they continued to have conflicts with their adolescents.

It would be incorrect, however, to conclude from Barkley's study that the multifaceted intervention outlined in this book will only help 15–20% of the families with adolescents diagnosed as having ADHD. This book outlines an intervention that includes not only the components used by Barkley but also medication, direct school-based interventions, and a broader home-based intervention with a greater emphasis on cognitive restructuring. In addition, I recommend 20 sessions whereas Barkley's study involves eight sessions. Of course, the effectiveness of our intervention awaits empirical research, but I am optimistic that it will help more than 20% of the adolescents with ADHD.

CONCLUSION

This chapter has discussed how to intervene to change the structural problems of families with ADHD adolescents. Chapters 10 and 11 discussed other aspects of family intervention. In addition to all of the family interventions, the practitioner may occasionally choose to incorporate individual or group interventions with the adolescent into the overall treatment plan. Such interventions might include anger management training, social skills training, or supportive individual psychotherapy. Even though the evidence for the effectiveness of these interventions is not compelling, they may sometimes be worth incorporating into a broader, family-based therapy. In this book I do not provide the practitioner with detailed instructions for conducting these adjunctive interventions, because they are not unique interventions developed and tested especially for adolescents with ADHD. Readers interested in information about these interventions should consult Barkley (1998), Braswell and Bloomquist (1991), and Feindler and Guttman (1994) for further discussion of these topics.

CHAPTER THIRTEEN

○

Phasing Out and Follow-Up

As indicated in several places throughout this volume, my philosophy of treating individuals with ADHD across their life span is to provide a short burst of intensive, multimodal intervention at the point of diagnosis and/or referral and then fade treatment out to a regular series of follow-up sessions. Additional intensive bursts of short-term intervention may take place at crucial developmental transition points if ADHD symptoms interact with environmental factors to create new crises in the individual's life. I call this approach the "dental checkup model of ADHD follow-up care" because it is analogous to dentists having their patients come in for checkups and cleanings twice per year, then receiving more intensive treatment if the checkup uncovers problems. The premise of this philosophy is that ADHD characteristics, based in genetics and neurobiology much of the time, often last a lifetime, although they may not continuously manifest themselves at the level of a clinical disorder throughout the individual's entire life. Until we can permanently alter the individual's genetic makeup or neurobiology, we need to teach individuals to cope with ADHD characteristics so that they do not create undue impairment.

Section II showed the reader how to identify the presence of ADHD, and earlier chapters in Section III showed the reader how to provide the intensive burst of multimodal intervention. How should the practitioner conduct the ongoing follow-up after the intensive burst of intervention? Because I know of no published, empirically based literature on how to conduct such long-term follow-up, I provide the reader with clinically based procedures, with the caveat that they have not been subjected to empirical scrutiny.

As therapy reaches the final phase, from sessions 16 to 20, I gradually increase the time between sessions. I typically make the interval between sessions 15 and 16, and 16 and 17, 2 weeks apiece and then see the adolescent and the family monthly for sessions 18, 19, and 20. As soon as the therapy reaches monthly intervals, the momentum of regular therapy stops and the patient is in follow-up. Afterward, I schedule a session every 3 months for the next year, then twice a year until the adolescent graduates from high school. At the point of high school graduation, I talk to the adolescent about his or her plans for the future and stop scheduling follow-ups, with an open-ended invitation for the adolescent to return for additional help at a later time if he or she needs or wants it. Of course, this represents my ideal approach, and a variety of practical circumstances, such as managed care authorization, finances, competing priorities, and lack of interest on the part of the adolescent or the parents, results in less frequent or premature termination of follow-up care.

When the adolescent continues to take medication through high school and beyond, this follow-up care ideally should be integrated with medical follow-up in one of several ways. The simplest approach is for a knowledgeable physician to conduct a psychosocial checkup and do the follow-up care on school and home issues. More commonly, the physician prompts, urges, or even requires the adolescent and the family to attend regular follow-up sessions with the mental health professional, in some cases making continued prescription of medication contingent upon attending such sessions.

Prior to each of the 3-month or 6-month follow-up sessions, I typically mail one parent, one teacher, and one adolescent self-report questionnaire to the family to complete and return. Most commonly, I use the Conners Parent Rating Scale—Revised Short Form, the TRF Attention Problems Scale or the Child Attention Profile, and the short form of the Conners–Wells Adolescent Self-Report Scale. I send sufficient copies of the teacher rating scale for all of the adolescent's current teachers; in September of each year, I sample the previous year's teachers because the new teachers have not yet had sufficient time to get to know the student. I may add the Conflict Behavior Questionnaire when family conflict was a major treatment target. This is the same battery of measures used for medication follow-ups. These measures can be rapidly scored at the beginning of the session and help the practitioner get a quick picture of how things are going.

The follow-up sessions, scheduled for 1 hour, are typically divided into a portion with the adolescent, a portion with the parents, and a portion with the family together. This format changes as the adolescent matures and grows older. With high school seniors and college students, I typically spend most of the time with the adolescent or young adult alone. At each follow-up, I review how the adolescent is coping in the areas that constituted the specific goals of the original intensive burst of therapy, and then I inquire more generally how the adolescent is doing in academic pursuits, peer relationships, family life, general life management skills, and for older adolescents, career/vocational functioning. I cast a wide net, screening for new problems or a resurgence of old problems. I give general advice for coping with minor problems that have arisen and reinforce the use of techniques learned during the original therapy for family conflict and academic success. If I uncover major new difficulties, I negotiate a contract for another short-term burst of family or individual therapy. I go out of the way to look for success stories of academic and social accomplishments, for which I heartily congratulate the adolescent and the family. Two case examples illustrate long-term follow-up.

CASE 1: ABE GELHART

Abe and his parents were first seen on a weekly basis for 15 sessions of family and individual therapy in 1994, when Abe was 11. At the time of entry into therapy, Abe, diagnosed with ADHD and ODD, had recently been released from a short stay in an inpatient unit. He had been admitted to the unit because of violent behavior at home and angry outbursts. Abe had a 110 Full Scale IQ and no learning disability, but he was classified as handicapped by ADHD under Section 504 and was receiving accommodation at school in fifth grade at entry into therapy. With the accommodation, Abe received A's and B's in school. He did, however, keep mostly to himself and did not have any close friends. Outside school, he was also a loner, with interests in the arts and reading, not sports or other things of common interest to boys his age. At that time, he had also been on Ritalin and Tofranil (imipramine), prescribed by a local psychiatrist. Abe, an only child, resided with his parents. His father was a lawyer, and his mother was a homemaker.

The goals of the initial course of therapy were to (1) teach Abe anger management skills, (2) help Mr. and Mrs. Gelhart further improve their parent management techniques to cope with Abe's angry outbursts, (3) help Abe maintain his good school performance, and (4) help Abe make and keep more friends. At the outset, Abe was having major anger outbursts at home three to four times a week, involving destruction of property once every other week. A combination of behavioral contracts, cognitive-behavioral anger management training, and helping the parents identify the triggers for Abe's outbursts and change the environment to minimize these triggers, helped Abe over the course of the 15 sessions to reduce the outbursts to one or two per month from three to four per week. School performance continued to be excellent, and Mr. and Mrs. Gelhart learned some new management techniques. Abe did not, however, change much with regard to reaching out to his peers and making friends.

The first seven sessions had been scheduled weekly, and the next eight were scheduled every other week. Afterward, I saw the family monthly for 6 months, and since that time I continue to see them approximately every 3 months. They have a type of managed care insurance that preauthorizes 6–10 sessions at a time, then requires a clinical review. In 1997, the insurance authorized six sessions for the entire year, but only four were needed. At a 3-month follow-up session in October 1996, the parents indicated that Abe had been having three to four major angry outbursts a week for the past month, a significant increase from one to two a month. Abe, now 14 and in seventh grade in a new school, concurred that he was feeling stressed out by school, and particularly one teacher who was giving him long and difficult writing assignments. He admitted that after holding his anger in all day at school, he let it out on his parents at home. Even though his parents consistently followed through on the contract to take away video game and computer privileges, it was insufficient to correct the problem now. Abe's medicine remained Ritalin and Tofranil, but the doses had been increased to keep pace with his increased growth, and the current problems did not appear to be medication-related issues.

It turned out that the new school was not following through on the Section 504 plan from elementary school because until now, Abe did not appear to need any accommodations. We decided that there was a need for a school meeting to revitalize and update the previous Section 504 plan, emphasizing adjustment of the quantity and difficulty level of assignments, establishing regular parent–teacher communication, and closer monitoring of Abe's functioning. I called the school social worker, who agreed to set up a school meeting. I attended the school meeting, where teachers agreed to make some accommodation. I scheduled another therapy session 2 weeks after the school meeting. At this session, I worked out a plan whereby Abe would signal his parents nonverbally with a sign on the refrigerator when he came home from school which indicated whether he had had a good or bad day. If he signaled that he had had a bad day, his mother would give him a lot of space for 1 hour. We reviewed the behavioral contract and anger management techniques. At the next session, 1 month later, Abe reported that the teacher had adjusted his assignments and that he had only had two outbursts in the past month. I will now schedule two more sessions at monthly intervals, then return to meeting every 3 months.

Comment

This case illustrates how a crisis arose upon Abe's entry into a new school, which led to an escalation of the original presenting problem: angry outbursts. Steps were taken at the regular follow-up to cope with the crisis, and several more frequent sessions were conducted. Then, as the crisis subsided, I returned to the less frequent follow-up mode, which I will continue for some time. I was able to accomplish these goals working within the constraints imposed by a managed care insurance company.

CASE 2: LISA BECKLEY

Mrs. Beckley first brought Lisa for an ADHD/LD evaluation and therapy when she was 16 and in 11th grade, in February 1994. At that time Lisa was inconsistent in completing her schoolwork, was arguing frequently with her mother, and had a tumultuous relationship with her natural father, who was divorced from her mother. Lisa also had a variety of chronic medical problems, including migraines, asthma, and frequent colds and infections, which caused her to miss a great deal of school. The migraines, which lasted 2 to 3 days, were particularly debilitating, and when Lisa did not have a migraine, she always had a chronic, dull aching headache. Lisa had a tendency to be highly emotionally overreactive, a tendency she learned and/or inherited from her mother, who easily decompensated into hysteria at the first sign of an impending crisis. Mother and daughter set each other off, resulting in major confrontations over rules such as curfew, driving, and household responsibilities. They vacillated between periods of extreme closeness, during which they confided often in each other, and periods of extreme anger and distance, during which they maliciously put each other down in the most obnoxious ways. They were hypersensitive to the nuances of each other's communication and could read things into the slightest inflection of voice tone or phrasing.

Lisa was an only child who resided with her mother. Her mother was engaged to a very understanding man, whom Lisa liked a lot. Her mother and father had been divorced for 5 years and had virtually no communication. They did not, however, badmouth each other in front of their daughter. The father had been diagnosed as Bipolar and ADHD but refused to accept these diagnoses or pursue any treatment. The mother was episodically depressed, meeting criteria for Major Depressive Disorder (although she was not suicidal), had major financial difficulties, and was generally a needy but gracious, warm, and loving person.

I diagnosed Lisa as having ADHD, Combined Type, and a Sadness Problem which was not yet a clinical Mood Disorder. Her Full Scale IQ was 102, and her WIAT achievement scores were all within 5 standard score points of her Full Scale IQ. Thus, she did have a comorbid learning disability, and any school-related difficulties were secondary to ADHD and missing a great deal of school due to medical problems. I recommended a combination of family/individual therapy and medication. A child psychiatrist started Lisa on Ritalin, which was titrated to 15 mg twice a day, weekdays only at that time. Lisa accepted taking Ritalin and was relieved to receive the ADHD diagnosis, although she mainly saw her mother's behavior as her primary problem. Ritalin helped her with schoolwork. Occasionally, she had hyperemotional reactions to Ritalin about 1 hour after ingesting her dose, but she felt the benefits outweighed this side effect.

I conducted 18 sessions of a flexible combination of family and individual therapy between the initial diagnosis in February 1994, and December 1994. Sessions were supposed to be either weekly or every other week, but often the interval was stretched to 3 weeks. The primary goals were (1) conflict resolution between Lisa and her mother; (2) teaching mother and daughter to regulate their communication and keep their relationship on an even keel; (3) helping Lisa come to terms with her relationship with her father, who refused to participate in any of the sessions; and (4) maintaining good school performance.

Frankly, at the time I did not consider the case to be going well. I did my best to teach this mother–daughter dyad positive communication skills and self-control techniques and to use cognitive restructuring to help them put their extreme beliefs of ruination, autonomy, and unfairness in perspective, but they continued to have knock-down arguments, often instigated by minor nuances in each other's communication patterns. They would exhibit improved communication in the session but would be unable to consistently apply what they learned at home. Lisa did improve her school grades from C's and D's to mostly A's and B's, and we did conduct one school meeting at the beginning of 12th grade to help her get off to a good start that fall. But, the case abruptly stopped in December 1994, when Lisa ran away from her mother's house to live with her father after a really bad argument with her mother.

A therapist never knows the impact he or she has had on clients, and I underestimated my help to this family. In August 1995, Lisa, then 18, contacted me herself and asked to come in. She was living with her mother again, had graduated from high school the previous spring by the skin of her teeth, and was planning to go to a local community college that fall. She asked for my help in getting herself organized to cope with ADHD and succeed academically in college. She had not been taking Ritalin for some time and wanted to restart it. She presented as a much more mature, self-assured older adolescent, who somehow had learned to deal better with her mother and to distance from her father, whose influence she now considered negative. She had a boyfriend and a part-time job, was driving, and was starting to think about career goals: She wanted to be a pilot. We agreed to schedule several individual sessions at 2-week intervals, to work primarily on school-related goals. Her mother supported the idea of the therapy and, amazingly, agreed with her daughter's assessment that the mother–daughter relationship was now excellent. In the next three sessions I helped Lisa with planning her studies, balancing her social life and her academics, monitoring the effects of Ritalin and deciding how to get the maximum benefit out of medication while in college, and reacting to the breakup with her boyfriend. At the end of the third session, she was adjusting well to college and we agreed to have a follow-up in 2 months. At the 2-month follow-up, she was getting A's and B's in college, taking her Ritalin regularly, getting along with her mother and her mother's fiance, and busy with her social life. She was happy and upbeat, with a newfound confidence. We left open the possibility of having another session, but she did not see the need at that time.

I next heard from Lisa one year later, during her second year in community college. She had stopped taking her Ritalin during the past semester, studied less, and her grades had been inconsistent. She was increasingly concerned about her future and was feeling torn in many directions by career goals, social life, work, and studies. She was living with her mother, who was now remarried and going to college herself. Lisa felt her life was "out of balance" and she very much wanted my help to achieve a balance and learn to manage her time better. Her medication had not been regulated in 2 years, and she was having "peaks and valleys" from short-acting Ritalin. We agreed to meet every other week. I referred her to an adolescent medicine specialist to regulate her medication. I met with Lisa four times and helped her achieve balance in her life and manage her schoolwork better. She did not return for therapy afterwards.

Two years later, Lisa scheduled a session. She now presented as a poised, impeccably attired young lady who had completed community college and was working as an assistant designer in an advertising firm. She was doing well socially, had individuated from her mother and was living on her own, and felt full of self-confidence as she looked forward to a career in commercial art and advertising. She had stopped taking Ritalin, but had been prescribed Prozac for the past 6 months. She reported that Prozac helped her a great deal with moodiness and impulsivity. She was considering returning to college to complete her Bachelor's degree and wanted my assistance in coping with her studies. Only time will tell how Lisa does in the future, but as of the present, she is coping effectively with ADHD.

Comment

The ongoing follow-up for Lisa was not planned in the orderly fashion suggested in this chapter but turned out to follow a similar pattern. In fact, this was one of the cases that caused me to formulate the plan for long-term follow-up. This case also taught me that even when we do not think we have had a positive impact on the presenting problems brought in by adolescents and their families, we may have helped in ways we do not always realize. That Lisa returned on her own at ages 18 and 20 suggests she got something out of the original therapy. That the mother and daughter eventually changed their communication patterns suggests they got something out of the family therapy, although clearly other factors were also operating.

The first series of follow-up sessions in 1995 were focused on the transition into college, and when Lisa successfully negotiated that transition, we stopped regular sessions. However, as she matured further and life became more complicated, she came to realize she needed additional help and returned twice. This case illustrates nicely how a therapeutic relationship established in midadolescence in one context can be helpful as the adolescent with ADHD transitions into adulthood, through periodic booster sessions at critical developmental transition points.

CONCLUSION

If the practitioner conducts ongoing follow-up sessions with his or her adolescent clients and their families over a number of years, new problems can be prevented from escalating into major conflicts, and periodic bursts of additional therapy can be applied as needed. This discussion of follow-up concludes the presentation of the comprehensive treatment program for adolescents with ADHD and their families. Practitioners might best regard the interventions outlined in the chapters in this section as a menu for successfully treating adolescents with ADHD. Each item on the menu—ADHD education, medication, school interventions, family interventions—is complicated and difficult. If any aspect of the treatment is carried out poorly, it will detract from the others and the overall success of the case.

The remaining two chapters serve different purposes. Chapter 14 consists of two stories written by adolescents with ADHD describing their struggles to cope with the disability. The Epilogue then briefly raises important questions which remain to be answered.

CHAPTER FOURTEEN

———— O ————

Two Adolescents Tell Their Stories

In this chapter Michael and Chris tell their stories of growing up and living with ADHD. Readers will see their trials and tribulations, their successes and failures, and the many ways in which their parents, teachers, professionals, and other caring adults helped them cope with ADHD. These stories are designed not only to be helpful to health care and mental health professionals but also to parents and adolescents coping with ADHD. I recommend that the therapist give a copy of this chapter to families during the family ADHD educational phase of the comprehensive intervention outlined in this book.

MICHAEL'S STORY
BY MICHAEL GINSBERG

A note to the reader: ADHD was once thought to be a problem predominantly found in boyhood, but recent studies suggest that many girls are also affected by the disorder. These girls are often overlooked, as ADHD tends to manifest itself differently in the two genders.

I have tried to avoid the use of pronouns such as "he" and "she" as much as possible, but there are times a singular pronoun must be used. I considered using "he or she," but I found it unwieldy; I considered using "s/he," but I felt that the slash would be distracting to the eye; and I even considered using "it," but decided against that idea as it is especially important to remember that ADHD children are still kids. I grudgingly decided on using the male pronoun as referring to either a male or a female. I kindly ask the reader to understand my decision, and it should be emphasized that I do not intend to shun girls at all.

Growing up is never an easy job. All children have their crosses to bear as they approach adulthood. The process is harder for some than others, but for a kid with ADHD, the entire experience can be an ordeal. Unlike other disorders and disabilities, ADHD does not manifest itself physically, which leads to a lack of understanding from others. For example, the wheelchairs used by the physically disabled serve as a signal to others that their occupants cannot walk.

On the other hand, it is impossible to discern the neurotransmitter deficiencies and minor structural differences in the brains of ADHD children at a glance. They look normal, they seem intelligent, and they sometimes even outperform their peers. This makes it seem that ADHD is nonsense or an excuse for poor behavior. Also, because ADHD children tend to behave differently from other children, other children tend to scorn their ADHD peers. A disorder which is so subtle is both a blessing and a curse. It is a blessing in that it does not necessarily place concrete limitations on the abilities of the individual in question, but it is a curse in that others tend not to understand it.

When I was born in 1977, ADHD was virtually unheard of. There was no sign on that hot July day that I was any different than the tens of other babies born that day. I looked just like any other newborn child: healthy, vigorous, and slightly purple with an egg-shaped head. It was several months until my parents began to notice that I was not behaving like their other children. I had very irregular sleep patterns and I would wake up in the middle of the night shrieking unusually often for a baby. My parents figured that I was just colicky, so they just waited for it to pass.

But it didn't pass. I was so active that my parents finally got me a sturdy indoor wooden climber and slide in the living room. I would climb up and slide down over and over and over again. I never seemed to tire of this exercise. In fact, according to my mother, I once kept at it for 4 straight hours, just going up and down, barely making a sound, but having the time of my life.

I was just 3 years old when my brother left for college. My aunt and my mother designed a special bedroom for me. An accurate description of the design would take up several pages, but suffice to say that it served as a gymnasium, a playroom, and a bedroom. Today, the exact same room serves as a study, a library, a spot for private reflection, and a bedroom. The furniture in the room was designed to be virtually indestructible and completely safe, even for the most rambunctious child. I still managed to break things and hurt myself.

First School Experiences

In nursery school and kindergarten, the teachers told my parents that I was "in a world of my own" or that I "marched to the beat of my own drummer." While I was never maliciously bad, I was very impulsive, and that got me into trouble quite often. I remember one incident in particular that occurred in kindergarten. My elementary school's playground was bordered by a woods on one side, and the children took advantage of the natural construction materials there to build "forts," which were manned by respective "clubs," that did mock "battle" with each other. I desperately wanted to join one of these clubs, but the other kids didn't like me as I was too talkative (I still am) and very impulsive (I still am), and I had a very violent temper (I've managed to fix that problem). One day, I strayed too close to a fort and was greeted by its "guardians," who all wielded small sticks and twigs as swords. Determined not to be outdone, I immediately picked up a large branch and hit the closest guardian in the eye (by mistake). Fortunately, no permanent damage was done to her eye, and she and I were able to look back and laugh at the incident several years later. Still, I was in deep trouble that day.

My creative mind was always at work as well. I remember once during music class when we were instructed to pantomime stirring a cauldron for a Halloween song. I decided that because nobody uses cauldrons any more (presumably including modern-day witches) I would simply turn the dials on a pantomime electric mixer. Not surprisingly, that action drew a strange look from the music teacher.

Academically my lower elementary school career was rocky, to say the least. I had still not been diagnosed with ADHD, so I was not on medication. School served as a theater of my disability. I had a terrible time learning to read. For 2 years my parents, my teachers, and even a few friends tried to get me to read. Finally, one day, my teacher sat me down in a small group of other kids with a simple book. Out of the blue, I read the first page fluently and conversationally. The teacher was shocked and had me continue. I read the rest of the book effortlessly. Within a week, I had jumped a year ahead of my classmates in reading. Suddenly, the problem was not getting me to read but getting me to stop.

My teacher in second grade was wonderful. She understood me and was the first to suspect that I might have "minimal brain dysfunction," now called ADHD. She started a program with weekly reports to my parents about my performance, behavior, relations with the kids, and so on. Her teaching style was warm and nurturing. She made frequent jokes, and allowed us to have a great deal of fun. She was firm but fair. Basically, because she had no children of her own, she loved her students as if they were hers. I loved her so much that I returned to see her a few times. Most recently, I visited her with all my college acceptance letters. It is the only way I know to express my gratitude to her.

Still, my writing was messy, I was disorganized, and my work was inconsistent. Despite her support and encouragement, my relations with the other kids were poor. They excluded me, made fun of me, and picked on me.

Disaster Strikes in Third Grade

All hell broke loose in third grade when I was assigned a teacher who was rigid, old-fashioned, and shortsighted. By constantly disciplining me in front of the class, she gave tacit approval to the other kids picking on me.

They jumped at the opportunity. They told me I was subhuman, that I was fat (I was a little chunky), that I gave off noxious fumes, and that I was a girl (they called me "Michelle"). Soon, I was believing them in a subconscious way. Every night I'd go home and check to make sure I still had a penis, that I could pass within 10 feet of people without their passing out, and that I was not some hideous monster covered in rolls of quivering fat. I remember often coming home and reporting that rather than having made a new friend, I had made a new enemy.

This alarmed my parents. None of my siblings had ever gone through this. I should have been making friends and enjoying myself, not making enemies and dreading each day of school.

My parents were called in again and again to see the principal. He told them that I had some serious problems and that he was going to refer me to the school psychologist. My parents searched for professional guidance. I had a medical evaluation with a pediatric neurologist who declared there was nothing wrong with me. In the meantime, I had no idea what all the commotion was about. In retrospect, I wish that my parents had been a little more candid with me, but I forgive them for that. They started me in counseling with a child psychologist who based her therapy on Freud. I enjoyed the therapy, which seemed to be based on play more than anything else, but I don't believe it really helped me.

Meanwhile, back at school, the third-grade teacher had put me at a desk that faced out the window, near the "cubby holes" the kids used. She felt that the isolation (I was in a corner) might spare me some of the taunting. It didn't work.

First of all, I was facing out a window, which made paying attention impossible because I could not see the teacher and because I was looking outside, and paying attention to everything but the teacher—which is a common problem for any ADHD kid. Also, if one of the other kids wanted to make fun of me, all he had to do was come over, pretend to use his cubby hole, and torment me. This kept up for a few weeks until I unexpectedly reached one of the most important turning points in my life.

One day, when the teacher was out of the room, my classmates ordered me to drop to all fours and beg like a dog. I complied with their request, hoping that I might gain their acceptance by doing what they told me to do. Suddenly, there was a sharp pain in my side and I was knocked onto my back. The same kid that had kicked me stepped on me. I struggled back to my hands and knees amid a sudden shower of blows being dealt from about 20 third-graders. I sheltered my head and tried to defend myself. I was so helpless at the moment that I did not even think to fight back, which would have been fruitless. Most of my memory of those awful moments is a blur, and I feel great pain when I recall it. In fact, there are tears in my eyes as I write this, and I almost *never* weep from emotion today. I remember looking up at the jeering faces of my attackers as they continued their assault. I was too confused and scared to cry out, and the beating continued. I remember feeling ashamed of being beaten up like this, and then I started to fight back. I was still on the floor, but I was struggling, driven by my raging emotions and my sheer hatred of the boys and girls who were attacking me. Finally, my rage and anger caused me to let forth a blood-curdling cry which attracted the attention of the principal, who happened to be walking by the room at the moment. I am thankful that he was there, for if not, I might have been seriously injured. When the principal broke up the mob, I was curled up on the floor, crying. The physical pain that I was suffering was bad, but the emotional welts hurt immeasurably more than my bruises.

When I went back to thank my second-grade teacher a few months ago, I visited my old third-grade room where this particular incident had taken place. I could not bear to look at the spot where I had lain on the floor that day, even almost a decade later, and I am not a very emotional man. As I look back on that traumatic day, I find it hard to believe that a group of third-graders could have been so brutal.

Time to Switch Schools

That same day the principal called my parents in for another conference and suggested that I be certified under the designation of emotionally impaired. My parents would not agree to this inaccurate label. They said that I was not emotionally impaired but, rather, I had other problems. Clearly, I was not a troublemaker or a bully, but rather I was misunderstood. The principal stated that I was not "learning disabled" and therefore strongly suggested that my parents withdraw me from his (*his!*) school as soon as possible (this was in mid-January) as there was nothing else the school could do. He also phoned around to all the other public schools in the district and blacklisted me. Why he should have wished to trap my family and me into a situation like that is beyond me.

To my knowledge, no disciplinary action was ever taken against any of the children who were involved in the beating. In fact, my parents were the only ones even notified of the incident.

My parents immediately removed me from that obnoxious environment and had me tested at several private schools. We had no choice after the principal of my old school had called around and blacklisted me. My test scores were excellent and described a high IQ. I was accepted by all of them for the following September. The only midyear opening was in a progressive school with a very loose curriculum and we grabbed it. I loved the freedom and the openness. I did not have to do much math or spelling . . . my weaknesses. The class was structured more like a kindergarten class than anything else. We were given a great deal of freedom over the course of the day to explore any of the educational materials in the room. I even learned to play chess there (and I am a lousy player to this day). The lack of structure appealed to me, obviously, but not to my parents.

The following fall my parents put me in a more structured independent school. My parents knew that consistent expectations and individual care would be beneficial for me.

The ADHD Diagnosis

Also, that summer, my parents took me to a psychiatrist who diagnosed me with ADHD and put me on Ritalin. He told my parents not to worry about me and assured them that I would indeed turn out to be a successful man. He cautioned them that I would need to take the Ritalin for the rest of my life. However, he assured us that the benefits reaped would far outweigh the inconvenience of having to take the pill. Just like he said, everything started to change.

When the school year began, I actually paid attention. I was placed in accelerated math, I seldom got in trouble, and I made a few friends who continue to be my friends, even though the majority of the kids treated me with little more respect than the kids in public school.

In addition, my parents enrolled me in a swim team program to help me burn off some of my excess energy. Of course, ADHD reared its ugly head again when my coaches told my parents that if I "would just listen and concentrate," I would be a much better swimmer. We extended my Ritalin dosages to last through practice, which helped solve that problem.

Fourth grade did not start off quite so smoothly. For the first month or so, I got in a fight at least once a week. After the fourth time I had gotten in a fight (and hit my best friend) I realized that I would have to come up with a better way of dealing with my emotions.

The popular view is that "letting it out" is the best way to handle emotions. I had a problem with this method because, invariably, something would get broken or someone would get hurt in the process of venting my emotions.

To avoid causing any more damage to friends, friendships, or property, I simply began to ignore my emotions. For a while I took it too far and I forgot how to be human, but I have now learned to find a medium between the Freudian "id" and "superego" (if I may be forgiven for referring to Freud).

At this time I also solidified my commitment to Boy Scouts, in which I had been active for several years. I decided that I would become an Eagle Scout and Senior Patrol Leader (the head scout) of my troop. My parents had to help me hold to that commitment, but I reached my goal in seventh grade.

As fourth grade ended, I was beginning to make friends, I followed directions, and the other kids even started to treat me with some respect. By the end of fifth grade, I was ready and eager to return to public school.

Middle and High School

My education in private school had prepared me for the idea of having more than one teacher, but the idea of having a locker . . . well, I believe that there might still be a "condemned" sign on my old locker from sixth grade. The academics were also still a little rocky. I would do assignments and then get zeros because the teacher could not read my handwriting. I recently looked over an old assignment from sixth grade. My answers were correct—and well-stated—but I had a zero because it was "illegible—can't read." The sheer frustration caused by such reports often brought me to tears; it is just not fair to work so hard on something and then be slapped in the face with it. One time, I completed a rather lengthy English assignment with a flair and a polish, but it was a few days late, and I got a C. Often, my assignments were found on the floor of the bus, in the hallway, or buried in my notebooks. I was being graded on my disability rather than my abilities.

The spring of eighth grade my parents began the process of certifying me as ADD under IDEA or Section 504. After a vicious struggle with the school district, I was certified and the few accommodations I requested were granted. They included use of a computer for written assignments, occasional flexibility on late assignments, seating near the front of the room, and an additional set of books so that I would not have to remember which ones to carry home each day. I never had a serious problem getting a teacher to cooperate, and my case manager was wonderful. Soon, I began helping other kids to get certified.

Freshman year in high school was relatively successful and I achieved a 3.579 grade point average. Meanwhile, I continued to suppress my emotions. Sophomore year was the great breakthrough we had been waiting for. Junior year finished with another 4.0, but with three Advanced Placement courses and two accelerated/honors classes in addition to Forensics and Advanced Conditioning for Swimming. As a senior, I took AP English, AP Calculus, AP Physics, and AP Spanish, and *I graduated at the top of my class.*

Success at College

I applied to 10 universities, with Harvard being my first choice (more accurately, Harvard was, as far as I was concerned, my *only* choice) and I was accepted to 8 of those 10 universities. Harvard was one of the two universities to which I was not admitted. Believe it or not, that was probably the best thing that ever happened to me. I am now a proud student at Stanford University, and I believe that I am far happier there than I ever could have been at Harvard.

The nice thing about having the 504 certification is that it remained with me when I went to Stanford. At Stanford, I have the same accommodations that I had in high school, with an exception. I also have a note taker in classes where I request it. A note taker is another student in the class who is paid $50 a quarter to take notes as he usually would but go to the Disability Resource Center and photocopy them and put them in a file for me. I use a note taker for fast-paced classes where I can't pay attention to the professor and take notes at once. Note takers are also used for physically disabled students, like me when I broke my right hand and couldn't write. There was minimal fuss in getting the necessary accommodations at Stanford and I am very happy with the services I have received there.

I have just completed my first quarter at Stanford as I write this in January 1997, and I came out with a B+, an A, and an A+. I'm also the president of the Learning Disabled Students of Stanford, active in Disabled Students of Stanford (the two organizations are linked), and a member of a political party on campus and a service organization.

Academically, I have overcome the petty faults that caused me so much grief in the past. My handwriting is no better than it was in second grade, except that I have given up on cursive, which helps a little. In fact, after looking back on some of my papers from that time, it could be argued that my handwriting is worse. I now own a laptop computer, which I take to all essay exams. I either carry my printer with me or give my answers to the professor on a disk. I find it ironic that such a minor flaw once caused so much trouble, especially as I highly doubt that my handwriting will result in "zero—can't read" in the "real-world," and particularly as I intend to be a physician.

I have also made a decision to try to spare as many other students as possible the nightmare I had to endure. Pursuant to this goal, I have become active in CH.A.D.D., as well as taking part in projects like this book.

The scars from the past are still there, however. Others often see me as cold and not very trusting. I tend to view a friendly overture with suspicion and caution, a residual instinct from elementary school, and I often prefer to spend time alone than with others. Curiously, many friends on campus are blind or wheelchair-bound. An odd side note is that two of the blind students also have ADHD.

Organizational Strategies

I discovered several organizational strategies that helped me to turn in my assignments on time in high school. These tips are not guaranteed, nor are they particularly ingenious, but they tend to work.

First and foremost was a correctly used Trapper Keeper (made by Mead) or a similar product. For the benefit of those who are not familiar with this invention, it is a large three-ring binder which can hold smaller "portfolios" or folders. Each folder is dedicated to a particular class and holds handouts, assignments, etc. In middle school, I usually jammed papers into random folders, rather than putting them in their correct places, resulting in frequent loss of handouts ("but, Mrs. Olson,* you never gave me one!"), and subsequent (and embarrassing) discovery of said handouts. In high school I actually started to place each paper carefully in its correct folder, which saved me time and embarrassment.

My second strategy is an assignment book. Unfortunately, like the Trapper Keeper, this only works when correctly used. It is important to write the assignments down, *and to remember to look at them later*. A small digital recording device or a tape player also functions nicely in the same capacity. In addition, wristwatch alarms are useful as a reminder to take medicine.

My only problem with the assignment book, as I hinted earlier, is that I frequently do not bother to look at it, and thus forget something. My remedy to this problem is to write important reminders on the back of my hand (in ballpoint pen). Not only is it extremely difficult to forget one's hand or to leave it somewhere (though I am sure I will someday find a way) but the reminder is constantly there, in plain view, and unavoidable. A warning: This method may not work for swimmers, as the chlorine will bleach the ink. I also sometimes leave little notes attached to my car keys, where I cannot possibly miss them.

Life at a university is an entirely different challenge. I have adapted quite well, I think. First and foremost, it is important to keep a neat and orderly desk. This facilitates the finding of various materials when they are needed. I use my lower drawer as a file cabinet (it is just the right size), and the other two to store various materials. The shelves over my desk are also organized into four areas. One houses class folders (notes, syllabuses, assignments, and the like); one houses books for pleasure and reference, as well as a few coffee mugs and some silver I have appropriated from the dining hall (I promise to return it at the end of the year); another compartment houses audiovisual equipment (i.e., my portable CD player), computer parts, and CDs; and the fourth compartment holds textbooks and paper (both looseleaf and computer paper). By holding to these divisions, I have been able to stay organized. My desk is normally spotless because everything has a place (contrast this to my three non-ADHD roommates, whose desks have attained a rudimentary level of consciousness) and a chemical model of methylphenidate even graces one of the corners. As long as everything is put away as soon as it is used, things stay clean. I even find time to make my bed every day (I only sleep under the comforter, so it's a 30-second job).

I have discovered several study techniques as well. In high school one

---

*I have never had a teacher by that name (for the record).

set of rules applies. First, never attempt to do homework while off medicine. Second, study for 40 minutes, and then take a 10-minute break. Third, just sit down and *do the work*; the toughest part is getting started, and after that it's easy. Fourth, experiment a little. For instance, some people study better with quiet music in the background, whereas others prefer silence.

In college, the rules should be modified. I prefer not to use my desk in my room as a study area. Because I also use the desk for purposes other than business, I try to do my studying at the library in the center of campus. The geographical change has a psychological affect on me in that it serves as a signal that it is time to work. Also, the dead silence of the library is a great boon to my efficiency, especially when compared to the bedlam that is dorm life at Stanford. I suggest that a student find a place to study (it need not be a library; a clearing in the woods or a secluded park bench would serve nicely) and use it. When a suitable study area is located, inspect it. Is there a drinking fountain, elevator, phone, door, etc., nearby? Is it normally crowded, or will there always be an empty space? The list of questions varies from situation to situation. The most important thing is that the study area is comfortable for studying, otherwise concentration is impossible.

Assignments are easier to keep track of in college, because there aren't as many. It helps to keep a schedule for the day as a reminder of when to study. However, because problem sets tend to be due on the same day every week, the routine quickly falls into place.

Closing Advice

It is important to eat well (this can be a problem for those taking methylphenidate because we do not get hungry and then we forget to eat), get plenty of sleep, and stay in good physical shape. Also, school nights are school nights, and social events should be kept to a bare minimum until Friday and Saturday.

I have to work longer and harder than my colleagues here at Stanford, because every second of schoolwork is a struggle. Still, ADHD is a part of both *what* I am and *who* I am. I wouldn't give it up for the world. Ultimately, the secret to defeating ADHD is to *not* try to defeat it. The trick is to learn to live *with* it. ADHD is a challenge and challenges can be fun, if you rise to meet them.

Good luck . . . and *have fun*.

CHRIS'S STORY
BY CHRIS EDNEY AND PAT EDNEY

"Wow what's that thing?" "It looks like a bike but has the wheels of a trike. It is very interesting, I think I will have to look at it and daydream a bit." These, arbitrary thoughts, have been my life for a number of years. This above all things has made school tough for me. My right brain wanders and takes the left brain with it. It's fun but gets me in trouble sometimes. I will give you a synopsis of my struggles and victories.

In the beginning, there was Mom and Dad (Pat and John), then came me, Chris. Noticeable to all upon my arrival on a cold wintry evening was how alert I was for my age. I am told that my eyes were wide open, wandering around the room, taking in everything. After trying to have children for 6½ years, my parents' lives were changed drastically overnight. I was adopted at 5 days old. Two years later my Mom and Dad conceived twins. I would then have a brother, Matt and sister, Jenny to keep on track!

I was quiet and easy to take places. I was spitting out words at age 7 months, and started stringing two words together at 10 months, including my famous "I want." By 12 months I was making complete sentences. At 14 months I became the largest mass-media target because I would repeat commercials to my parents in the store such as, "No, no mommy don't get those Pampers, get Huggies, they are not soggy and they don't leak." I was also saying, "I'm fascinated with electricity" and "We are moving to Mississippi." Singing was among my many other talents. When the guitarist at church started his solo I immediately launched into my own personal rendition of "El Vira."

Curiosity and Mischief

As a young'n I required very little sleep. I would arise at o'dark thirty, sometimes even earlier. In these wee hours of the morn in complete solitude I would leap over two gates at my bedroom door. There was lawlessness in the house. I would start the washing machine, spread toothpaste and Vaseline over the walls. Peanut butter would find its way all over the counters and cupboards and I would raid the refrigerator and make much mess. Spilleth upon the floor much milk and maketh many a pop tart that fell upon the counter as crumbs and then I would leave my artistic imprint upon the countertops with sugar and flour. Could they have sold this as a Piccaso?

Curiosity was a large part of my life. I was constantly taking things apart and would rarely get them back together again. This included timers, clocks and radios. At the ripe age of 3, convicted of talking too much, I was then sentenced, and kicked out of preschool after my first day. I enjoyed opening the windows and drawers and meandering up and down the halls. I even had a difficult time sitting in a circle quietly. Turning on and off the faucet also intrigued me. One morning after watching *The Lost Boys* (a movie about modern-day vampires) with my babysitter (I was not supposed to have watched TV at all that night), I decided to keep all the vampires away by spreading a bottle of garlic powder and garlic salt over every square inch of the floor, counters, and of course all the appliances.

Not surprisingly, my parents were not believers. My dad says though, "It must have worked because we have never been bothered by vampires."

Due to my curious nature, the hospital reserved a place for me in the emergency room. Drinking rug cleaner, eating a whole bottle of vitamins, cutting the corner of my eyelid, falling off of a chair (I was spinning on it at a velocity close to the speed of sound), and breaking my clavicle are some of my claims to fame (or perhaps shame). To my surprise, I ended up starting the sprinkler system during one of my brother's soccer games. During a critical point of the game it went off on the opposing team's side. I just had to see how that intriguing knob worked!

I was in and out of three different preschools. I don't exactly have fond memories of this period because I spent much of my time sitting in the time-out chair. Only occasionally would I assert myself and have my personal Jihad (or a holy war) to prove my point. I do remember distinctly that it was at the Montessori school that I was allowed to use a knife (whoopee!) to cut potatoes (and occasionally my fingers). I then found that I was fascinated with knives, firearms, and pyrotechnics (wow!).

The ADHD Evaluation

It was time, at this point, to get my head "checked" (I personally had absolutely no problems with it so far, and had actually grown quite fond of it). My parents (I think they were not fond of it, or possibly wanted to get me a new one) had difficulty making eye contact with me and problems getting my attention. (Wow! this is deep.) They felt at times they were talking to a brick wall (or some other similarly impenetrable structure). So I was abducted by aliens and evaluated at a " highly reputable" place in "Omaha" (Or maybe it was in Roswell, New Mexico). They proceeded to give me an IQ test and concluded that I was very bright and that my parents just needed to discipline me more frequently (I didn't think so). Well, my mom had just completed her master's in education with emphasis in learning disabilities and understood what battery of tests is supposed to be given. She was not happy with this clinic and decided to go for a second opinion. My parents took me to see a pediatric neurologist. I was in the room for only 5 minutes and he told my mom and dad that he thought I had ADD but wanted to confirm his diagnosis with a battery of other tests (Come on, let me study for one of these tests.) I then went to a private clinical psychologist. Upon completing the sessions, her conclusion coincided with the neurologist's. I was placed on Ritalin after the psychologist persuaded my parents. My parents were advised to tell me I was not taking Ritalin but was taking vitamins. When I found out what it was, I lost it. I was enraged and felt I had been betrayed, especially by my mom because she was the one who gave me my medicine. The anger didn't last long. My parents stated that they felt a need to wait for the right maturity level because I have a tendency to blow things out of proportion (I deny it) and either overexaggerate or play it down. I guess they were right.

Elementary School

Kindergarten would be my next epic adventure. Due to my high IQ I did not qualify for "special" services so I was placed in a regular classroom. My parents searched to find a school in a good district with a low student-to-teacher ratio. I remember this year as pivotal. My teacher was rigid; it was like juvenile hall. We were made to feel guilty if we could not learn as fast as she wanted us to. She would not slow down to accommodate us. She was like a lead weight dragging us down. I learned to be independent from the crowd. I was different, and people don't like what is different. I could be my own person. I had no friends.

I pretty much sailed through first, second, third, and fourth grade. My first-grade teacher was remarkable. She was enthusiastic and taught with a hands-on approach. She communicated well with my parents (so I am told). She found ways to stimulate our creativity and always let my parents know about upcoming tests, projects, or anything out of the ordinary with a phone call. Even though my second-, third-, and fourth-grade teachers did not know a lot about ADD, they were willing and able to learn. The class size would increase at my current school the following year. My parents decided that because the class size was increasing to the same amount as a private school it was time to make a change. The environment would be more structured and I would not have to make another move until after eighth grade (I thought).

Dangerous Games

Danger intrigued me. I was fearless. I enjoyed lighting matches and sometimes would drop them off the balcony. I would light small objects like leggos on fire or just play with candles. If there were any fireworks left over to be had, I would find them. I loved mixing up different potions. I remember my soda and vinegar mixture because it exploded all over my parents' brand-new coffee table. Dad set up a pyrotechnics time about every other week. This is when I could light as many matches as I wanted under direct supervision. My dad got me involved in a gun safety course. This was his way of seeing to it that my fascination for knives and guns were experienced in a positive light.

Nonpurposeful destruction seemed to loom over me (I know it's not a word). I tried to mix a special potion to clean the hood of my mom's car but it ended up taking off the paint. I tried to spray paint a box so I put it up against our blue house and sprayed it black ... you know what happened! One time when mom was having a backyard party she just got everything all cleaned up and left to go get ice. While she was away I decided to feed the birds and spread dog food over most of our deck. The birds were very hungry!

Creativity has always been a strong quality for me. One time when I was mowing, I was getting a little bored just going back and forth, back and forth, so I decided to do the design of a fish hook. It actually gave the yard a unique look.

Reading is another positive activity for me. Over the years I have enjoyed reading about topics such as snakes, horses, planes, dinosaurs, and oceanography. My current topics include scuba diving, Hummers, and mountain biking. Oh and yes, I sometimes perseverate on these subjects.

Like perseveration, my free flight of ideas can be good at times but on other occasions can hinder me and/or cause frustration to others around me. One day my cousin (thanks John!) kept track on paper of the topics I covered on the way home from school. Within 7 minutes I covered 20 different topics.

With free flight of ideas comes my distraction. Consequently, I need to hear directions, for chores or other tasks, as well as see the steps on paper to meet with success. Demonstrations have proven helpful, too. I remember well the time we visited my brother and sister in the hospital. They were in incubators. I became fascinated with the dials trying to see how far I could turn them. As quickly as that thought and action came and went I climbed on a chair and pulled the chord to alert the hospital staff of a code 99 (cardiac arrest). I remember that the nurse said to my mom as we departed, "Good luck, honey."

It was in fifth grade that kids began really to notice that I was different. In this year we would change rooms just like in junior high. I was dealing with four different (and unique) teachers instead of one. Trying all the while to remember my papers, write assignments down, turn projects in on time, write legibly, and read out loud. To all the misguided I appeared so stupid. Kids tortured me constantly, and you know how ruthless kids can be. I was fascinated with how things would explode and periodically would talk about this. I am not a harmful person but the other kids did not understand this. On occasion I was put in a big storage room, left alone to do my work so I wouldn't be distracted (oh yea, whatever). I was the outsider, alone in the multitudes. If you hammer someone long enough you drive their self-esteem down. Even though some of the teachers were trying to understand ADHD, there was not much information at that time and they were getting frustrated (I think they gave up). They felt they could no longer meet my needs.

The Decision to Home School

Frustration led to my reevaluation. Because the original psychologist had retired, we chose a psychologist who came "highly recommended." She gave me a battery of tests, including writing a paragraph. Because I sat in the room for 1 hour and refused to write a paragraph, she concluded that I had Oppositional Defiant Disorder. She did say that my academics were basically fine but that I needed a little extra help in math. But she had the nerve to suggest that I should be taken out of my home and placed in a psychiatric facility for 2 or 3 weeks. Well, that conclusion did not meet with my parents' approval. It was their feeling that we should get a second opinion. The psychiatrist who gave the second opinion said that even though I needed a change of schools, I did not need to go to a hospital (good idea). Upon checking with our school district for placement we found that they agreed I needed extra help and was not a behavior problem, but that the only placement they had available was in a behaviorally disturbed classroom (oh joy, not). This recommendation also did not sit well with my parents. After much deliberation, discussion, and the frustration of feeling backed into a corner with no choices, we decided to school at home.

Home schooling would be my life for the next 3 years (sixth, seventh, eighth grade). It had its ups and downs, but for the most part it was a good experience. We got more subjects done in a shorter period. There was no waiting and I did not get shot down. Mom was accepting of me. At times I have felt it shot my social life in the foot. In reality it was during my home schooling that I had the opportunity to develop interests like horseback riding and scuba diving and from these interests had more friends than I ever did at school. At times we had big power struggles (the other Cold War). I met my match. No matter how much I puffed up my chest and tried to look big, bad and scary, Mom would puff up more. I would have to complete a certain amount of schoolwork before I had rights, even if it took me until midnight. I thought I had it figured out, if I sat down and waited for the rest of my life, she would eventually stop waiting for me. But for the most part we had more positive interactions. She told me it took her the first 3 months to convince me that I was smart and not dumb and could learn whatever I put my mind to learning. She believed in me. I began to believe in myself. I could be whatever I wanted to be.

Success with Home Schooling

Home schooling allowed my mom to help me enhance my strengths, teach me compensating skills for my weaknesses, and incorporate my interests into our curriculum. We used the same curriculum as the private school I would have been going to. I stayed on regular doses of medication. For my academics my mom combined a visual and hands-on approach with the auditory, always seeming to have a backup way of explaining any new concept. The computer assisted my fine motor coordination problems. I didn't have to erase so much and therefore I could be proud of the work I produced. A trainer put me on a physical fitness program to aid in my gross motor skills. I met with him twice a week. Head phones, timers, and music assisted in maintaining my attention. For memory and processing difficulties we learned to slow the process down by going from my head to the tape recorder to the computer. Or from my head to my mom the secretary, then she would read it back while I typed on the computer. This made a substantial difference in broadening my spelling and writing skills. (When I was in the psychologist's office the reason I had so much difficulty writing the paragraph wasn't because I was trying to be obstinate but because I have a hard time getting started and have processing problems). Brainstorming and mind mapping have also been useful tools. For organization I learned to use the Franklin planner. It contains my assignment sheets, calendar, pens and pencils, and telephone numbers. A five-subject spiral notebook contains my notes and pockets to hold my papers and projects. We also worked on 10 social skills: proximity, anger, eye contact, tone of voice, manners, body language, friendship, responding to teasing, how to greet someone, and when to interrupt. We used the Boys Town system and only worked on two at a time.

Horseback Riding Builds Self-Esteem

Home schooling allowed me to pursue a challenging interest: horseback riding. Through horseback riding I gained a sense of power and control. I was praised for having a natural talent (even by a professional rider). I had the ability to put my own style into my riding. Team sports just didn't seem to work for me. I attempted to play soccer and baseball but seemed to be more interested in running after the butterflies and stopping to talk to the opposite team's players than being involved in the game. No one poked fun at me in the barn. It was a safe environment. My trainer was strict but cared about me and took pleasure in my success. Oh yes, there were times when my distractions or impulsiveness would get in the way. For instance, when I tacked up my horse and left him on cross-ties for an hour and a half (oops!) after someone asked me to go wandering on the trails, I just forgot about my horse! Or at one of my shows when I made an impulsive move and cut my horse's tail off (only 2½ feet!). I did a perfect job of cropping his tail. To my great surprise, my trainer did not at first notice what I had done. When I entered the arena for my stadium jumping round and saluted the judge, you could hear the booming voice of my trainer saying, "*Oh my god!*" Actually ADHD was beneficial for this sport. I had to keep noticing everything and the bursts of energy helped me greatly for cross country when I needed it. What an adrenaline rush! Because of home schooling I could afford to travel and be gone on a Friday, Saturday, and Sunday. I just made my time up earlier in the week. Horseback riding changed my life in a positive way.

The effect of home schooling on the rest of our family and friends ended up positive but met with many skeptics at first. In reality, Mom had more time to spend with my younger brother and sister because we were not doing homework every night. In the past, our homework evenings had turned into battles, so being free of those exchanges made for more peace on the homefront. I think (wait, I know) my siblings were jealous that I got to stay home.

A Return to School: Big Trouble

In my seventh-grade year, after one year of home schooling, my parents attempted to send me to another private school. This was a very structured, small private school. I thought I was ready. I thought it was peculiar, though, that on my first day there was no one assigned to walk me around to my classes. I remember being very anxious about going back to school after all the relentless teasing I had experienced before. Even with this being a new experience, most of the day went smoothly until about 2:30 P.M. (14:30 hours for all you military types). Then I had gym class. As I was changing out of my gym clothes I felt insecure, because a group of five to six rather large boys cornered me in an area by my locker. I didn't want to change in front of them, because they seemed very focused on me. They were intent on making fun of me. They called me faggot, dipshit, and jackoff and assorted other names. One even said, "Why don't you go in one of the stalls and masturbate?" I told them to back off about nine or ten times and they didn't. Feeling cornered and threatened with harm I boldly stated, "Well I am the jackoff with the knife, so back off." I pulled the knife out of my bag, opened the blade and waved it around, never touching anyone. All those kids told the coach and I gave it up and took the consequences. My parents were immediately called and I was instantly expelled. My parents took it before the board (I would not have gone back). The decision was that I would never be admitted to that school again. The school agreed not to put this incident on my record, but I know that the school had to expel me. I would like to add that the students were never disciplined for their verbal assault and threatening demeanor toward me. (*"The wrongs we rue, we cannot undue, but I forgave you long ago"*—Robert Service.) Although my parents were very upset with what happened, they did support me.

Sometimes we do not understand why something happens but there must have been a reason. I must not have been ready to go back at this point. I returned to home schooling for the next couple of years. We spent a good deal of time preparing so I could enter high school. More than ever I was bound and determined to get into a good private school.

I went to a psychologist for about a year. My parents felt we would work on social skills and other behaviors. To their surprise they were spending $90 a week for me to go in and complain or as they say "get into my negative mode." It was not a worthwhile experience and very costly. I made no progress in these areas so we ended the sessions.

Finally: Success at School

What an ecstatic moment when I found out I was accepted to Creighton Prep. Creighton Prep is a challenging private college prep school here in Omaha, Nebraska. I am a junior maintaining an 82% average. I have asked for few, if any, accommodations. I take my medicine on a regular basis. In a school where you get demerits if your shirt isn't tucked in, I am well below average with demerits. My success has been due in part to the structure of the school, using a Franklin planner, living out of my rather large Kelty®™ (thanks you guys at Kelty) backpack, putting in a lot of extra hours studying, and having a college student occasionally come to my house in the evening just to keep me on track. Because I have a difficult time getting to my locker and remembering what to bring to class or take home in the evening I organize my life around my backpack. I just keep all books, day planner, and notebooks in my backpack. People joke about the size of the bag, saying I must have a few freshmen in there. I had to build a wall around myself to protect against the hurt of teasing. I learned I can't let it get to me. I like it at Prep. The atmosphere, besides being 19% oxygen and 21% nitrogen, is accepting, of who I am, what I do and what I love.

The Understanding Teacher

Most of my teachers at Prep have been very understanding and cooperative. They have spent time learning about ADHD. I owe one teacher in particular, my former German teacher, many thanks for taking the time to believe in me. He didn't just believe in me, but in all his students. He did not single me out. He treated all students equally. He was interested in his students as people. He would pull our interests into the subject material, and when writing essays, he encouraged us to incorporate them and he likewise would share his. He became a part of the class. He was like a student with an extended role as a teacher. He got down to our level. He was strict and demanded a lot out of us. He gave lots of homework. He would always yell in class or be silly. He was so energetic and made the experience fun. You wanted to go to his class. Dr. Hajo Drees was that charismatic adult in my life. I ended up with a 95% in his class and was able to go to Germany with him, his wife, and her sister and 13 other students last summer. He landed a job at a university. It's so hard to say good-bye. The first meeting my mom had with the teachers my freshman year, Dr. Drees, who grew up in Germany, came up to my mom and said he thought he had ADHD. He said he understood and not to worry, that I would be OK. I know he was right! *Vielen Dank, Hajo, Sie hatten meinen leben verbessert* (Thank you, Hajo, you made my life better).

In the End, There Was Poetic Justice

As I reflect on my school years I think about how many times I was told I wasn't responsible or I lacked motivation. There is no magical age when you become responsible or have motivation. Motivation and responsibility come with success. It's the people who believe in you who allow you to meet with success.

First off, I want to thank those people who did not believe in me, for it has been my driving force to go back and prove them wrong. I cannot wait until I can walk across Creighton Prep's stage and receive my diploma. I will have proof then that I did it.

In my heart now I already know I've made it. There have been people who believed in me, and it is them I want to thank. I dedicate this chapter to them. And now I have a poem for all.

"Prophets"

I've watched them come,
And I've watched them go.
Their ideas, and prophecies of his demise.
Poor child,
He will never be anything, but a trouble maker.
Labeled behaviorally disturbed, and called many things that are worse.
Stupid child,
They wanted nothing to do with him,
They think its his destiny to fail,
All their false ideas backed with false degrees.
Put him at St. Joe's, because he can never make it through high school.
Failure
Maybe one day this child will get the respect he deserves,
and I pray that his scars heal.
The pity I feel for this boy, is so real,
Because once a long time ago I was that boy
and he has done so much more then they said I could.

Epilogue

I conclude this volume by raising some of the issues you, readers, ideally will address through research and clinical efforts. These questions reflect many of the topics throughout the book where I used that phrase, "more research is needed."

1. How can we better help adolescents to come to accept ADHD and related conditions, and be open to taking steps to learn about and cope with them? We need to develop measures of adolescent acceptance of ADHD and study the developmental changes in acceptance that we know clinically occur over the course of adolescence. We need to build on the ideas discussed in Chapter 7 of using adolescents to help other adolescents deal with ADHD (e.g., peer coaching). In Chapter 7 I briefly described the teen forum conducted at the CH.A.D.D. National Conference. Similar programs need to be available around the country, and we need to research their effectiveness. I also described books and videotapes written for adolescents. We need to evaluate their effectiveness in reaching ADHD teenagers. This kind of research might actually be done with the assistance of ADHD college students who have reached a stage in their life where they are coping well with their disability and want to give something back to their younger peers.

2. How can we improve our diagnostic procedures for use with adolescents? There are many specific questions within this area. Should we make the diagnostic criteria for ADHD developmentally sensitive if we do view ADHD as a dimensional disorder? How can we better operationalize "impairment" from an educational and a psychosocial perspective? How should we better integrate and understand rating scale data from multiple teachers? Are there versions of continuous performance tests that will prove more sensitive with older adolescents? A great deal of psychometric research is needed to answer these questions.

3. What is the long-term effectiveness of stimulant medication with adolescents, in particular dextroamphetamine spansule and Adderall? Can we develop measures of problems in daily living and administer them periodically over weeks, months, and years, to tap whether adolescents consistently medicated with stimulants do better in the long run than those who are not so medicated? We need research to determine whether the results of the medication research on family interaction with younger children generalize to adolescents, and to what extent medication improves driving behavior and reduces the adolescent's tendency to engage in such high-risk behaviors as unprotected sexual relations or failure to wear seatbelts.

4. How can we "beef up" such psychosocial treatments as the family interventions described in this book to reach a greater proportion of the families than Barkley, Guevremont, et al. (1992) found were helped in the one controlled evaluation of such interventions with ADHD adolescents? What is the effectiveness of the entire 20-session intensive intervention outlined in this book? What accommodations can be demonstrated to be effective in schools? There is virtually no research on this topic with adolescents.

5. What types of interventions will more effectively help parents regain control over those adolescents who flagrantly violate street and house rules and engage in delinquent, conduct-disordered behaviors in the community?

6. What are the separate, common, and synergistic effects of medication and the various psychosocial interventions discussed in this book? Careful comparative research needs to be done to address these issues.

7. More theoretically, how do the variables discussed in the behavioral family systems model interact with the basic neurobiological tendencies of the individual to cause an adolescent's ADHD to manifest as mild, moderate, or severe? Can we demonstrate that Barkley's version of Patterson's performance theory of ODD in ADHD youngsters is in fact correct? What is the correct way to integrate the concept of temperament into our thinking about ADHD? Is response inhibition truly the central organizing construct for ADHD? And what is the central organizing construct for ADHD, Inattentive Type? Although less immediately compelling than the diagnostic and treatment questions, these theoretical questions are equally important to our ultimate ability to understand and deal with ADHD in adolescents.

And so I end this journey through the world of ADHD in adolescents. In order to remind the reader why we are doing this in the first place, I would like to end with a poem written by Charlotte Booth, an adolescent with ADHD. Charlotte was diagnosed with ADHD while in fifth grade. Now she is an honor roll student. At the time of her diagnosis, she wrote the following poem:

"Trapped"
by Charlotte Booth

I feel trapped
like I'm in a cage
screaming
screaming
trapped
trapped

My heart is confused
I am changing
life changing
feelings changing
all new things
coming
coming at
me

I feel safe
in the cage
but
trapped
while
safe

Life is different
I am different
HELP!

APPENDIX

———————— O ————————

Medication Research

This appendix is a supplement to Chapter 8 regarding medication. We believe that the practitioner should become an informed consumer who can critically assess the latest research concerning the effectiveness of medication. In this appendix, I review in some detail research on the effectiveness of medication with adolescents diagnosed as having ADHD. The information presented here is based primarily on three sources: (1) comprehensive reviews of the outcome literature by Joseph Biederman and his colleagues, one of the leading ADHD research teams in the field (Spencer et al., 1996; Wilens & Biederman, 1992); (2) a critical review and discussion of the literature on stimulant medication with adolescents (Smith, Pelham, Evans, et al., 1998; Smith, Pelham, Gnagy, & Yudell, 1998); and (3) the original studies cited by these reviewers.

Spencer et al. (1996) based their review on a Medline search of all manuscripts published in the English language in peer-reviewed journals with at least minimally explicit methodology (e.g., use of rating scales to document response). They categorized the results of each controlled study into three categories: (1) robust (> 50% of the subjects responded positively); (2) moderate (30% to 50%); (3) poor (< 30%); or (4) mixed (not categorizable). They used more stringent response criteria for open, uncontrolled medication trials: (1) robust (> 70%); (2) moderate (50% to 70%); (3) poor (< 50%); (4) or mixed (not categorizable). They broke down their results by (1) type of medication (stimulants, tricyclic antidepressants, non-tricyclic antidepressants, antipsychotics, other drugs), (2) age (preschoolers, latency-age children, adolescents, adults), and (3) ADHD plus comorbidities (conduct/aggression, depression/anxiety, tic disorders, mental retardation). I focus most heavily here on the results for adolescents, referring as necessary to the broader sets of results.

EFFECTIVENESS OF STIMULANT MEDICATION

There was an average of 70% overall positive response rate of the 5,608 children and adolescents and 160 adults participating in 155 studies of stimulant medica-

425

tion (methylphenidate, amphetamine, pemoline). The positive effects were obtained on measures of overactivity, impulsivity, and inattentiveness, as well as on-task behavior, academic performance, and social functioning in family and peer interactions. These effects occurred at home, at school, and in the clinic and were clearly dose-dependent. Twenty-three to 27% of the children and adolescents did not respond to stimulants or could not tolerate them because of adverse side effects. In an earlier, often quoted study (Sprague & Sleator, 1977), it had been found that the higher doses required to ameliorate behavior had an adverse impact on performance on cognitive tasks, raising concerns about the nature of the dose-related improvements and the use of higher doses. In this review of the literature, attempts to replicate and extend Sprague and Sleator's (1977) findings were reviewed; these similar studies found dose-related improvements in behavior and cognitive functioning, failing to replicate the adverse impact on cognitive performance at higher doses found by Sprague and Sleator. Rachel Gittelman Klein (1987) also reviewed dose effects of methylphenidate on children with ADHD and found that cognitive function showed a linear dose response in about half the studies and variable results on different cognitive tasks in the other studies—but there was no corroboration for a decrease in learning with increased doses.

The vast majority of the studies were conducted with latency-age children (147, or 87%). Only seven (4%) of the studies reviewed by Spencer et al. (1996) were done specifically with adolescents (Brown & Sexson, 1988; Coons, Klorman, & Borgstedt, 1987; Evans & Pelham, 1991; Klorman, Coons, & Borgstedt, 1987; Leser & Leser, 1977; MacKay, Beck, & Taylor, 1973; Safer & Allen, 1975; Varley, 1983). All these studies evaluated methylphenidate in doses ranging from 10 to 60 mg per day (0.3–1.0 mg/kg), over periods ranging from 3 weeks to 2 years. Six of the seven studies reported a robust response to methylphenidate, and one reported a moderate response. Four of the seven studies were controlled trials; three were open trials. Dose-dependent effects were obtained in studies using multiple doses. No evidence of abuse or tolerance was found, but several studies noted a mild increase in heart rate and blood pressure. Six of the studies were conducted primarily with Caucasian males, and one was conducted exclusively with African American males (Brown & Sexson, 1988).

Critical Analysis

Smith, Pelham, Evans, et al. (1998) critically analyzed the published placebo-controlled, double-blind studies of stimulant treatment for adolescents with ADHD and found that contrary to the more optimistic conclusions of Spencer et al. (1996), who also included open trials in their review, only about 50% of the adolescents responded well enough to recommend continued use of stimulants (Evans & Pelham, 1991; Fischer & Newby, 1991; Klorman et al., 1987; Pelham et al., 1991; Varley, 1983). They pointed out that we do not know why there is a 20% lower positive response rate in adolescents versus children with ADHD (50 % vs. 70%). They suggested that although there may be a true difference in the effectiveness of stimulants as children move into adolescence, a number of methodological factors in the nature of the research done to date could plausibly account for this difference in response rate: (1) the small samples in the adolescent studies, coupled with the extreme heterogeneity of presenting problems of adolescents with ADHD may have limited the power to detect medication effects; (2) longitudinal studies have suggested that the core symptoms of ADHD lessen as children move into adolescence, lessening the severity of behavior at baseline, thus making it more difficulty to show improvement due to medication (e.g., a ceiling effect); (3) the lack of developmentally sensitive measures; and (4) the increased variability in the environment of adolescents (e.g., high school is more complicated than elementary school) coupled with the decreased time that adults rating adolescents spend with the adolescents may have decreased effect sizes in medication trials; and (5) perhaps the adolescents in the studies with the lower response rates were receiving relatively low doses of stimulant medication.

Two New Studies

Studying medication effects longitudinally in one cohort of subjects medicated both as children and adolescents would help us understand whether medication effects diminish developmentally and why. Two open trials that followed groups on medication from childhood to adolescence found overall response rates of 70% to 100% continuing over time (MacKay et al., 1973; Safer & Allen, 1975). Smith, Pelham, Gnagy, et al. (1998) conducted the first controlled, double-blind placebo follow-up study of the stability of stimulant medication effects from childhood to adolescence, attempting to avoid the methodological pitfalls discussed earlier as much as possible. Sixteen individuals with ADHD, IQ above 80, and no learning disabilities who completed both the child (mean age = 10.2) and adolescent (mean age = 12.7) versions of the Pittsburgh Summer Treatment Program (STP) served as participants. The STP is an intensive behavior therapy program including a token economy, intensive feedback, and structured training in social, recreational, and academic skills. The activities were geared to be developmentally appropriate but parallel in nature for the children and adolescents. Daily activities included 3 hours of classroom activities, 3 hours of therapeutic recreation, therapeutic group discussions, and cooperative tasks. Children and adolescents attend the STP for 9 hours a day, 5 days a week, for 8 weeks. From the third through the eighth weeks of the program, the participants were evaluated on a medication protocol that alternated medication conditions on a daily basis, using placebo or methylphenidate, such that each subject received each medication condition a mode of six times. Although several different methylphenidate doses were compared throughout the program, this study focused on placebo days versus 0.3 mg/kg days for the 16 participants who attended the program as children and again as adolescents.

Dependent measures included (1) daily counselor and teacher ratings on the Iowa Conners Rating Scales, which yield Inattention/Overactivity and Oppositional/Defiant scores; (2) the frequencies of four composite scores of 17 negative behaviors recorded reliably by trained observers throughout the day (noncompliance, conduct problems, negative verbalizations, and disruptive classroom behavior); (3)

the amount and accuracy of work completed in the classroom; and (4) the percentage of time the youngsters were on-task in the classroom. The dependent measures were converted to a common metric of individual medication effect sizes for analysis. The effect size represents the difference between the means of the placebo and medication conditions divided by the standard deviation in the placebo condition. Eight individual dependent measure effect sizes and an overall effect size were compared between childhood and adolescence.

Analyses indicated that the overall medication effect size was significantly smaller in the adolescents (mean = 0.59) than in the children (mean = 0.82). Two of the eight individual effect sizes changed significantly in the same direction as the overall effect size (noncompliance and disruptive classroom behavior), indicating that medication decreased noncompliance and disruptive classroom behavior less when the participants were adolescents compared to when they were children. The individual medication effect size for the accuracy of the classroom work was higher for the adolescents (mean = 0.63) than for the children (mean = 0.27), indicating that the participants benefited more from medication when they were adolescents than when they were children on this variable. For all the other measures, including the Iowa Conners, several behavioral observation categories, and the amount of classwork completed, the effect size of medication was comparable during the two periods.

In addition, when considering overall medication response, 14 of the participants were positive medication responders both as children and adolescents at the same dose in terms of mg/kg. There was an average increase in the absolute total daily dose of methylphenidate of 18.2 mg for the adolescents: 5 mg of this increased was due to weight gain; 13.2 mg due to receiving a third dose in adolescence and not in childhood.

This study indicates that response to stimulant medication is relatively stable as children move into adolescence, with 93% of the participants responding positively to methylphenidate during childhood and adolescence, and only 3 of 12 dependent variables showing changes in effect size with regard to medication. Smith, Pelham, Gnagy, et al. (1998) point out that interestingly, when the variables were aggregated without respect to domain or presenting problem, there was approximately a one-fourth standard deviation decrease in effect size from childhood to adolescence; this significant change is consistent with the decrease from 70% to 50% in response rate found from their review of the literature. Given the rigor of the controls in this study, the authors argue that the decrease in effect size looked at in this way probably represents developmental changes in the tasks faced by adolescents compared to children, and the increasing need for psychosocial and educational interventions to improve performance on these tasks. Of course, these results were obtained with a concurrent, comprehensive behavior therapy program in effect and might be underestimates of similar medication effects obtained in the absence of such a highly structured psychosocial intervention.

The limited number of controlled studies of stimulant medication conducted with adolescents have not yet given the practitioner much guidance about selection of the optimal dose. Based on the research with children, Spencer et al. (1996) concluded that basically progressively higher doses lead to incrementally better functioning, and the earlier work suggesting an "inverted U-shaped" (e.g., quadratic) relationship between dose and outcome failed to replicate. As noted earlier, the relatively few controlled studies of stimulant medication with adolescents have found that methylphenidate is superior to placebo but have suffered from methodological deficiencies that make it impossible to reach definitive conclusions about dose/response relationships. Smith, Pelham, Evans, et al. (1998) conducted a controlled, double-blind medication/placebo study with a large sample of 46 adolescents designed to compare the effectiveness of three wide-spaced doses of methylphenidate on social behavior of adolescents diagnosed as having ADHD. Smith et al. (1998) designed their study and analysis to test out three hypotheses about dose/response relationships: (1) linear effects—improvement increases in direct proportion to increased dosages; (2) plateau effect—once an improvement is found, there is no further change at higher doses (e.g., all doses are superior to placebo but equal to each other); and (3) quadratic effect—there is an inverted U-shaped curve such that above a certain dose, higher doses have deleterious effects. These adolescents were participants in the same STP described previously for their study on the stability of medication, and similar dependent measures were used. From the third to the eighth weeks of the program, the adolescents received three doses per day of either placebo, 10 mg, 20 mg, or 30 mg of methylphenidate 4 days a week. Medication conditions lasted 1 day and were randomly assigned such that each youngster experienced each dose for a mode of 6 days. Dependent measures included (1) the Iowa Conners; (2) side effects ratings; (3) the frequency of 19 behaviors observed throughout the day, grouped into four scales: (a) conduct disorders—intentional aggression, destruction of property, stealing, lying, leaving the area without permission; (b) defiance to adults—abusive verbalizations to staff, threats to staff, noncompliance, swearing, and intentional disruptions; (c) impulsivity—interruptions, using materials or possessions inappropriately, and rule violations; and (d) teasing peers—teasing peers, threatening peers, and horseplay; and (4) the success ratio—a ratio obtained from the record of 19 rows of negative behaviors and 8 columns of time intervals in a day indicating the percentage of cells in which there was no negative behavior.

There was a significant effect of medication on all of the eight dependent measures. Trend analysis suggested that the linear trend was a reasonable fit to the data for six of the eight measures (excluding Impulsivity and the Success Ratio); the plateau trend was a good representation of the data for four of the eight dependent measures, but the quadratic trend was not a good representation of the data for any of the dependent measures.

The medication effect size was computed for each subject for each dose, as were differences between effect sizes as one increased from each dose to the next highest one. The number of subjects whose medication effect exceeded a threshold of 0.5 effect size for each dose was determined. Then, number of subjects with differences between threshold for adjacent doses greater than 0.5 (continuing returns) were computed. Positive response rates ranged from 24% to 87%, depending on the measure selected, averaging about 68%. Forty-nine percent reached the threshold of 0.5 at 10 mg, 15% at 20 mg, and 11% at 30 mg. An average of 21% of the subjects showed continuing therapeutic returns when the dose was raised from 10 to 20 mg, and 22% showed continuing returns when the dose was raised from 20 mg to 30 mg. These continuing returns are clearly lower than the 50% likelihood of improving social behavior when the 10 mg dose is compared to placebo.

Side effects of severe loss of appetite and dull or tired affect, withdrawal, and picking were reported especially at the higher doses.

These results clearly supported the effect of methylphenidate on social behavior in adolescents with ADHD and suggested that the linear effect was a good representation of the data. However, the effect size and continuing returns analyses also revealed dropoff in the size of further medication effects at higher doses. Smith, Pelham, Gnagy, et al. (1998) describe this type of dose–response curve as asymptotic, a compromise between the linear and the plateau trends. The type of trend that best explained the data also varied with the dependent measure domain. Rating scale measures showed clearer linear effects and observational data showed clearer asymptotic effects. In the past, other studies finding linear effects have relied on rating scale data. Thus, the type of dose–response effect obtained in part must be a function of the type of dependent measure examined, posing an interesting dilemma for clinicians. As Smith, Pelham, Evans, et al. (1998) point out, a decision about which dose schedule to use might depend on the availability of extensive norms for these measures, so clinicians can pick a dose that normalizes scores on ecologically valid measures. In any case, taking the side effects and overall results into account, this study suggests conservatism concerning robust dosing of methylphenidate, indicating that optimal balances of positive effects and/or side effects may be best obtained at the lower or moderate dose levels.

Most of the research done with stimulant medication in adolescents has relied primarily on teacher and parent ratings rather than ecologically valid measures such as classroom assignments and test scores. The work of Pelham, Smith, and their colleagues at Western Psychiatric Clinic in Pittsburgh is a refreshing exception to this trend. Additional research similar to Smith, Pelham, Evans, et al.'s (1998) study in classroom settings is sorely needed. In particular, more attention needs to be paid to the fine tuning of medication for different academic activities, classroom structures, and teachers. The average adolescent encounters five to eight different teachers a day. Classes vary in degree of difficulty. There is no reason to believe that a single dose of medication would be ideal for every class. We need more information about the dose ranges that work well for lecture versus laboratory classes, for example, in order to combine dosing recommendations with hand-scheduling recommendations, to maximize performance across the entire school day for the adolescent.

The largest trial of medication effects, the multimodal treatment trial, is currently being carried out at six centers in the United States (Abikoff & Hechtman, 1996). This trial will enroll 576 children (ages 7–9 years) and follow them for 2 years on the treatment arm into which they are assigned. Prolonged follow-up will, it is hoped, be carried into the adolescent years. The study is designed to compare medication treatment alone with three other groups: (1) an extensive psychosocial treatment arm including parent counseling, social skills training, and educational interventions; (2) a combination of the psychosocial treatment arm and the medication treatment arm; and (3) a community-treated referral group. For those participants in one of the medication treatment arms, there is an attempt to optimize the medication treatment for each subject using the stimulant (or other medication) to which they had the best response. Results from this study have not as yet been published but promise to provide important data on the response rates to different medications and on the changes in response to these medications as children progress into adolescence.

Concluding Comment

There have been no published studies of the effectiveness of the other stimulants in adolescents. I have recently learned of two not yet published studies of pemoline with adolescents (J. Biderman, personal communication, May 12, 1998; B. Smith, personal communication, January 12, 1998). A single study of Adderall in school-age children also recently appeared (Swanson et al., 1998).

EFFECTIVENESS OF NONSTIMULANT MEDICATIONS

Antidepressants

Spencer et al. (1996) reviewed 29 studies which have evaluated the efficacy and safety of tricyclic antidepressants (TCAs) in children, adolescents, and adults with ADHD. Twenty-seven (93%) of the studies reported moderate ($N = 9$) or robust ($N = 18$) response rates. Twenty-six of these studies were conducted primarily with latency-age children. Eight studies (three controlled and five open) included adolescents, but only one was done exclusively with adolescents (Gastfriend et al., 1985). Seven of these eight studies reported a robust response in adolescents. The breakdown of studies for specific TCAs was as follows: (1) imipramine—12 studies; (2) desipramine—9 studies; (3) amitiptyline—3 studies; (4) nortriptyline—4 studies; and (5) clomipramine—1 study. Wide-ranging doses from 5 up to 200 mg/day (0.4 to 6.3 mg/kg) were used in these studies, but response rate was surprisingly equally positive at all dose ranges. TCAs had the greatest positive effect of behavioral symptoms rated by parents and teachers, but a much more variable impact on neuropsychological measures. In 13 studies, TCAs were compared to stimulants: five studies found stimulants to be superior to TCAs, five found them to be equal, and three found TCAs to be superior to stimulants.

Other antidepressants such as monoamine oxidase inhibitors, fluoxetine, venlafaxine, and bupropion were also evaluated in 11 studies, several of which included some adolescents (Spencer et al., 1996). Response rate was robust in 50% and moderate in 50% of these studies, but specific effects for adolescents are not clear at the present time.

There has been concern about the cardiac effects of TCAs. Four cases of sudden death in desipramine-treated children (no adolescents) were identified (Barkley, 1998), and even though the risk may be low, it is conservative to regard TCAs as second-line treatments for ADHD until more is known.

Regarding other antidepressants, there have not been any controlled trials with individuals with ADHD, but there has been one open trial of Wellbutrin (bupropion) with ADHD adults, where it was found to be helpful (Spencer et al., 1996).

Clonidine

Clonidine is thought to act on alpha-adrenergic receptors in the brain stem, decreasing sympathetic outflow from the central nervous system. In ADHD, clonidine has been used when other medications do not work or are counterindicated (e.g., ADHD plus Tic Disorders), and particularly for children with Sleep Disorders and in the evening when an additional dose of methylphenidate could interfere with sleep. Spencer et al. (1996) reviewed four studies with children which evaluated the effects of clonidine and reported beneficial effects, usually of moderate robustness in 50% to 70% of the subjects. In addition, two double-blind, placebo controlled trials examined the effects of clonidine on ADHD symptoms in children with Tourette's Disorder; these studies found that there was significant improvement in both hyperactive–impulsive behavior and motor tics, but not in other measures ("Clonidine for Treatment of ADHD," 1996). The most common adverse effects of clonodine have been irritability and sedation, but hypotension and bradycardia can occur. At least five unexplained sudden deaths were reported in children who were taking clonidine, but no cause and effect relationship has been clearly established yet ("Clonidine for Treatment of ADHD," 1996). In addition, one open trial examined the effect of another similar drug, guanfacine, in children and adolescents, reporting beneficial effects (Spencer et al., 1996).

In summary, although clonidine may sometimes be effective in treating ADHD, particularly with comorbid tics or sleep problems, the controlled trials are inadequate, none have been done exclusively with adolescents, and there are major unresolved safety issues. Clonidine is, therefore, a medicine of last resort for adolescents with ADHD.

Concluding Comment

The evidence suggests that all the nonstimulant medications are not generally as effective for ADHD as the stimulants, and of those evaluated, we only have solid evidence of effectiveness for the TCAs in adolescents.

LONG-TERM EFFECTIVENESS

In contrast to the vast literature on the short-term effectiveness of medication with ADHD, little research has examined the long-term effectiveness of medication. It is hoped that the multimodal treatment trial mentioned earlier will help to change this picture (Abikoff & Hechtman, 1996). Of the existing long-term studies, Weiss, Kruger, Danielson, and Elman (1975) compared the adolescent outcome of children who received stimulant medication for 3 to 5 years in childhood with those who did not receive any medication. No significant differences were found. Hechtman, Weiss, and Perlman (1984) compared prospectively followed ADHD children when they were between 19 and 25 years of age. One group had received 3 to 5 years of stimulant medication; the other had not received any medication. The study is described in detail in Weiss and Hechtman's (1993) book, *Hyperactive Children Grown Up*. There were few significant differences between the groups in adulthood on education completed, job status, psychiatric history, substance abuse, and anti-social behavior. The group that had received stimulant medication remembered their childhood more positively and had better social skills, better self-esteem, and fewer car accidents than did the group that did not have stimulant medication. In addition, there were no differences between the groups on height, weight, blood pressure, or pulse, suggesting that long-term treatment with stimulant medication did not have an adverse impact on growth or cardiovascular functioning.

The difficulties in doing controlled studies of the long-term effectiveness of medication are immense. Getting subjects to remain on controlled doses for long periods may be difficult enough; getting members of control groups not to take any medication could be even more difficult. Experimentally controlling for a variety of confounding life events is virtually impossible, although statistical controls may be possible given a sufficient sample size. Deciding on appropriate outcome measures for long-term studies is equally complicated. To date, investigators have looked at static, cumulative outcome measures such as employment status, education, and psychiatric status. It may be that quality-of-life measures, such as the number of problems in daily living per week, month, and year, are more appropriate. It may also be that individuals with ADHD need to remain on adequate doses of medication for several years to produce long-term outcomes.

To put this issue in its proper perspective, the difficulties of looking at long-term outcome of treatments for childhood disorders are not limited to ADHD. There is little research on the long-term outcomes of any treatments for any childhood psychiatric disorders. Thus, when critics of the use of medication dismiss it because of the lack of evidence of long-term effectiveness (Armstrong, 1995), their criticisms should be viewed within the context of the difficulties of conducting such research and not considered evidence against using medication or attempting to conduct the appropriate research.

Despite these difficulties, a recent study has provided the first double-blind, placebo-controlled evaluation of the effectiveness of stimulant medication over an 18-month period. Even though the study was done with 6- to 11-year-old children, I describe it here because of its importance to the field. Working in Sweden, Gilberg et al. (1997) conducted a randomized, double-blind placebo-controlled trial of amphetamine sulfate (short-acting amphetamine) on 62 children, ages 6 to 11, meeting the DSM-III-R criteria for ADHD. Treatment was not restricted to children with "pure" ADHD (i.e., 42% had comorbid diagnoses). The comorbid diagnoses included pervasive developmental disorders ($N = 7$), mild mental retardation ($N = 10$), Oppositional Defiant Disorder ($N = 8$), Conduct Disorder ($N = 1$), separation anxiety disorder ($N = 3$), and tic disorders ($N = 3$). Children underwent five phases: (1) baseline evaluation (month 0), (2) a 3-month period when the dosage of amphetamine was titrated to an optimal level in a single-blind condition (months 1–3), (3) randomization at the end of month 3, (4) a 12-month period of treatment with either amphetamine or placebo in double-blind fashion (months 4–15), and (5) a 3-month period of single-blind placebo. Dosages of amphetamine were titrated from 5 mg twice daily up to the optimal dose, with an allowed maximum of 60 mg a day; the mean dose at the beginning of the double-blind treatment phase was 17 mg a day.

In this type of study, the investigators expected that a number of youngsters would drop out of the placebo condition, and they decided to offer such subjects an open trial on medication. Therefore, they made the duration of participation in the double-blind treatment one of their dependent measures. They also used Conners Parent and Teacher Rating Scales and WISC-R IQ scores as other dependent measures; the analyses of these measures are based on reduced samples because of the dropout rates. The IQ tests were given at the beginning of the study and at the 15-month point; the Conners Rating Scales were given at months 0, 3, 6, 9, 12, 15, and 18.

During the 12-month double-blind placebo period, 71% of the placebo group and 21% of the amphetamine group stopped treatment or went to an open medication trial; this was a highly significant difference strongly supporting the effectiveness of medication. On the Conners Parent and Teacher Rating Scales, there were highly significant improvements from baseline to the 3-month measurement point during the initial titration phase; during the double-blind phase, the placebo group deteriorated and returned to its baseline scores whereas the active drug group maintained its improvements. Comparable results were obtained for boys and girls and for children with pure ADHD as well as children with ADHD plus comorbid conditions. Interestingly, the 9- to 11-year-olds improved more than did the younger children on parent and teacher rating scales. Also, the amphetamine group gained a mean of 4.5 IQ points on the WISC-R, whereas the placebo group gained 0.7 IQ points; this difference was highly significant.

The analysis of side effects is very important in such a long-term study. Gilberg et al. (1997) did a very careful analysis of side effects, examining the number of children in the amphetamine and placebo group who exhibited the following side effects before and after treatment: difficulty falling asleep, early awakening, disturbed sleep, increased need for sleep, headaches, abdominal pain, diarrhea, constipation, dry mouth, nausea/vomiting, tics, stereotypies, anxiety, dysthymia, euphoria, palpitation, dizziness, decreased appetite, increased appetite, and hallucinations/delusions. In addition, they compared expected and actual height of the children before and after treatment.

No side effects occurred in more than 50% of the children in either the amphetamine or the placebo group, and many side effects were in fact reported to be occurring in the placebo group. The only side effect that occurred in significantly more of the amphetamine (42%) than the placebo (12%) group was a decreased appetite. A careful analysis was done of tics as a side effect. Of four children diagnosed with Tic Disorders before entering the study, three did not show an increase in tics on amphetamine and one did. The 18 children who begin to exhibit tics during the study were distributed across the placebo and drug group, and amphetamine did not cause an increase in tics. In fact, tics decreased in several of the children while on amphetamine. Finally, there was no significant relationship between height development and duration of amphetamine treatment.

The results of this study provide clear-cut evidence in a prospective, controlled study of the long-term positive effects of stimulant medication in helping children with ADHD. More children remained on medication for the duration of the study, and these children received significantly more improved parent and teacher ratings than did those in the placebo condition. The medication group also improved more on Full Scale IQ than did the control group. A careful analysis of side effects illustrated that there were no long-term adverse reactions associated with being on amphetamine. This study provides some of the most compelling evidence to date of the long-term benefit and safety of treatment with stimulant medication.

CONCLUDING COMMENT

No other intervention for ADHD has been subjected to the same degree of empirical scrutiny as medication. Stimulant medications continue to emerge as having the strongest support for their effectiveness in general and their effectiveness with adolescents in particular. With the Gillberg et al. (1997) study, we are beginning to have controlled evidence of the long-term effectiveness of stimulant therapy, although we clearly need a lot more such research, particularly with adolescents.

Unfortunately, with perhaps the single exception of the work by Pelham and his associates reviewed earlier, all the medication research with adolescents has relied primarily on teacher and parent rating scales rather than more ecologically sound dependent measures. With regard to dosing of methylphenidate in adolescents, increasing doses up to 1.0 mg/kg seem to produce linearly increasing improvements in functioning, whereas doses above 1.0 mg/kg either produce no further improvement or sometimes decrements in performance. Although we have some compelling research of the impact of stimulant medication on family interactions for younger children (Barkley, 1998), no such research exists yet for parent–adolescent interactions. Surprisingly, methylphenidate is the only stimulant systematically evaluated in the published studies with adolescents. There is a great need for carefully conducted trials of dextroamphetamine spansule, Adderall, and pemoline in adolescents using classroom performance and family interaction measures.

References

Abikoff, H. B., Gittelman-Klein, R., & Klein, D. (1977). Validation of a classroom observation code for hyperactive children. *Journal of Consulting and Clinical Psychology, 45,* 772–783.

Abikoff, H. B., & Hechtman, L. (1996). Multimodal therapy and stimulants in the treatment of children with Attention Deficit Hyperactivity Disorder. In E. D Hibbs & P. S. Jensen (Eds.), *Psychosocial treatments for child and adolescent disorders: Empirically based strategies for clinical practice* (pp. 341–369). Washington, DC: American Psychological Association.

Abikoff, H. B., & Klein, R. G. (1992). Attention-Deficit Hyperactivity Disorder and Conduct Disorder: Comorbidity and implications for treatment. *Journal of Consulting and Clinical Psychology, 60,* 881–892.

Achenbach, T. M. (1991). *Manual for the Child Behavior Checklist/4–18 and the 1991 profile.* Burlington, VT: University of Vermont Department of Psychiatry.

Achenbach, T. M. (1996). Subtyping ADHD: A request for suggestions about relating empirically based assessment to DSM-IV. *The ADHD Report, 4,* 5–9.

Achenbach, T. M., & Edelbrock, C. S. (1983). *Manual for the Child Behavior Profile and Child Behavior Checklist.* Burlington, VT: Author.

Adams, W., & Sheslow, D. (1990) *Wide Range Assessment of Memory and Learning (WRAML).* Wilmington, DE: Wide Range.

Alexander-Roberts, C. (1995). *ADHD and teens: A parent's guide to making it through the tough years.* Dallas, TX: Taylor.

Amen, A. J., Johnson, S., & Amen, D. G. (1996). *A teenager's guide to ADD: Understanding and treating Attention Deficit Disorder through the teenage years.* Fairfield, CA: MindWorks Press.

Amen, D. G., & Amen, A. J. (1995). *A teenager's guide to ADD: Understanding and treating Attention Deficit Disorder through the teenager years audio cassette tapes.* Fairfield, CA: MindWorks Press.

American Psychiatric Association. (1994). *Diagnostic and statistical manual of the mental disorders* (4th ed.). Washington, DC: Author.

American Academy of Pediatrics. (1996). *Diagnostic and statistical manual for primary care (DSM-PC), Child and Adolescent Version.* Elk Grove, IL: Author.

Anastopoulos, A. D. (1993). Assessing ADHD with the Child Behavior Checklist. *The ADHD Report, 1*(3), 3–4.

Anastopoulos, A. D., Barkley, R. A., & Sheldon, T. L. (1996). Family based treatment: Psychosocial intervention for children and adolescents with Attention Deficit Hyperactivity Disorder. In E. D. Hibbs & P. S. Jensen (Eds.), *Psychosocial treatments for child and adolescent disorders: Empirically based strategies for clinical practice* (pp. 267–284). Washington, DC: American Psychological Association.

Anastopoulos, A. D., & Costabile, A. A. (1995). The Conners continuous performance test: A preliminary examination of its diagnostic utility. *The ADHD Report, 3,* 7–8.

Angold, A., & Costello, E. L. (1993). Depressive comorbidity in children and adolescents: Empirical, theoretical, and methodological issues. *American Journal of Psychiatry, 150,* 1779–1791.

Arcia, E., & Conners, C. K. (1998). Gender differences in ADHD. *Journal of Developmental and Behavioral Pediatrics, 19,* 77–83.

Armstrong, T. (1995). *The myth of the ADD child.* New York: Dutton Press.

Atkeson, B. M., & Forehand, R. (1979). Home-based reinforcement programs designed to modify classroom behavior: A review and methodological evaluation. *Psychological Bulletin, 86,* 1298–1308.

Barkley, R. A. (1981). *Hyperactive children: A handbook for diagnosis and treatment.* New York: Guilford Press.

Barkley, R. A. (1987). *Defiant children.* New York: Guilford Press.

Barkley, R. A. (1990). *Attention-deficit hyperactivity disorder: A handbook for diagnosis and treatment.* New York: Guilford Press.

Barkley, R. A. (1991a). *Attention-deficit hyperactivity disorder: A clinical workbook.* New York: Guilford Press.

Barkley, R. A. (1991b). The ecological validity of laboratory and analogue assessment methods of ADHD symptoms. *Journal of Abnormal Child Psychology, 19,* 149–178.

Barkley, R. A. (1994). Impaired delayed responding: A unified theory of Attention-Deficit Hyperactivity Disorder. In D. K. Routh (Ed.), *Disruptive behavior disorders in childhood* (pp. 11–57). New York: Plenum Press.

Barkley, R. A. (1995a). A closer look at the DSM-IV criteria for ADHD: Some unresolved issues. *The ADHD Report, 3*(3), 1–5.

Barkley, R. A. (1995b). Sex differences in ADHD. *The ADHD Report, 3*(1), 1–6.

Barkley, R. A. (1995c). *Taking charge of ADHD: The complete, authoritative guide for parents.* New York: Guilford Press.

Barkley, R. A. (1996a). ADHD and life expectancy. *The ADHD Report, 4,* 1–4.

Barkley, R. A. (1996b). Gender is already implicit in the diagnosis of ADHD: Shouldn't it be explicit? *The ADHD Report, 4,* 3–7.

Barkley, R. A. (1996c, November). *Medication controversy: Why now?* Paper presented at the Eighth Annual Conference of Children and Adults with Attention Deficit Disorder, Chicago, IL.

Barkley, R. A. (1996d). 18 ways to make token systems more effective for ADHD children and teens. *The ADHD Report, 4,* 1–5.

Barkley, R. A. (1997a). *ADHD and the nature of self-control.* New York: Guilford Press.

Barkley, R. A. (1997b). Behavioral inhibition, sustained attention, and executive functions: Constructing a unifying theory of ADHD. *Psychological Bulletin, 121,* 65–95.

Barkley, R. A. (1997c). *Defiant children: A clinician's manual for assessment and parent training* (2nd ed.). New York: Guilford Press.

Barkley, R. A. (1998). *Attention-deficit hyperactivity disorder: A handbook for diagnosis and treatment* (2nd ed.). New York: Guilford Press.

Barkley, R. A., Anastopoulos, A. D., Guevremont, D. G., & Fletcher, K. E. (1991). Adolescents with ADHD: Patterns of behavioral adjustment, academic functioning, and treatment utilization. *Journal of the American Academy of Child and Adolescent Psychiatry, 30,* 752–761.

Barkley, R. A., Anastopoulos, A. D., Guevremont, D. G., & Fletcher, K. E. (1992). Adolescents with Attention Deficit Hyperactivity Disorder: Mother–adolescent interactions, family beliefs and conflicts, and maternal psychopathology. *Journal of Abnormal Child Psychology, 20,* 263–288.

Barkley, R. A., DuPaul, G. J., & McMurray, M. B. (1990). A comprehensive evaluation of attention deficit disorder with and without hyperactivity. *Journal of Consulting and Clinical Psychology, 58,* 775–789.

Barkley, R. A., Edwards, G. H., & Robin, A. L. (in press). *Defiant teens: A clinician's manual for assessment and family training.* New York: Guilford Press.

Barkley, R. A., Fischer, M., Edelbrock, C., & Smallish, L. (1990). The adolescent outcome of hyperactive children diagnosed by research criteria: I. An 8-year prospective follow-up study. *Journal of the American Academy of Child and Adolescent Psychiatry, 29,* 546–557.

Barkley, R. A., Fischer, M., Edelbrock, C., & Smallish, L. (1991). The adolescent outcome of hyperactive children diagnosed by research criteria: III. Mother–child interactions, family conflicts, and maternal psychopathology. *Journal of Child Psychology and Psychiatry, 32,* 233–255.

Barkley, R. A., Fischer, M., Newby, R., & Breen, M. (1988). Development of a multi-method clinical protocol for assessing stimulant drug response in ADHD children. *Journal of Clinical Child Psychology, 17,* 14–24.

Barkley, R. A., Guevremont, D. G., Anastopoulos, A. D., DuPaul, G. J., & Shelton, T. L. (1993). Driving-related risks and outcomes of Attention Deficit Hyperactivity Disorder in adolescents and young adults: A 3- to 5- year follow-up survey. *Pediatrics, 92,* 212–218.

Barkley, R. A., Guevremont, D. G., Anastopoulos, A. D., & Fletcher, K. E. (1992). A comparison of three family therapy programs for treating family conflict in adolescents with Attention-Deficit Hyperactivity Disorder. *Journal of Consulting and Clinical Psychology, 60,* 450–462.

Barkley, R. A., McMurray, M. B., Edelbrock, C. S., & Robbins, K. (1990). Side effects of methylphenidate in children with Attention Deficit Hyperactivity Disorder: A systemic, placebo controlled evaluation. *Pediatrics, 86,* 184–192.

Barkley, R. A., Murphy, K. R., & Kwasnik, D. (1996). Motor vehicle driving competencies and risks in teens and young adults with Attention Deficit Hyperactivity Disorder. *Pediatrics, 98,* 1089–1095.

Barrickman, L. L., Perry, P. J., Allen, A. J., Kuperman, S., Arndt, S. V., Herrmann, K. J., & Schumacher, E. (1995). Bupropion versus methylphendiate in the treatment of attention-deficit hyperactivity disorder. *Journal of the American Academy of Child and Adolescent Psychiatry, 34,* 649–657.

Baumgaertel, A., Wolraich, M. L., & Dietrich, M. (1995). Comparison of diagnostic criteria for Attention Deficit Disorder in a German elementary school sample. *Journal of the American Academy of Child and Adolescent Psychiatry, 34,* 629–638.

Beck, A. T. (1976). *Cognitive therapy and emotional disturbances.* New York: International Universities Press.

Becker, W. C. (1964). Consequences of different kinds of parental discipline. In M. L. Hoffman & L. W. Hoffman (Eds.), *Review of child development research* (pp. 169–208). New York: Russell Sage Foundation.

Bellak, L. (1985). ADD Psychosis as a separate entity. *Schizophrenia Bulletin, 11,* 523–527.

Bellak, L. (1994). The schizophrenic syndrome and attention deficit disorder: Thesis, antithesis, and synthesis? *American Psychologist, 23,* 25–29.

Bellak, L., Kay, S. R., & Opler, L. A. (1987). Attention deficit disorder psychosis as a diagnostic category. *Psychiatric Developments, 3,* 239–263.

Biederman, J., Faraone, S. V., Doyle, A., Lehman, B. K., Kraus, I., Perrin, J., & Tsuang, M. T. (1993). Convergence of the Child Behavior Checklist with structured interview-based psychiatric diagnoses of ADHD children with and without comorbidity. *Journal of Child Psychology and Psychiatry, 34,* 1241–1251.

Biederman, J., Faraone, S. V., & Lapey, K. (1992). Comorbidity of diagnosis in Attention-Deficit Hyperactivity Disorder. *Child and Adolescent Psychiatric Clinics of North America, 1,* 335–360.

Biederman, J., Faraone, S. V., Mick, E., Moore, P., & Lelon, E. (1996). Child Behavior Checklist findings further support comorbidity between ADHD and major depression in a referred sample. *Journal of the American Academy of Child and Adolescent Psychiatry, 35,* 734–742.

Biederman, J., Faraone, S. V., Mick, E., Wozniak, H., Chen, L., Ouellete, C., Marrs, A., Moore, P., Garcia, J., Mennin, D., & Lelon, E. (1996). Attention-Deficit Hyperactivity Disorder and juvenile mania: An overlooked comorbidity? *Journal of the American Academy of Child and Adolescent Psychiatry, 35,* 997–1008.

Biederman, J., Faraone, S. V., Milberger, S., Curtis, S., Chen, L., Marrs, A., Ouellette, B. A., Moore, P., & Spencer, T. (1996). Predictors of persistence and remission of ADHD into adolescence: Results from a four-year prospective follow-up study. *Journal of the American Academy of Child and Adolescent Psychiatry, 35,* 343–351.

Biederman, J., Faraone, S. V., Milberger, S., Guite, J., Mick, E., Chen, L., Mennin, D., Marrs, A., Ouillette, C., Moore, P., Spencer, T., Norman, D., Wilens, T., Kraus, I., & Perrin, J. (1996). A prospective 4-year follow-up study of Attention-Deficit Hyperactivity and related disorders. *Archives of General Psychiatry, 53,* 437–446.

Biederman, J., Milberger, S., Faraone, S. V., Kiely, K., Guite, J., Mick, E., Ablon, S., Warburton, R., & Reed, E. (1995a). Family-environment risk factors for Attention-Deficit Hyperactivity Disorder. *Archives of General Psychiatry, 52,* 464–470.

Biederman, J., Milberger, S., Faraone, S. V., Kiely, K., Guite, J., Mick, E., Ablon, S., Warburton, R., Reed, E., & Davis, S. G. (1995b). Impact of exposure to parental psychopathology and conflict on adaptive functioning and comorbidity in children with Attention-Deficit Hyperactivity Disorder. *Journal of the American Academy of Child and Adolescent Psychiatry, 34,* 1495–1503.

Bowen, J., Fenton, T., & Rappaport, L. (1990). Stimulant medication and Attention-Deficit Hyperactivity Disorder: The child's perspective. *American Journal of Diseases of Childhood, 145,* 291–295.

Bowring, M., & Kovacs, M. (1992). Difficulties in diagnosing manic disorders among children and adolescents. *Journal of the American Academy of Child and Adolescent Psychiatry, 31,* 611–614.

Braswell, L., & Bloomquist, M. L. (1991). *Cognitive-behavioral therapy with ADHD children: Child, family, and school interventions.* New York: Guilford Press.

Bronowski, J. (1977). Human and animal languages. In *A sense of the future* (pp. 104–131). Cambridge, MA: MIT Press. (Reprinted from 1967, *To honor Roman Jakobson, Vol. 2.* The Hague, Netherlands: Mouton)

Brown, R. T., & Sexson, S. B. (1988). A controlled trial of methylphenidate in black adolescents: Attention, behavioral, and physiological effects. *Clinical Pediatrics, 27,* 74–81.

Brown, T. E. (1996). *Brown Attention Deficit Disorder Scales Manual.* San Antonio, TX: Psychological Corporation.

Carey, W. B., & McDevitt, S. C. (1995). *Coping with children's temperament: A guide for practitioners.* New York: Basic Books.

Carlson, G. A. (1990). Annotation: Child and adolescent mania—diagnostic considerations. *Journal of Child Psychology and Psychiatry, 31,* 331–341.

Casat, C. D., Pleasants, D. Z., & Van Wyck Fleet, J. (1987). A double-blind trial of bupropion in children with attention deficit disorder. *Psychopharmacology Bulletin, 23,* 120–122.

Chamberlain, P. (1996). Intensified foster care: Multi-level treatment for adolescents with conduct disorders in out-of-home care. In E. D. Hibbs & P. S. Jensen (Eds.), *Psychosocial treatments for child and adolescent disorders: Empirically based strategies for clinical practice* (pp. 475–496). Washington, DC: American Psychological Association

Children and Adults with Attention Deficit Disorder. (1996). *ADD and adolescence: Strategies for success from CH.A.D.D.* Plantation, FL: Author.

Clonidine for treatment of Attention-Deficit/Hyperactivity Disorder. (1996). *The Medical Letter, 38*(989), 109–110.

Cohen, M. D. (1996). Summary of IDEA/Section 504. In Children and Adults with Attention Deficit Disorder, *ADD and adolescence: Strategies for success* (pp. 52–53). Plantation, FL: Children and Adults with Attention Deficit Disorder.

Conger, J. J. (1977). *Adolescence and youth: Psychological development in a changing world.* New York: Harper.

Conners, C. K. (1995). *Conners Continuous Performance Test version 3.0 user's manual.* North Tonawanda, NY: Multi-Health Systems.

Conners, C. K. (1996). Letter to the editor. *The ADHD Report, 4,* 13.

Conners, C. K. (1997a). *Conners Parent Rating Scale—revised.* North Tonowanda, NY: Multi-Health Systems.

Conners, C. K. (1997b). *Conners rating scales—revised technical manual.* North Tonowanda, NY: Multi-Health Systems.

Conners, C. K., & Wells, K. (1997). *Conners–Wells Adolescent Self-Report Scale.* North Tonowanda, NY: Multi-Health Systems.

Coons, H. W., Klorman, R., & Borgstedt, A. D. (1987). Effects of methylphenidate on adolescents with a childhood history of Attention Deficit Disorder: II. Information processing. *Journal of the American Academy of Child and Adolescent Psychiatry, 26,* 368–374.

Corman, C. (1995). *New data supports use of the T.O.V.A. test over competing software.* Unpublished marketing letter, Universal Attention Disorders, Inc., Los Alamitos, CA.

Corman, C., & Greenberg, L. (1996). *Guidelines for medication titration with the TOVA.* Unpublished marketing manuscript, Universal Attention Disorders, Inc., Los Alamitos, CA.

Davila, R., Williams, M., & MacDonald, J. (1991). *Clarification of policy to address the needs of children with attention deficit disorders within general and/or special education.* Washington, DC: U.S. Department of Education.

Davis, L., Sirotowitz, S., & Parker, H. G. (1996). *Study strategies made easy.* Plantation, FL: Specialty Press.

Derogatis, L. R. (1983). *SCL-90-R manual II.* Towson, MD: Clinical Psychometric Research.

Dixon, E. B. (1995). Impact of adult ADD on the family. In K. F. Nadeau (Ed.), *A comprehensive guide to Attention Deficit Disorders in adults* (pp. 236–259). New York: Brunner/Mazel.

Downey, K. K., Pomerleau, C. S., & Pomerleau, O. F. (1996). Personality differences related to smoking and adult Attention Deficit Hyperactivity Disorder. *Journal of Substance Abuse, 8,* 129–135.

Drug Enforcement Administration. (1995). *Drug Enforcement Administration yearly aggregate production quotas.* Washington, DC: Author.

DuPaul, G. J. (1991). Parent and teacher ratings of ADHD symptoms: Psychometric properties in a community-based sample. *Journal of Clinical Child Psychology, 20,* 2425–2453.

DuPaul, G. J., Anastopoulos, A. D., Power, T. J., Reid, R., Ikeda, M. J., & McGoey, K. E. (in press). Parent ratings of attention deficit hyperactivity disorder symptoms: Factor structure and normative data. *Journal of Psychopathology and Behavioral Assessment.*

DuPaul, G. J., Anastopoulos, A. D., Shelton, T. L., Guevremont, D. G., & Metevia, L. (1992). Multimethod assessment of Attention-Deficit Hyperactivity Disorder: The diagnostic utility of clinic-based tests. *Journal of Clinical Child Psychology, 21,* 394–402.

DuPaul, G. J., Guevremont, D. G., & Barkley, R. A. (1991). Attention Deficit–Hyperactivity Disorder in adolescence: Critical assessment parameters. *Clinical Psychology Review, 11,* 231–245.

DuPaul, G. J., & Stoner, G. (1994). *ADHD in the schools: Assessment and intervention strategies.* New York: Guilford Press.

D'Zurilla, T. J., & Goldfried, M. R. (1971). Problem solving and behavior modification. *Journal of Abnormal Psychology, 78,* 197–226.

Elder, G. H. (1962). Structural variations in the childrearing experience. *Sociometry, 25,* 241–262.

Ellis, A., & Grieger, R. (1977). *Handbook of rational emotive therapy.* New York: Springer.

Evans, S. W., & Pelham, W. E. (1991). Psychostimulant effects on academic and behavioral measures for ADHD junior high students in a lecture format classroom. *Journal of Abnormal Child Psychology, 19,* 537–552.

Evans, S. W., Pelham, W. E., & Grudberg, M. V. (1995). The efficacy of notetaking to improve behavior and comprehension of adolescents with Attention Deficit Hyperactivity Disorder. *Exceptionality, 5,* 1–17.

Feindler, E. L., & Guttman, J. (1994). Cognitive-behavioral anger control training. In C. W. LeCroy (Ed.), *Handbook of child and adolescent treatment manuals* (pp. 170–199). New York: Lexington Books.

First, M. B., Gibbon, M., Williams, J. B., & Spitzer, R. L. (1995). *SCID Screen Patient Questionnaire computer program.* North Tonowanda, NY: Multi-Health Systems.

Fischer, M., Barkley, R. A., Edelbrock, C. S., & Smallish, L. (1990). The adolescent outcome of hyperactive children diagnosed by research criteria: II. Academic, attentional, and neuropsychological status. *Journal of Consulting and Clinical Psychology, 58,* 580–588.

Fischer, M., & Newby, R. G. (1991). Assessment of stimulant response in ADHD children using a refined multimethod clinical protocol. *Journal of Clinical Child Psychology, 20,* 232–244.

Fischer, M., Newby, R. G., & Gordon, M. (1995). Who are the false negatives on continuous performance tests? *Journal of Clinical Child Psychology, 24,* 427–433.

Forehand, R., Wierson, M., Frame, C., Kempton, T., & Armistead, L. (1991). Juvenile delinquency and persistence: Do attention problems contribute to conduct problems? *Journal of Behavior Therapy and Experimental Psychiatry, 22,* 261–264.

Forgatch, M., & Patterson, G. (1989). *Parents and adolescents living together: Part II. Family problem solving.* Eugene, OR: Castalia.

Fowler, M. (1995). *CH.A.D.D. educator's manual* (2nd ed.) . Plantation, FL: Children and Adults with Attention Deficit Disorder.

Friedman, H. S., Tucher, J. S., Schwartz, H. E., Tomlinson-Keasey, C., Martin, L. R., Wingard, D. G., & Criqui, M. H. (1995). Psychosocial and behavioral predictors of longevity: The aging and death of the "Termites." *American Psychologist, 50,* 69–78.

Fuster, J. M. (1989). *The prefrontal cortex.* New York: Raven Press.

Fuster, J. M. (1995). Memory and planning: Two temporal perspectives of frontal lobe function. In H. H. Jasper, S. Riggio, & P. S. Goldman-Rakic (Eds.), *Epilepsy and the functional anatomy of the frontal lobe* (pp. 9–18). New York: Raven Press.

Gastfriend, D. R., Biederman, J., & Jellinek, M. S. (1985). Desipramine in the treatment of attention deficit disorder in adolescence. *Psychopharmacology Bulletin, 21,* 144–145.

Gaub, M., & Carlson, C. L. (1996). Meta-analysis of gender differences in AD/HD. *Attention, 2,* 25–30.

Gephart, H. T. (1997). A managed care approach to ADHD. *Contemporary Pediatrics, 14,* 123–139.

Gillberg, C., Melander, H., von Knorring, A., Janols, L., Thernlund, G., Hagglof, B., Eidevall-Wallin, L., Gustafsson, P., & Kopp, S. (1997). Long-term stimulant treatment of children with Attention Deficit Hyperactivity Disorder Symptoms. *Archives of General Psychiatry, 54,* 857–864.

Gittelman Klein, R. (1987). Pharmacotherapy of childhood hyperactivity: An update. In H. Y. Metzer (Ed.), *Psychopharmacology: The third generation of progress* (pp. 1215–1224). New York: Raven Press.

Goldstein, S. (1991). *It's just attention disorder* [Videotape]. Salt Lake City, UT: Neurology, Learning, and Behavior Center.

Goldstein, S. (1997). *Managing attention and learning disorders in late adolescence and adulthood.* New York: Wiley.

Goldstein, S., & Goldstein, M. (1990). *Managing attention disorder in children.* New York: Wiley.

Gordon, M. (1987). How is a computerized attention test used in the diagnosis of Attention Deficit Disorder? In J. Loney (Ed.), *The young hyperactive child: Answers to questions about diagnosis, prognosis, and treatment* (pp. 53–64). New York: Haworth Press.

Gordon, M. (1993a). Do computerized measures of attention have a legitimate role in ADHD evaluations? *The ADHD Report, 1*(6), 5–6.

Gordon, M. (1993b). *I would if I could: A teenager's guide to ADHD/hyperactivity.* DeWitt, NY: GSI Publications.

Gordon, M. (1995a). *How to operate an ADHD clinic or subspecialty practice.* Dewitt, NY: GSI Publications.

Gordon, M. (1995b). *The down and dirty guide to adult ADD.* DeWitt, NY: GSI Publications.

Gordon, M. (1996). Must ADHD be an equal opportunity disorder? *The ADHD Report, 4,* 1–3.

Gordon, M., Barkley, R. A., & Murphy, K. R. (1997). ADHD on trial. *The ADHD Report, 5*(4), 1–4.

Gordon, M., & Irwin, M. (1997). *The diagnosis and treatment of ADD/ADHD: A no-nonsense guide for primary care physicians.* DeWitt, NY: GSI Publications.

Gordon, M., & Keiser, S. (1998). *Accommodations in higher education under the Americans with Disabilities Act (ADA).* New York: Guilford Press.

Gordon, M., & Mettlemen, B. B. (1987). *Technical guide to the Gordon Diagnostic System (GDS).* DeWitt, NY: GSI Publications.

Gordon, M., & Mettlemen, B. B. (1988). The assessment of attention: I. Standardization and reliability of a behavior-based measure. *Journal of Clinical Psychology, 44,* 682–690.

Gordon, T. (1970). *Parent effectiveness training.* New York: Wyden.

Greenberg, L. M. (1996). Response to Dr. Conners' letter to the editor. *The ADHD Report, 4,* 13–16.

Greenberg, L. M., & Waldman, I. D. (1993). Developmental normative data on the Test of Variables of Attention (T.O.V.A.). *Journal of the American Academy of Child and Adolescent Psychiatry, 34,* 1019–1030.

Grilo, C. M., Becker, D. F., Walker, M. L., Levy, K. N., Edell, W. S., I McGlashan, T. H. (1995). Psychiatric comorbidity in adolescent inpatients with substance use disorders. *Journal of the American Academy of Child and Adolescent Psychiatry, 34,* 1085–1091.

Grotevant, H. D., & Cooper, C. R. (1983). *Adolescent development in the family*. San Francisco, CA: Jossey-Bass.

Hallowell, E. M., & Ratey, J. J. (1994a). *Answers to distraction*. New York: Random House.

Hallowell, E. M., & Ratey, J. J. (1994b). *Driven to distraction*. New York: Random House.

Hart, E. L., Lahey, B. B., Loeber, R., Applegate, B., & Frick, P. J. (1995). Developmental changes in Attention-Deficit Hyperactivity Disorder in boys: A four-year longitudinal study. *Journal of Abnormal Child Psychology, 23,* 729–749.99.

Hartmann, T. (1993). *Attention deficit disorder: A different perception*. Novato, CA: Underwood-Miller Press.

Hechtman, L. T. (1992). Long-term outcome in Attention-Deficit Hyperactivity Disorder. *Child and Adolescent Psychiatric Clinics of North America, 1,* 553–565.

Hechtman, L. T., Weiss, G., & Perlman, T. (1984). Young adult outcome of hyperactive children who received long-term stimulant treatment. *Journal of the American Academy of Child and Adolescent Psychiatry, 23,* 261–269.

Henggeler, S. W., & Borduin, C. M. (1990). *Family therapy and beyond: A multisystemic approach to treating the behavior problems of children and adolescents*. Pacific Grove, CA: Brooks/Cole.

Henggeler, S. W., Schoenwald, S. K., Borduin, C. M., Rowland, M. D., & Cunningham, P. B. (1998). *Multisystemic treatment of antisocial behavior in children and adolescents*. New York: Guilford Press.

Herjanic, B., & Reich, W. (1982). Development of a structured psychiatric interview for children: Agreement between child and parent on individual symptoms. *Journal of Abnormal Child Psychology, 10,* 307–324.

Hibbs, E. D., & Jensen, P. S. (Eds.). (1996). *Psychosocial treatments for child and adolescent disorders: Empirically based strategies for clinical practice*. Washington, DC: American Psychological Association.

Jacobson, N. S., & Truax, P. (1991). Clinical significance: A statustical approach to defining meaningful change in psychotherapy research. *Journal of Consulting and Clinical Psychology, 59,* 12–19.

Kashden, J., Fremouw, W. J., Callahan, T. S., & Franzen, M. D. (1993). Impulsivity in suicidal and nonsuicidal adolescents. *Journal of Abnormal Child Psychology, 21,* 339–353.

Kavanaugh, J. (1988). *New federal definition of learning and attention disorders*. Speech given at the 15th annual conference of the New York branch of the Orton Society, New York, N.Y.

Kazdin, A. E. (1996). Problem solving and parent management in treating aggressive and antisocial behavior. In E. D. Hibbs & P. S. Jensen (Eds.), *Psychosocial treatments for child and adolescent disorders: Empirically based strategies for clinical practice* (pp. 377–408). Washington, DC: American Psychological Association.

Kelley, M. L. (1990). *School–home notes: Promoting children's classroom success*. New York: Guilford Press.

Kelly, K., & Ramundo, P. (1993). *You mean I'm not lazy, stupid, or crazy*. Cincinnati, OH: Tyrell & Jerem Press.

Kendall, P. C., & Treadwell, K. R. H. (1996). Cognitive-behavioral treatment for childhood anxiety disorders. In E. D. Hibbs & P. S. Jensen (Eds.), *Psychosocial treatments for child and adolescent disorders: Empirically based strategies for clinical practice* (pp. 23–42). Washington, DC: American Psychological Association.

Kilcarr, P. J., & Quinn, P. O. (1997). *Voices from fatherhood: Fathers, sons, and ADHD.* New York: Brunner/Mazel.

Klorman, R., Coons, H. W., & Borgstedt, A. D. (1987). Effects of methylphenidate on adolescents with a childhood history of attention deficit disorder. I. Clinical findings. *Journal of the American Academy of Child and Adolescent Psychiatry, 26,* 363–367.

Koepke, T. (1986). *Construct validation of the parent–adolescent relationship inventory: A multidimensional measure of parent–adolescent interaction.* Unpublished doctoral dissertation, Wayne State University, Detroit, MI.

Koepke, T., Robin, A., Nayar, M., & Hillman, S. (1987, August). *Construct validation of the parent–adolescent relationship questionnaire.* Paper presented at the annual meeting of the American Psychological Association, New York, NY.

Lahey, B. B., & Carlson, C. L. (1992). Validity of the diagnostic category of attention deficit disorder without hyperactivity: A review of the literature. In S. E. Shaywitz & B. Shaywitz (Eds.), *Attention deficit disorder comes of age: Towards the twenty-first century* (pp. 119–144). Austin, TX: Pro-Ed.

Latham, P. H., & Latham, P. S. (1997). Legal rights. In S. Goldstein (Ed.), *Managing attention and learning disorders in late adolescence and adulthood* (pp. 315–326). New York: Wiley.

Latham, P. S., & Latham, P. H. (1992). *Attention deficit disorder and the law: A guide for advocates.* Washington, DC: JKL Communications.

Latham, P. S., & Latham, P. H. (1993). *ADD and the law.* Washington, DC: JKL Communications.

Leser, R. J., & Leser, M. P. (1977). Responses of adolescents with minimal brain dysfunction to methylphenidate. *Journal of Learning Disabilities, 10,* 223–228.

MacKay, M. C., Beck, L., & Taylor, R. (1973). Methylphenidate for adolescents with minimal brain dysfunction. *New York State Journal of Medicine, 73,* 550–554.

Mannuzza, S., Klein, R. G., Bessler, A., Malloy, P., LaPadula, M. (1993). Adult outcome of hyperactive boys. *Archives of General Psychiatry, 50,* 565–576.

Mannuzza, S., Klein, R., Bonagura, N., Malloy, P., Giampino, T. L., & Addalli, K. A. (1991). Hyperactive boys almost grown up: V. Replication of psychiatric status. *Archives of General Psychiatry, 48,* 77–83.

Markel, G., & Greenbaum, J. (1996). *Performance breakthroughs for adolescents with learning disabilities or ADD.* Champaign, IL: Research Press.

Martin, C. S., Earleywine, M., Blackson, T. C., & Vanyukov, M. M. (1994). Aggressivity in attention, hyperactivity and impulsivity in boys at high and low risk for substance abuse. *Journal of Abnormal Child Psychology, 22,* 177–203.

Mash, E. J., & Terdal, L. G. (Eds.). (1997). *Behavioral assessment of childhood disorders* (3rd ed.). New York: Guilford Press.

Mercer, C. D., & Mercer, A. R. (1993). *Teaching students with learning problems* (4th ed.). Columbus, OH: Merrill.

Milberger, S., Biederman, J., Faraone, S. V., Chen, L., & Jones, J. (1997). Attention Deficit Hyperactivity Disorder is associated with early initiation of cigarette smoking in children and adolescents. *Journal of the American Academy of Child and Adolescent Psychiatry, 36,* 37–44.

Milberger, S., Biederman, J., Faraone, S. V., Murphy, J., & Tsuang, M. T. (1995). Comorbidity within attention deficit hyperactivity disorder is not an artifact of overlapping symptomatology. *American Journal of Psychiatry, 152,* 1793–1800.

Monitoring the Future Study. (1995). Ann Arbor: University of Michigan.

Moffitt, T. E., & Silva, P. A. (1988). Self-reported delinquency, neuropsychological deficit, and history of attention deficit disorder. *Journal of Abnormal Child Psychology, 16,* 553–569.

Murphy, K., & Barkley, R. A. (1995). Preliminary normative data on DSM-IV criteria for adults. *The ADHD Report, 3*(3), 6–7.

Murphy, K., & Barkley, R. A. (1996a). Updated adult norms for the ADHD Behavior Checklist for Adults. *The ADHD Report, 4,* 12–16.

Murphy, K., & Barkley, R. A. (1996b). Prevalence of DSM-IV symptoms of ADHD in adult licensed drivers: Implications for clinical diagnosis. *Journal of Attention Disorders, 1,* 147–161.

Nadeau, K. (1994). *Survival guide for college students with ADD or LD.* New York: Magination Press.

Nadeau, K. (1995). *A comprehensive guide to adult Attention Deficit Disorder.* New York: Brunner/Mazel.

Nadeau, K. (1996). *Adventures in fast forward.* New York: Magination Press.

National Advisory Committee on Handicapped Children. (1968, January 31). *Special education for handicapped children* (First annual report). Washington, DC: U.S. Department of Health, Education and Welfare.

Nayar, M. (1985). *Cognitive factors in the treatment of parent–adolescent conflict.* Unpublished doctoral dissertation, Wayne State University, Detroit, MI.

O'Dell, S. (1974). Training parents in behavior modification: A review. *Psychological Bulletin, 81,* 418–433.

Orvaschel, H., & Puig-Antich, H. (1987). *Schedule for Affective Disorders and Schizophrenia for School-Age Children—epidemiologic 4th version.* Ft. Lauderdale, FL: Nova University, Center for Psychological Study.

Parker, G. (1979). Parental characteristics in relation to depressive disorders. *British Journal of Psychiatry, 135,* 155–160.

Parker, G. (1983). *Parental overprotection: A risk factor in psychosocial development.* New York: Grune & Stratton.

Parker, G. (1990). The parental bonding instrument: A decade of research. *Social Psychiatry and Psychiatric Epidemiology, 25,* 281–282.

Parker, G., Tupling, H., & Brown, L. B. (1979). A parental bonding instrument. *British Journal of Medical Psychology, 52,* 1–10.

Parker, R. (1992). *Making the grade: An adolescent's struggle with ADD.* Plantation, FL: Specialty Press.

Pataki, C. S., Carlson, G. A., Kelly, K. L., Rapport, M. D., & Biancaniello, T. M. (1993). Side effects of methylphenidate and desipramine alone and in combination in children. *Journal of the American Academy of Child and Adolescent Psychiatry, 32,* 1065–1072.

Paternite, C. E., Loney, J., & Roberts, M. A. (1996). A preliminary validation of subtypes of DSM-IV Attention Deficit Hyperactivity Disorder. *Journal of Attention Disorders, 1,* 70–86.

Patterson, G. R. (1982). *Coercive family process.* Eugene, OR: Castalia.

Patterson, G. R., & Forgatch, M. (1987). *Parents and adolescent living together: Part I. The basics.* Eugene, OR: Castalia.

Pelham, W. E., Greenslade, K. E., Vodde-Hamilton, M., Murphy, D. A., Greenstein, J. J., Gnagy, E. M., Guthrie, K. J., Hoover, M. D., & Dahl, R. E. (1990). Relative efficacy of long-acting stimulants on children with Attention-Deficit Hyperactivity Disorder: A comparison of standard methylphenidate, sustained-release methylphenidate, sustained-release dextroampehtamine, and pemoline. *Pediatrics, 86,* 226–237.

Pelham, W. E., & Hoza, B. (1996). Intensive treatment: Summer treatment program for children with ADHD. In E. D Hibbs & P. S. Jensen (Eds.), *Psychosocial treatments for child and adolescent disorders: Empirically based strategies for clinical practice* (pp. 311–340). Washington, DC: American Psychological Association.

Pelham, W. E., Jr., Vodde-Hamilton, M., Murphy, D. A., Greenstein, J., & Vallano, G. (1991). The effects of methylphenidate on ADHD adolescents in recreational, peer group, and classroom settings. *Journal of Clinical Child Psychology, 20,* 293–300.

Phelan, T. (1998). Lessons from the trenches: Managing the teen with ADD. *Attention, 4,* 44–47.

Pomerleau, O. F., Downey, K. K., Stelson, F., & Pomerleau, C. S. (1995). Cigarette smoking in adult patients diagnosed with Attention Deficit Hyperactivity Disorder. *Journal of Substance Abuse, 7,* 373–378.

Prinz, R., & Kent, R. (1978). Recording parent–adolescent interactions without the use of frequency or interval-by-interval coding. *Behavior Therapy, 9,* 602–604.

Quay, H. C. (1996, January). *Gray's behavioral inhibition in ADHD: An update.* Paper presented at the meeting of the International Society for Research in Child and Adolescent Psychopathology, Los Angeles, CA.

Quinn, P. O. (1995). *Adolescents and ADD.* New York: Magination Press.

Rappley, M. (1996). The use of methylphenidate in Michigan. *The ADHD Report, 4*(3), 8–10.

Rappley, M. D., Gardiner, J. C., Jetton, J. R., & Houang, R. T. (1995). The use of methylphenidate in Michigan. *Archives of Pediatric and Adolescent Medicine, 149,* 675–679.

Rapport, M. D., & Kenney, C. (1997). Titrating methylphenidate in children with attention deficit/hyperactivity disorder: Is body mass predictive of clinical response. *Journal of the American Academy of Child and Adolescent Psychiatry, 36,* 523–530.

Reich, W., Welner, Z., Herjanic, B., & MHS Staff. (1997). *Diagnostic Interview for Children and Adolescents IV* (DICA-IV). *Windows version.* North Tonowanda, NY: Multi-Health Systems

Rey, J. M., & Plapp, J. M. (1990). Quality of perceived parenting in oppositional and conduct disordered adolescents. *Journal of the American Academy of Child and Adolescent Psychiatry, 29,* 382–385.

Reynolds, C. R., & Kamphaus, R. W. (1992). *BASIC: Behavior Assessment System for Children manual.* Circle Pines, MN: American Guidance Services.

Reynolds, G. R. (1985). Critical measurement issues in learning disabilities. *Journal of Special Education, 18,* 451–476.

Reynolds, G. R. (1990). Conceptual and technical problems in learning disability diagnosis. In G. R. Reynolds & R. W. Kamphaus (Eds.), *Handbook of psycho-*

logical and educational assessment of children: Intelligence and achievement (pp. 571–592). New York: Guilford Press.

Robin, A. L. (1976). Behavioral instruction in the college classroom. *Review of Educational Research, 46,* 313–354.

Robin, A. L. (1990). Training families with ADHD adolescents. In R. A. Barkley, *Attention-deficit hyperactivity disorder: A handbook for diagnosis and treatment* (pp. 462–497). New York: Guilford Press.

Robin, A. L., & Foster, S. L. (1989). *Negotiating parent–adolescent conflict: A behavioral–family systems approach.* New York: Guilford Press.

Robin, A. L., Koepke, T., & Moye, A. (1990). Multidimensional assessment of parent–adolescent relations. *Psychological Assessment: A Journal of Consulting and Clinical Psychology, 2,* 451–459.

Robin A. L., Kraus, D., Koepke, T., & Robin, R. (1987, August) . *Growing up hyperactive in single versus two parent families.* Paper presented at the annual meeting of the American Psychological Association, New York, N.Y.

Robin, A. L., Siegel, P. T., & Moye, A. (1995). Family versus individual therapy for anorexia: Impact on family conflict. *International Journal of Eating Disorders, 17,* 313–322.

Robin, A., & Vandermay, S. (1996). Validation of a measure for adolescent self-report of Attention Deficit Disorder symptoms. *Journal of Developmental and Behavioral Pediatrics, 17,* 211–215.

Rosenberg, J. (1996). From the newsroom to your living room—Talking to teens about methylphenidate abuse. In Children and Adults with Attention Deficit Disorder, *ADD and adolescence: Strategies for success from CH.A.D.D.* (pp. 70–71). Plantation, FL: Children and Adults with Attention Deficit Disorder.

Rourke, B. P. (1989). *Nonverbal learning disabilities: The syndrome and the model.* New York: Guilford Press.

Safer, D. J. (1996). Medication usage trends for ADD. In Children and Adults with Attention Deficit Disorder, *ADD and adolescence: Strategies for success from CH.A.D.D.* (pp. 16–18). Plantation, FL: Children and Adults with Attention Deficit Disorder.

Safer, D. J., & Allen, R. P. (1975). Stimulant drug treatment of hyperactive adolescents. *Diseases of the Nervous System, 36,* 454–457.

Safer, D. J., & Krager, J. M. (1985). Prevalence of medication treatment for hyperactive adolescents. *Psychopharmacology Bulletin, 21,* 212–215.

Safer, D. J., & Krager, J. M. (1988). A survey of medication treatment for hyperactive/ inattentive children. *Journal of the American Medical Association, 260,* 2256–2258.

Safer, D. J., & Krager, J. M. (1989). Hyperactivity and inattentiveness: School assessment of stimulant treatment. *Clinical Pediatrics, 28,* 216–221.

Safer, D. J., & Krager, J. M. (1994). The increased rate of stimulant treatment for hyperactive/inattentive students in secondary schools. *Pediatrics, 94,* 462–464.

Safer, D. J., Zito, J. M., & Fine, E. M. (1996). Methylphenidate usage for Attention Deficit Disorder in the 1990s. *Pediatrics, 98,* 1084–1088.

Schubiner, H. (1995). *ADHD in adolescence: Our point of view* [Videotape]. Detroit, MI: Children's Hospital of Michigan Department of Educational Services.

Schubiner, H. (1996). *ADHD/cocaine dependence: Stimulant trial.* Grant proposal submitted to the National Institute on Drug Abuse, Washington, DC.

Schubiner, H., Robin, A. L., & Neinstein, L. S. (1996). School problems. In L. S. Neinstein (Ed.), *Adolescent health care: A practical guide* (3rd ed., pp. 1124–1142). Baltimore: Williams & Wilkins.

Schubiner, H., Tzelepis, A., Isaacson, H., Warbasse, L., Zacharek, M., & Musial, J. (1995). Dual diagnosis of attention-deficit hyperactivity disorder and substance abuse: Case reports and review of the literature. *Journal of Clinical Psychiatry, 56,* 146–150.

Schwab-Stone, M., Fisher, P., Piacentini, J., Shaffer, D., Davies, M., & Briggs, M. (1993). The Diagnostic Interview Schedule for Children—Revised version (DISC-R): II. Test–retest reliability. *Journal of the American Academy of Child and Adolescent Psychiatry, 32,* 651–657.

Schweickert, L. A., Strober, M., & Moskowitz, A. (1997). Efficacy of methylphenidate in bulimia nervosa comorbid with Attention-Deficit Hyperactivity Disorder: A case report. *International Journal of Eating Disorders, 21,* 299–301.

Semrud-Clikeman, M. S., Biederman, J., Sprich-Buchminster, S., Lehman, B. K., Faraone, S. V., & Norman, D. (1992). Comorbidity between ADDH and learning disability: A review and report in a clinically referred sample. *Journal of the American Academy of Child and Adolescent Psychiatry, 31,* 439–444.

Silver, L. (1992). *Attention deficit hyperactivity disorder: A clinical guide to diagnosis and treatment.* Washington, DC: American Psychiatric Press.

Slombowski, C., Klein, R. G., & Mannuzza, S. (1995). Is self-esteem an important outcome in hyperactive children? *Journal of Abnormal Child Psychology, 23,* 303–315.

Smith, B. H., Pelham, W. E., Evans, S., Molina, B., Willoughby, M., Gnagy, E., Greiner, A., & Bukstein, C. (1997). *Dose effects of methylphenidate on the social behavior of adolescents diagnosed with Attention-Deficit Hyperactivity Disorder.* Manuscript submitted for publication.

Smith, B. H., Pelham, W. E., Jr., Evans, S., Gnagy, E., Molina, B., Bukstein, O., Myak, C., Greiner, A., Presnell, M., & Willoughby, M. (1998). Dosage effects of methylphenidate on the social behavior of adolescents with Attention Deficit Hyperactivity Disorder. *Experimental and Clinical Psychopharmacology, 6,* 187–204.

Smith, B. H., Pelham, W. E., Jr., Gnagy, E., & Yudell, R. (1998). Equivalent effects of stimulant treatment for ADHD during childhood and adolescence. *Journal of the American Academy of Child and Adolescent Psychiatry, 37,* 314–321.

Snyder, D. (1997). *Marital Satisfaction Inventory Manual—Revised.* Los Angeles: Western Psychological Association.

Snyder, J., Dishion, T. J., & Patterson, G. R. (1986). Determinants and consequences of associating with deviant peers during preadolescence. *Journal of Early Adolescence, 6,* 29–43.

Solden, S. (1995). *Women with Attention Deficit Disorder.* Grass Valley, CA: Underwood Press.

Spencer, T., Biederman, J., Steingard, R., & Wilens, T. (1993). Bupropion exacerbates tics in children with attention deficit hyperactivity disorder and Tourette's syndrome. *Journal of the American Academy of Child and Adolescent Psychiatry, 32,* 211–214.

Spencer, T., Biederman, J., Wilens, T., Harding, M., O'Donnell, B. A., & Griffin, S. (1996). Pharmacotherapy of Attention-Deficit Hyperactivity Disorder across the Life Cycle. *Journal of the American Academy of Child and Adolescent Psychiatry, 35*, 409–432.

Spires, H. A., & Stone, D. P. (1989). The directed notetaking activity: A self-questioning approach. *Journal of Reading, 33*, 36–39.

Spitzer, R. L., Williams, J. B., Gibbon, M., & First, M. B. (1990). *Structured Clinical Interview for DSM-III-R—Non-patient edition.* Washington, DC: American Psychiatric Press.

Spivack, G., Platt, J. J., & Shure, M. (1976). *The problem-solving approach to adjustment.* San Francisco: Jossey-Bass.

Sprague, R., & Sleator, E. (1977). Methylphenidate in hyperkinetic children: Differences in dose effects on learning and social behavior. *Science, 198*, 1274–1276.

Steinberg, L., Fletcher, A., & Darling, N. (1994). Parental monitoring and peer influences on adolescent substance use. *Pediatrics, 93*, 1060–1064.

Steinberg, L., Lamborn, S. D., Darling, N., Mounts, N. S., & Dornbusch, S. M. (1994). Over-time changes in adjustment and competence among adolescents from authoritative, authoritarian, indulgent, and neglectful families. *Child Development, 65*, 754–770.

Stern, S. B. (in press). Anger management in parent–adolescent conflict. *The American Journal of Family Therapy.*

Swanson, J. M., Wigal, S., Greenhill, L., Browne, R., Waslik, B., Lerner, M., Williams, L., Flynn, D., Agler, D., Crowley, K., Fineberg, E., Baren, M., & Cantwell, D. P. (1998). Analog classroom assessment of Adderall in children with ADHD. *Journal of the American Academy of Child and Adolescent Psychiatry, 37*, 519–526.

Thorley, G. (1984). Review of follow-up and follow-back studies of childhood hyperactivity. *Psychological Bulletin, 96*, 116–132.

Varley, C. K. (1983). Effects of methylphenidate in adolescents with attention deficit disorder. *Journal of the American Academy of Child Psychiatry, 22*, 351–354.

Vincent-Roehling, P., & Robin, A. L. (1986). Development and validation of the Family Beliefs Inventory: A measure of unrealistic beliefs among parents and adolescents. *Journal of Consulting and Clinical Psychology, 54*, 693–697.

Vuchinich, S., Wood, B., & Angelelli, J. (1996). Coalitions and family problem solving in the psychosocial treatment of preadolescents. In E. D. Hibbs & P. S. Jensen (Eds.), *Psychosocial treatments for child and adolescent disorders: Empirically based strategies for clinical practice* (pp. 497–518). Washington, DC: American Psychological Association.

Waldman, I. D., & Greenberg, L. M. (1992). *Inattention and impulsivity discriminate among disruptive behavior disorders.* Unpublished manuscript, University of Minnesota, Minneapolis, MN.

Webb, D. (1987). *Discriminant and concurrent validity of the structural scales of the Parent Adolescent Relationship Questionnaire.* Unpublished doctoral dissertation, University of South Carolina, Columbia, SC.

Wechsler, D. (1991). *Wechsler Intelligence Scale for Children—III (WISC-III).* San Antonio, TX: Psychological Corporation.

Wechsler, D. (1992). *Wechsler Individual Achievement Test (WIAT).* San Antonio, TX: Psychological Corporation.

Wechsler, D. (1997a). *WAIS-III/WMS-III technical manual.* San Antonio, TX: Psychological Corporation.

Wechsler, D. (1997b). *Wechsler Adult Intelligence Scale—III (WAIS-III)*. San Antonio, TX: Psychological Corporation.

Wechsler, D. (1997c). *Wechsler Memory Scale—III*. San Antonio, TX: Psychological Corporation.

Weiss, G., & Hechtman, L. T. (1993). *Hyperactive children grown up* (2nd ed.). New York: Guilford Press.

Weiss, G., Kruger, E., Danielson, R., & Elman, M. (1975). Effect of long-term treatment of hyperactive children with Methylphenidate. *Canadian Medical Association Journal, 112,* 159–165.

West, S., McElroy, S., Strakowski, S., Keck, P., & McConville, B. (1995). Attention deficit hyperactivity disorder in adolescent mania. *American Journal of Psychiatry, 152,* 271–274.

Wielkiewicz, R. M. (1990). Interpreting low scores on the WISC-R third factor: It's more than distractibility. *Psychological Assessment: A Journal of Consulting and Clinical Psychology, 2,* 91–97.

Wilens, T. E., & Biederman, J. (1992). The stimulants. *Psychiatric Clinics of North American, 15,* 191–222.

Wilens, T. E., Spencer, T., Biederman, J., Woznak, J., & Connor, D. (1995). Combined pharmacotherapy: An emerging trend in pediatric psychopharmacology. *Journal of the American Academy of Child and Adolescent Psychiatry, 34,* 110–112.

Wilson, J. M., & Marcotte, A. C. (1996). Psychosocial adjustment and educational outcome in adolescents with a childhood diagnosis of Attention Deficit Disorder. *Journal of the American Academy of Child and Adolescent Psychiatry, 35,* 579–587.

Wolraich, M. L., & Baumgaertel, A. (1996). The prevalence of Attention Deficit Hyperactivity Disorder based on the new DSM-IV criteria. *Peabody Journal of Education, 71,* 168–186.

Woodcock, R. W., & Johnson, M. B. (1989). *Woodcock–Johnson Psycho-Educational Battery—Revised, Tests of Achievement*. Allen, TX: DLM Teaching Resources.

Wozniak, J., Biederman, J., Kiely, K., Ablon, J. S., Faraone, S. V., Mundy, E., & Mennin, D. (1995). Mania-like symptoms suggestive of childhood-onset bipolar disorder in clinically referred children. *Journal of the American Academy of Child and Adolescent Psychiatry, 34,* 867–876.

Young, R. C., Biggs, J. T., Ziegler, V. E., & Meyer, D. A. (1978). A rating scale for mania: Reliability, validity, and sensitivity. *British Journal of Psychiatry, 133,* 429–435.

Zeigler Dendy, C. A. (1995). *Teenagers with ADD: A parents' guide*. Bethesda, MD: Woodbine House.

Zentall, S. S. (1985). A context for hyperactivity. In K. D. Gadow & I. Bialer (Eds.), *Advances in learning and behavioral disabilities* (Vol. 4, pp. 273–343). Greenwich, CT: JAI Press.

Zimetkin, A. J., Nordahl, T. E., Gross, M., King, A. C., Semple, W. E., Rumsey, J., Hamberger, S., & Cohen, R. M. (1990). Cerebral glucose metabolism in adults with hyperactivity of childhood onset. *New England Journal of Medicine, 323,* 1361–1366.

Zimetkin, A. J., & Rapoport, J. L. (1987). Neurobiology of attention deficit disorder with hyperactivity: Where have we come in 50 years? *Journal of the American Academy of Child and Adolescent Psychiatry, 26,* 676–686.

Index

——————— O ———————